About the authors

Dr Jonathan Brostoff is Honorary Consultant Physician and Reader in Clinical Immunology at the Middlesex Hospital Medical School in London. After training as a general physician he became interested in allergy, and for many years has studied the way the immune system works, and how it produces allergic diseases such as asthma and excema. His research into allergy aroused his interest in the related topic of food intolerance, and he has an ongoing programme of research in this area. Dr Brostoff is recognised as a leading international authority on food allergy and intolerance, and is co-author of the principal medical textbook on this subject.

Linda Gamlin trained as a biochemist and worked in research for several years, before turning to journalism. She specializes in writing about the immune system, allergy and other health matters.

THE COMPLETE GUIDE TO

FOOD
ALLERGY AND
INTOLERANCE

THE COMPLETE GUIDE TO
FOOD
ALLERGY AND
INTOLERANCE

DR. JONATHAN BROSTOFF
AND LINDA GAMLIN

BLOOMSBURY

For
David Burnie
and
Deanna and Joshua Brostoff

First published 1989

This edition published 1992

Copyright © Jonathan Brostoff and Linda Gamlin 1989; 1992

Bloomsbury Publishing Limited, 2 Soho Square, London W1V 5DE

British Library Cataloguing in Publication Data

A CIP catalogue record for this book is available from the British Library

ISBN 0 7475 1260 4

2 4 6 8 10 9 7 5 3

Designed by Malcolm Smythe
Illustrations by Elsa Godfrey
Typeset by Hewer Text Composition Services, Edinburgh
Printed and bound in Great Britain by
Cox & Wyman Ltd, Reading, Berkshire

Contents

Acknowledgments

The authors would like to thank Dr Michael Radcliffe for his many helpful comments on the manuscript. We are also grateful to Dr Katherine Sloper, Dr Jonathan Maberly, Dr Stephen Davies, Dr David Freed, Dr Hugh Cox, Dr Gail Darlington, Dr David Pearson, Dr David Bender, Dr Robert Gardner, Dr Celia Gibb, Dr Ronald Finn, Dr Len McEwan, Dr Ian Menzies, Dr John Hunter, Dr William Bynum, Dr Ellen Grant, Dr Joseph Miller, Dr Theron G. Randolph, Dr John Mansfield, Dr Harry Morrow-Brown, Dr Ronald Williams, Dr Jeff Reardon, Sheila Burnie, Maureen Minchin, Moira Mole and Brian Hammond who gave us their help, comments and advice at various times during the preparation of this book. Special thanks are due to David Burnie for his considerable help in preparing the manuscript.

Authors' note

This book is designed to be read by two different types of reader – those who like to read straight through from beginning to end, and those who prefer to 'dip in' to topics that interest them. With the second group in mind, we have included numerous page references to point the way to related topics or explanations of technical terms. Those reading straight through should ignore these cross-references. We hope that everyone, including the dippers-in, will read Chapter One as this sets the scene for the rest of the book.

We have had to use some technical terms in writing this book, but all these are explained, and the index can be used to find the place in the text where the explanation is given.

Note to the second edition

When the first edition was published, no one was quite sure if the world was waiting with bated breath for a detailed, comprehensive book about food and chemical sensitivity, or whether the slim volumes already available were what readers preferred. The many very positive reactions we received have reassured us that people *do* find it useful to have all this information packed into one book, are not intimidated by scientific data, and like to hear both sides of the controversial issues. It has been encouraging to discover how many readers have been helped by the book. 'It saved my life . . .' was one reaction, from a reader whose case history appears in this new edition. Whatever your experience with the book – good or bad – do please write and tell us. (The publisher's address appears opposite the contents page.) All comments, criticisms and suggestions will be helpful in preparing the next edition. As before, thanks are due to many doctors and other professional people for their help, but we would particularly like to mention Dr John Hunter and Sheila Burnie for their expert advice.

Chapter One

ANOTHER MAN'S POISON

What is food allergy, and what is food intolerance? How do the two differ? The best way to answer this question is to tell the stories of Jane and Susan.

Jane's story

Jane's health problems began as a baby. She had colic and vomited often, and at the age of three months developed eczema on her face and arms. Her mother had hay-fever every summer and her father had suffered from asthma as a child – both complaints are common allergies. Even before Jane was born, their family doctor was well aware that they were an **atopic** family – in other words, they were prone to allergies. As Jane grew older she developed asthma and hay-fever, although only mildly. Her asthma seemed to get worse when there was a cat in the room. Using extracts of grass pollen and cat fur, and inserting minute amounts of them under her skin (a **skin-prick test**), the doctor found that she was indeed allergic to both these substances – her arm came up in a red, itchy bump where the extract had entered the skin.

Once or twice during her early years, Jane's mouth and tongue swelled up enormously after eating, and she had to be rushed to hospital. After thinking carefully about what she had eaten on these occasions, Jane's mother concluded that it was peanuts that had caused this alarming reaction. The doctor used skin-prick tests again, and they confirmed that Jane had a food allergy – she was extremely sensitive to peanuts. Other skin-prick tests were negative, so it seemed that she could eat most foods safely.

Even though Jane avoided peanuts carefully from then on, there were occasional problems. One day when Jane was about eight, and her parents were holding a party, she handed round a bowl of nuts to the guests. Later she rubbed her eyelids, and they soon began to swell and itch furiously. Although her hay-fever and asthma subsided as Jane grew older, her sensitivity to peanuts remained the same.

As an adult, Jane had a successful career which involved a great deal of travelling and eating out. Wherever she ate she had to be careful to avoid anything with peanuts – even the slightest trace of them. All was well until Jane, now in her thirties, ordered some cheesecake in a restaurant. She had asked the waiter if the brown powder on the surface of the cheesecake contained any nuts, and he assured her that it was pure chocolate. Usually it was – but the chef had run out of chocolate that day and had been forced to use something else. Unfortunately for Jane, that something else was finely grated nuts, including some peanuts.

Within seconds of taking her first mouthful of cheesecake, Jane's mouth was itching. Her tongue began to swell and her breathing became difficult. She could no longer speak, and, as the swelling blocked her windpipe, she began to turn blue. Within minutes she had collapsed on the floor.

The colleagues she was dining with were horrified and had no idea what to do, but a stranger at the next table intervened. By an extraordinary, and lucky, chance he was a doctor. Grabbing a spoon from the table, he pushed the handle over the edge of her tongue and managed to open up the blocked windpipe. As he did so, Jane gradually turned from blue to pink, but she was still in a state of collapse (known as **anaphylactic shock**) and her face was still horribly swollen. Meanwhile, someone had telephoned the hospital, and another doctor arrived with the life-saving medicines that Jane needed. These were injected and she slowly regained consciousness.

Thereafter, Jane was even more careful about avoiding peanuts in her food. She realized that she could easily have died had it not been for the presence of a doctor. By scrupulously avoiding peanuts she has remained well.

Susan's story

Susan is about the same age as Jane. She was reasonably well as a child, apart from frequent colds and chest infections. At the age of 21, however, she suffered a bad bout of diarrhoea when travelling abroad. Although she recovered from this, her bowels never really returned to normal. A mild form of diarrhoea stayed with her so that she needed to go several times a day, often at the most inconvenient moment. As the years passed this problem gradually got worse, and unpleasant pains began in the lower part of her stomach. When she finally consulted her doctor about this problem, she was told that this was **irritable bowel syndrome**, or **IBS**, and that she should try to relax more.

For many years Susan also suffered headaches, but thought little of them – she simply took aspirin when she felt one coming on. One day, just after her twenty-eighth birthday, she experienced a strange sort of headache that was on the left side of her head only. She took some aspirin, but the pain did not go away – indeed it became more intense, and she began to feel slightly sick. Eventually she had to draw the curtains and go to bed because she could not bear the light. There were more of these attacks over the next few months and Susan eventually went to see her doctor again. He told her that these were migraines, and again recommended that she should try to worry less and learn to relax. Although she followed his suggestions, the migraines continued, and so did her bowel problems.

Over the next few years, Susan had to give up alcohol and chocolate as these always seemed to bring the migraine attacks on. But despite avoiding these items, her migraines continued to become more frequent. She also felt excessively tired, especially first thing in the morning, and she sometimes felt light-headed and confused, or very edgy and irritable. To add to these problems, she began to get odd little pains in her knees. These gradually grew worse, and by the time she was 34 she could no longer run up the stairs without pain, and she was forced to give up jogging and riding a bicycle because these activities made her knees so much worse. The pains spread to some of her other joints and she began to feel that there was something seriously wrong, because she was ill most of the time.

Susan had previously accepted her doctor's diagnosis that most of her problems were due to her 'nerves', but at this point she began to have doubts. She was now married, and had a good job that she enjoyed. Apart from her health problems she had few worries – indeed she felt more settled and happy than at any time in her life – so why was her health getting worse instead of better? She went to see her doctor again, and he gave her a thorough examination, but could find nothing wrong. He repeated his earlier diagnosis, and suggested that her joint pains were also psychosomatic.

A few months later, Susan read a magazine article about something called 'food allergy', which seemed to cause the sort of symptoms she had. She asked her doctor's opinion about this and found he was very dismissive of the idea – as far as he could see, her symptoms were nothing like those of food allergy. Another year went past in which Susan became steadily worse. Then a new doctor joined the practice, and when she next rang for an appointment, it was suggested that she see him instead, as he had a special interest in patients like herself. When Susan went to see the other doctor, he explained that symptoms such as hers could sometimes be caused by food, although there were other potential causes as well. He went on to explain why his colleague had dismissed the idea of her having food allergy – the condition he treated was quite different and he preferred to use the name 'food intolerance'. While he could not guarantee that this was her problem, it was certainly a possibility. He suggested that she try a special diet which avoided all the foods she normally ate. Susan began the diet on a Monday with high hopes, but by Tuesday she felt very ill indeed. Her tiredness was far worse, and she experienced a severe migraine attack – the worst one she had ever suffered – that lasted through Wednesday as well. On Thursday she felt completely 'washed out' from the migraine, and Friday was little better. In desperation, she rang the doctor, but he told her that this sort of reaction often occurred – in fact it was a positive sign that foods were the source of the problem, so she should persevere with the diet.

On Saturday, Susan woke up quite early before her alarm clock went off – which was most unusual, because she normally had great difficulty in waking up. As she got out of bed, she noticed that her knees did not give their customary painful twinge. She tried walking downstairs and then running up them again. To her amazement, she found that the pains she had endured for two years had suddenly vanished.

As the day went on, she realized that she felt altogether different – she was no longer tired, her head felt clearer, and there was no headache or migraine, unlike most weekends. Indeed she felt better than she had done for many years. Over the next few days, it became obvious that her bowels were also a great deal better.

When she returned to the doctor, Susan was jubilant – she simply couldn't believe how much better she felt. Even her irritability, which she had thought was just part of her personality, had now vanished. The doctor explained that she must now reintroduce foods, one at a time, to see what effect they had. Over the next two months, she tried out all the foods she normally ate. Some of these had no effect, but others made her very ill – milk, wheat, rye, barley, yeast, oranges, lemons, beef and tomatoes were the main culprits. By avoiding all these foods, and adding some other, more unusual foods into her diet instead, Susan remained well. Migraines, which had previously afflicted her once or twice a week, were now a thing of the past.

After eight months, the doctor suggested that she try out some of the incriminated foods, to see what effect they had. She found that she still reacted to milk, but was fine on the other foods. The doctor advised her not to eat them more than once every four days. A year later, Susan discovered that she could now drink milk again without ill-effects. Interestingly, she discovered that she could also drink alcohol, in moderation, and eat chocolate, as they no longer seemed to trigger off migraines. By this stage, she had begun to forget what a migraine felt like!

ALLERGY AND INTOLERANCE

Both Jane and Susan were clearly being made ill by the food they ate. But their symptoms were very different – and so was the treatment they received from the medical profession. Food allergy – which caused Jane's dramatic illness – is a recognized complaint, whose underlying mechanism is fairly well understood. Food intolerance, on the other hand, is not regarded as a sound diagnosis by the majority of doctors. Most would agree that there *is* such a thing as food intolerance (although they might use a different name for it), but they would argue that it affects relatively few people. Like Susan's doctor, they would regard the majority of patients with vague, multiple symptoms, including headache or migraine, fatigue and diarrhoea, as suffering from emotional and mental problems that expressed themselves in ill-health.

This book deals with both food allergy (Jane's problem) and food intolerance (Susan's problem), but it concentrates most attention on food intolerance, since this is the area that has been sadly neglected by conventional medicine. (The reasons for this neglect, and for the continuing controversy over food intolerance, will be examined later, in Chapter Six.)

The meaning of 'allergy'
The medical controversy about adverse reactions to food is compounded by a long-running dispute over the meaning of **allergy**. For a word that is scarcely more than 80 years old, it has had a very chequered career. A Viennese doctor, Baron Clemens von Pirquet, first used it in 1906 to mean 'altered reactivity'. Von Pirquet was a paediatrician and he felt the need for a new medical term to describe certain reactions in his young patients. These changed reactions included the development of immunity to infection, on the one hand, and marked reactions to certain foods, pollen or insect stings, on the other. He was principally concerned with reactions involving the **immune system**, the set of cells that protect our bodies from infection. But he apparently intended his newly coined word to mean *any* altered response to the environment. In this context, **environment** means all the external things that can affect the body, whether in food or water, in the air we breathe, or in things that come into contact with our skin. Von Pirquet also introduced the word **allergen** to describe the substances that brought about these changed reactions.

At that stage, very little was known about how some of these reactions might arise. The following decades brought greater understanding, and the meaning of allergies was narrowed down – the development of immunity to disease was dropped from the definition, because it was obviously something quite different from adverse reactions to food, pollen or bee stings.

In 1925, the definition of allergy was narrowed down still further. Experiments had shown that many adverse reactions to pollen or food could be transferred from one person to another by injecting a small amount of blood serum into the skin. The area around the injection site became very sensitive to the allergen. This, and other evidence, indicated that the immune system really was at work in these cases, as von Pirquet seems to have suspected. Most of those working in the field decided to limit the definition. Henceforth, a disease could only be described as an allergy if the immune system was demonstrably involved.

The way to demonstrate immune system involvement was by a **skin-prick test**. This involved making a purified extract of the allergen. A small amount of the extract was then inserted under the skin, by scratching or pricking it. If the area came up in a bump with a large area of red, itchy skin around it, then an **immune reaction** had occurred.

It had become clear that patients with certain diseases were likely to give positive skin-prick tests. These diseases were **hay-fever**, **asthma** (breathlessness with wheezing episodes), and **non-seasonal** or **perennial rhinitis** (constant runny or congested nose). Also linked with positive skin-prick tests, although to a lesser extent, were **urticaria** or **hives** (a rash that resembles nettle-stings) and one type of **eczema** (areas of red, itchy, flaky skin). Moreover, these five disorders often seemed to go together, either in individuals or in families.

These became the only legitimate subjects for study as far as orthodox allergists were concerned, and they are still described as the **classical allergic disorders**. Included in their ranks was a type of reaction to food that was very violent and came on rapidly after eating the allergen, often within minutes. The symptoms produced included swelling of the lips, mouth and tongue, urticaria (nettle-rash), vomiting and, in severe cases, collapse or **anaphylactic shock** – the reaction that Jane experienced when she ate peanuts in the restaurant cheesecake. In these cases, too, there was almost always a positive reaction to a skin-prick test with the suspect food.

Not everyone was happy with the change in the definition of allergy. At the time this change was made, several doctors in the US were already studying what they called 'delayed' or 'masked' food allergies. In these cases, the symptoms were much more varied. They also took far longer to materialize and were less acute. Because they rarely gave positive skin-prick tests, they could not be included in the new definition of allergy.

While the doctors concerned with 'masked food allergy' protested at the redefinition of allergy announced by their colleagues, they lost out to the newly arisen orthodoxy. There was pressure on them to conform, both from the medical establishment and, in some cases, from large food manufacturers who were funding research, and were alarmed at the idea of whole sections of the populace discovering they could not eat wheat or milk – the two most common culprits as identified by the alternative allergists. There are very few processed foods that do *not* contain wheat or milk.

Some of the doctors involved in such unpopular research were highly respected medical scientists, with promising research careers ahead of them. But all this pressure eventually forced them out of the medical mainstream and into private practice, where they continued to use the term 'allergy' in their own way – to mean simply 'altered reactivity'. This tradition has continued in the USA, and many American doctors working in this field still use 'allergy' in this much broader sense. Other doctors, especially in Britain, prefer the less controversial terms 'food intolerance' or 'food sensitivity'.

Another trans-Atlantic difference should be pointed out here. The American doctors working in this field describe themselves as **clinical ecologists** because they are concerned with the effect of a great variety of environmental factors – such as pollens, synthetic chemicals and air pollutants – as well as food. Some of their British and Australian counterparts also use this title, but most reject it because of its perceived links with the worst sort of fringe medicine and bogus diagnostic methods. Nevertheless, most of the British doctors who study and treat food intolerance also consider other forms of allergy and sensitivity, including chemical sensitivity, a subject that is discussed in detail in Chapter Nine.

Enter IgE

A major advance in classical allergy – and one that helped to widen the rift with the unorthodox food allergists – was the discovery of **immunoglobulin E**, or **IgE**, in the 1960s. This type of immunoglobulin, or **antibody**, is the main villain in the classical allergic conditions. How it works will be considered in some detail in the next chapter, but it is worth describing briefly here.

An antibody is a protein molecule made by the body to help combat disease-causing bacteria and viruses. The antibody binds to a specific target, known as its **antigen**. This target is usually a chemical located on the virus or bacterium, so the net result is that the antibody binds to the invader. The bound antibodies are rather like accusing fingers, pointing at the invading microbe – their presence rouses the body's defensive cells (the **immune cells**) to attack the microbe.

What goes wrong in allergy is that the body makes IgE antibodies in response to an innocuous antigen, such as a food molecule. IgE antibodies are usually found on the surface of special immune cells known as **mast cells**, that occur in tissues throughout the body.

If the IgE molecules on the surface of a mast cell bind to their specific antigen, they stimulate the mast cell to release several chemical messengers. The normal purpose of these chemicals is to organize a more effective immune response, but in sufficient quantities they can produce the damaging symptoms of allergy. The antigen that causes such a reaction (*eg* a food molecule) is known as an **allergen**.

The discovery of IgE was a breakthrough for classical allergists. Laboratory tests showed raised levels of total IgE in most patients displaying classical allergic symptoms. If the patient knew what antigen caused their symptoms, then a radioallergosorbent test or **RAST** (described on p82) could be applied to measure IgE for that specific antigen. The RAST result usually confirmed that there was an excessive amount of IgE antibody that would bind the incriminated antigen. In a very short space of time, IgE became the touchstone of respectability for classical allergists. Some even changed the definition of allergy, yet again, to mean reactions involving IgE only. This definition is still used by a few allergists.

When immunologists tried RASTs on patients diagnosed as food-allergic, they found a basic division. Those like Jane, with immediate, violent reactions, even to a very small amount of the offending food, almost always had high levels of IgE for that food, confirming the status of such reactions as classical allergies. Those like Susan, with 'delayed' or 'masked' reactions to foods, rarely produced positive RAST results for their culprit foods. More recently, some studies have shown that a small IgE reaction in the gut wall could be a contributing factor in people like Susan, but IgE is certainly not the major cause of the problem.

A battle of words

'When *I* use a word it means just what I choose it to mean . . .' as Humpty Dumpty declared in Lewis Carroll's *Through the Looking Glass.* This sort of verbal anarchy should not be encouraged, but there is so little agreement over terms such as 'food allergy', 'food intolerance', and 'food sensitivity', (not to mention 'food idiosyncrasy', 'false food allergy', 'pseudo-food allergy' and 'food hypersensitivity') that anyone writing about this subject is forced to take Humpty Dumpty's line. There is no option but to select a set of suitable words and state clearly at the outset what is meant by them.

Food allergy is used in this book to mean any adverse reaction to food in which the immune system is demonstrably involved. A positive skin-prick test, as described above, is usually taken as adequate proof of immune-system involvement, although this should be backed up by RAST or other laboratory tests, where possible. Where skin-prick tests or RAST results are negative, this does not necessarily mean that the immune system is not involved. Although reactions involving IgE are the principal cause of such allergies, there are other possible mechanisms, some of which will be considered in Chapter Five. Different kinds of tests are needed for this type of allergy.

False food allergy here denotes a special type of non-immunological reaction, seen with particular foods, in which a substance in the food triggers the mast cells *directly*. The reaction is not really an allergy at all: the immune system is not at fault and the body does not over-produce IgE. But because the end result (the mast cells releasing their chemical messengers) is the same, the symptoms are exactly like those of food allergy.

Food intolerance, as used in this book, means any adverse reaction to food, other than false food allergy, in which the involvement of the immune system is unproven because skin-prick tests and other tests for allergy are negative. This does not exclude the possibility of immune reactions being involved in some way, but they are unlikely to be the major factor producing the symptoms.

Food sensitivity is employed as an umbrella term for food allergy, food intolerance and other adverse reactions to food, except where these are purely psychological in origin. As will become obvious, the dividing line between food allergy and food intolerance is sometimes blurred, so there is a need for a term that covers both.

Food aversion – the only non-controversial term in this list – means dislike and avoidance of a particular food for purely psychological reasons.

These definitions are ones that the majority of mainstream doctors practising in this field would feel reasonably happy with. But bear in mind, if comparing this book with other books or articles, that the same words may be used in an entirely different way. It is also important to remember that they are *theoretical* definitions, and there is a sizeable gap between theory and practice when it comes to diagnosing individual patients. In practice the designation of an illness as 'food allergy' or 'food intolerance' would not depend so much on skin-prick tests or other tests as on the type of symptoms that the patient shows. If the symptoms are among those traditionally associated with allergy, such as asthma or urticaria, and if foods are shown to be responsible, then the condition will probably be labelled as food allergy, even if skin-prick tests are negative, as they sometimes are in such cases. If, on the other hand, the symptoms are not of the allergic kind – as in Susan's case – then the label 'food intolerance' will be used. Skin-prick tests will not normally be carried out because they are most unlikely to give a positive result, so they will not contribute much to the diagnosis.

In theory, then, the distinction between allergy and intolerance is based on *causes*. In the doctor's surgery, however, the distinction is likely to be based on *symptoms*, because it is known that asthma or urticaria are probably true allergic reactions, while migraine or depression are not. With a symptom such as diarrhoea, the cause might be an allergic reaction, an intolerant one, or something else entirely. In such cases, special tests would be needed to make a diagnosis of 'food allergy'.

Where patients show a collection of symptoms that include, say, asthma *and* migraine, the diagnosis is more difficult. If all these symptoms clear up at once when certain foods are avoided, is it allergy or is it intolerance? This is not a question that can be easily answered at present, and for the purposes of this book we will use the umbrella term 'food sensitivity' to cover such situations.

DANNY

For a young man of 22, Danny had a surprising number of health problems. Afraid of losing his job as a trainee hotel manager, he pretended not to be as unwell as he really was. He only consulted the doctor when the red, itchy bumps that covered his skin (nettle-rash) became unbearable. It was with great reluctance that he admitted his other symptoms – regular bouts of indigestion and diarrhoea, aches in his joints, headaches and extreme fatigue. There was also some eczema and hay-fever, both of which he had suffered from as a child. Skin-prick tests showed that he was sensitive to grass pollen and cat fur, but not to any foods. Nevertheless, the doctor decided to try Danny on an elimination diet, excluding most of the foods that he usually ate. Within six days he returned to the surgery looking very pleased. He reported that his nettle-rash was gone, along with his headaches, joint pains and digestive problems. He felt far more fit and energetic as well. Under the doctor's supervision, he then reintroduced foods one at a time. Wheat, milk, eggs, tomatoes and oranges caused the problems. These brought on urticaria within a few hours, with tiredness, headache and aching joints later. Danny can avoid these foods most of the time and has remained well. His eczema also cleared up after a while, and his hay-fever is less troublesome than before. This sort of case is interesting because the diet apparently helps with symptoms that are thought to be due to allergic reactions, such as urticaria and eczema, as well as clearing up symptoms like headache, diarrhoea and joint pain. There are many cases of this type on record, making it difficult to draw a sharp dividing line between food allergy and food intolerance.

Changing ideas about food allergy

Until fairly recently, most conventional allergists believed that the sort of symptoms seen in a patient depended largely on the type of allergen involved: the part of the body affected would be the part that first encountered the allergen. Thus, allergens that fell on the skin or brushed against it, called **contactants**, would tend to produce skin reactions such as eczema. Inhaled allergens or **inhalants**, such as pollen or dust, would produce symptoms in the nose and airways. Food allergens, obviously, would produce symptoms in the lips, mouth, stomach and gut. It was all very logical.

Among the patients treated by allergists, there were always some whose allergens could not be identified. With these unfortunate patients, it was assumed that some other non-allergic mechanism was producing the symptoms. Asthma patients, for example, were given the label 'intrinsic asthma' if no allergen could be pinpointed. Like many of the labels used in medicine this is just a clever way of saying that no-one has any idea what is causing the disease. These insoluble cases were an indication that something was wrong with the traditional concept of allergies, although few doctors realized this at the time.

In the last 20 years the traditional picture of allergies has changed substantially, as conventional allergists have recognized that things are much less neat and logical than they originally seemed. Allergens do not necessarily cause their major symptoms at the place where they first encounter the body. They can enter the body by one route and then cause symptoms somewhere else entirely, because they are carried to that point in the blood. Thus foods can cause asthma or eczema, although they are likely to share the blame with inhalants or contactants respectively. Inhaled allergens can also cause skin reactions because they enter the bloodstream through the membranes of the nose or lung and are carried by the blood to the skin.

It has taken a long time – 40 years or more – for these new ideas about allergy to be accepted by orthodox allergists. This is largely because the discoveries were first made by the clinical ecologists in America and their counterparts elsewhere – they tended to attract those patients who had been declared incurable by more conventional doctors. Because of the long-running controversy over clinical ecology, the traditional allergists at first regarded their findings with great suspicion.

Even today, there are vestiges of the old ideas about allergy in the way conventional allergists think about food. The traditional concept of a food allergy is a severe reaction to food which is almost always immediate. The types of symptoms produced are fairly well defined and limited in number – the sort of symptoms seen in Jane's case. Although most conventional allergists now accept that foods may produce slower and less violent reactions, with more varied symptoms, such as asthma and eczema, these are not what spring to mind when the words 'food allergy' are used. The same tends to be true of family doctors, and this is sometimes a contributing factor in the disagreements and misunderstandings over food allergy.

Food intolerance

Jane could fairly be described as a 'typical' case of food allergy. But Susan is not a typical case of food intolerance because there is no such thing. Food intolerance cannot lay claim to any single set of symptoms. Every patient is different, both in the cluster of symptoms they show and in the foods that affect them. Nor is there a single, clear-cut mechanism underlying the symptoms, as there is with food allergy. The available evidence indicates that there may be half-a-dozen or more different factors that contribute to the illness. In other words, food intolerance is a complex subject, and few generalizations can be made.

Nevertheless there are certain features that characterize this type of food sensitivity, and distinguish it from food allergy. Whereas food allergy reactions are usually immediate, food intolerance reactions tend to be much slower. The culprits in food intolerance are foods that are eaten very regularly, especially items such as wheat and milk that are consumed at almost every meal. The slowness of the reaction, combined with the fact that the foods are eaten so often, contributes to the 'masking' effect observed by the first doctors to study these reactions – the link between food and symptoms is unlikely to be made when the body is subjected to a constant bombardment with the food.

Whereas food allergy reactions can be provoked by quite small amounts of the food – a smear of the food from a badly washed saucepan for some highly allergic individuals – much larger quantities are needed to provoke the symptoms of food intolerance. Food intolerance is also far more insidious than food allergy: it is often difficult to say when it began, because the symptoms are very mild at first but gradually get worse. There are exceptions to this rule however, for in some cases a bad bout of influenza or diarrhoea can spark off food intolerance. As in Susan's case, those with food intolerance tend to collect more and more new symptoms as the years go by, and become intolerant of more and more foods.

Food allergy usually persists for many years, often for a lifetime, even though the food is scrupulously avoided. Food intolerance, on the other hand, may well disappear if the food is not eaten for a few months. But it will tend to recur if the food is ever eaten regularly again.

The symptoms of food intolerance are extraordinarily varied and affect almost every body system. The illustration opposite summarizes the major symptoms that are generally agreed upon. Most doctors working in this field would probably wish to add various other symptoms to this list, and there is

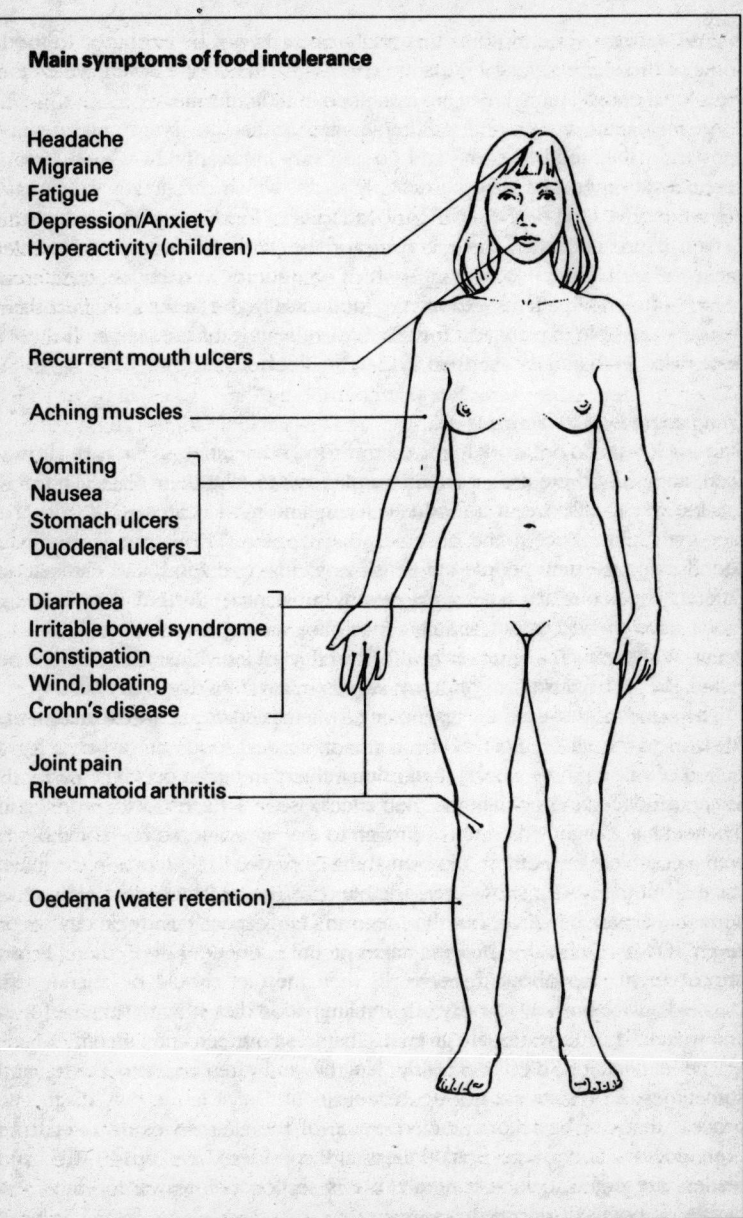

Main symptoms of food intolerance

Headache
Migraine
Fatigue
Depression/Anxiety
Hyperactivity (children)

Recurrent mouth ulcers

Aching muscles

Vomiting
Nausea
Stomach ulcers
Duodenal ulcers

Diarrhoea
Irritable bowel syndrome
Constipation
Wind, bloating
Crohn's disease

Joint pain
Rheumatoid arthritis

Oedema (water retention)

intense debate over symptoms that might or might not be attributed to food. Some of these controversial areas are considered in Chapter Seven, where the symptoms of food intolerance are described in more detail.

An important aspect of food intolerance is that the symptoms are not constant – they tend to come and go and vary in severity. Non-food factors may play an important part, particularly stress, which can greatly exacerbate the symptoms. One of the most curious facets of food intolerance is that the person concerned often has a craving for the particular food or foods that cause the problem. In such cases – which account for as many as 50 per cent of food-intolerant patients – eating the food initially gives a sense of great well-being. A possible explanation for this bizarre feature of the disease has now been discovered and is described in Chapter Twelve.

Diagnosing food intolerance

Skin-prick tests do not work in the case of food intolerance, as we have already seen, and sadly there are no other simple tests to take their place. The only reliable way to discover if a food is causing illness is to eliminate it from the diet, then reintroduce it and observe what happens. This is not as easy as it sounds, because few people are sensitive to just one food, and eliminating different foods one at a time rarely has any substantial effect. All the offending foods have to be cut out simultaneously for an improvement in health to occur. Without such a return to health, the effect of individual foods cannot be tested, simply because the symptoms vary so much from day to day anyway.

The standard test used for diagnosing food intolerance is the **elimination diet**, in which all or most of the commonly eaten foods are avoided for a period of one to three weeks. If an improvement in health occurs, then foods are reintroduced individually and their effect assessed. Every doctor working in this field has a slightly different approach to the elimination diet – some begin with a complete fast, others allow anything from two to 50 foods in the initial stage – but the results show a remarkable consistency. The patient often feels a great deal worse initially, but then recovers fairly spectacularly on day six or seven. Occasionally the process takes a little longer, but if there is no improvement after about three weeks then the diet should be abandoned. Detailed advice on how to carry out an elimination diet, how to prepare for it, and what to do afterwards, are given in Chapters Fourteen and Fifteen.

The elimination diet is a fairly lengthy and tiresome procedure, and sometimes the results are not entirely clear-cut. But it is the only diagnostic process that can be recommended. Some of the alternatives on offer from both doctors and fringe practitioners are considered on pp100–104, and readers are urged to look carefully at this section before wasting time and money on bogus diagnostic tests.

FOOD FOR THOUGHT

All of us, patients and doctors alike, are conditioned to think about food and other aspects of our environment in a particular way. As civilized inhabitants of temperate climes, we can indulge in the luxury of regarding 'nature' as safe and welcoming, and of thinking of food as entirely wholesome and beneficial. These attitudes are part of our culture, another luxury that we simply take for granted, like armchairs or motor cars. If we are to understand food intolerance, some of these accepted ideas need to be challenged.

Much of the medical prejudice against food intolerance is rooted in the idea that food – as long as it is part of a balanced diet – 'cannot be bad for you'. What is often forgotten is that our foods were not designed specifically for human consumption, but were drawn from a pool of wild plants and animals that were domesticated by the first farmers.

In the wild, most food items are reluctant food items. They do not want to be eaten, and their efforts to stay off the menu are part of what Charles Darwin called the 'struggle for existence'. Most animals can run away, or fight back, but plants do not have this option.

Their defence is based partly on thorns and prickles, but far more important than these is the array of invisible chemical weapons that pervade almost all plant tissues. Some of these simply taste bad, others cause vomiting or other ill-effects. A few even mimic the hormones of insects or mammals and thus disrupt their growth or sexual development.

Plant-eating animals have, in the course of their evolution, simply adapted to these chemicals in their food. They can detoxify them sufficiently to be able to feed on their chosen food or foods, and the plants can ward them off sufficiently to stay alive. It is rather like the situation between criminals and the police, where each side becomes increasingly cunning, better armed and more ruthless, but neither side ever wins and obliterates the other. The term 'biological arms race' aptly describes this situation.

Fruits and nuts

Although most foods do not want to be eaten, there are exceptions to the rule in the form of fruits and nuts. These contain the seeds of the plant and they rely on animals eating them to disperse the seed. The wild version of a fruit such as an apricot consists of a juicy, sweetish layer on the outside, with which the plant tempts birds and other animals. Inside is the seed, which is protected by a hard kernel or 'stone'. The idea is that the animal eats the fruit, but that the seed passes through its gut to the outside and is voided with the animal's droppings, some distance away from the parent plant.

The seed itself is highly nutritious – it contains all the food the young seedling will need to become established – so the plant must guard its seeds well. Animals who might be tempted to break the apricot stone open and eat the seed as well are deterred by toxins, principally cyanides (the chemicals that give almonds and apricot kernels their characteristic smell and flavour). As a final safeguard, the parent plant adds a chemical to the outer skin of the fruit that affects the animal's gut. It speeds up the movements of the gut, making it void the stone more rapidly, so that the damage done by the digestive juices is minimised. This is why so many fruits have a laxative effect.

Nuts are rather more generous to their animal partners. They rely on animals such as squirrels that hoard food for the winter months, and they operate a 'planned loss' strategy, whereby a great many of the seeds are actually eaten. The pay-off is that the squirrels not only disperse the seed, but also plant them in a suitable spot when creating their winter stores. Since they inevitably forget where some are planted, a proportion of the nuts survive and grow into trees.

Both nuts and fruits have a major problem to contend with, despite these cunning stratagems. There are a great many other living things that would like to eat them without providing any service in return. These range from small animals, that might nibble away at the fruit without dispersing it, to bacteria and fungi that would rot the nut as it lies in the soil.

A range of chemicals are present to keep these creatures at bay, many of them being selective toxins that affect one type of creature but not another. The 'poisonous berries' of many wild plants are poisonous only to mammals – birds relish them, and are of far more use to the plant in dispersal. The chemicals that stop bacteria and fungi from spoiling the fruit or nut are not always so specific. Although their main effect will be on microscopic life-forms, they may have minor untoward effects on larger animals as well – including human beings.

Clearly, there is a massive chemical arsenal in wild food, even in the foods that *want* to be eaten. In the course of our evolution, we have adapted to the challenge of eating these chemicals.

Eating everything

Being an omnivore – an animal who eats adaptably, taking whatever is available – is a high-risk, high-return strategy in the natural world. It opens up a huge range of foods, but it makes it impossible for the omnivore to adapt to the specific chemical toxins of a single food source. Rats are omnivores, which is why they are so remarkably successful and so very difficult to poison. When a rat encounters a new food it nibbles at it very cautiously, taking a tiny amount. Then it waits for a day or so. As long as it is not ill, it returns to eat some more.

At one time, the human approach to eating out would have been very similar. Until about 10,000 years ago our ancestors were hunter-gatherers whose food consisted of wild plants and animals. Like the rat, they would generally have approached new foods with extreme caution. They would also have been endowed, as we are today, with the best type of equipment for breaking down food toxins. That equipment resides in the liver, in the form of chemical compounds called **enzymes** that can break down foreign molecules. A powerful set of detoxification enzymes is something every good omnivore needs.

We are still omnivores today, although we do not rely much on wild foods. Farming changed our way of eating fundamentally, but it was not a change that happened overnight. The process took thousands of years, beginning with the collecting of wild grasses where these were growing abundantly. The wealth of food available from this harvest allowed people to settle down in one place, whereas before they had always been nomadic. The grass seeds could be stored and eaten for a large part of the year, but other wild plants and animals were still a major element in the diet.

The transition to farming took place once people realized that they could *plant* some of the stored seed and thus grow more grasses and increase their food supply. In time, they would have started to select the seeds used for planting, choosing those from the best types of grass. The process of domestication and plant improvement had begun.

Staple crops

All this happened in the Middle East, about 12,000–10,000 years ago, when the earliest forms of wheat and barley were domesticated. The same sort of events occurred quite independently in the Far East between about 9,000 and 7,000 years ago, and in Central America over 7,000 years ago. Grass-derived crops, which we now call cereals, were important in both areas. In the Far East, rice became the main crop (or **staple**), while in the Americas it was maize, also known as corn. In Africa, domestication probably took place rather later, and the main cereal crops were millet and sorghum. South-east Asian farmers differed in relying on a root-crop, the yam, as their staple, and root-crops were also important in other parts of the world where grasses did not grow well. The potato became the main crop of the high Andes, and in tropical Africa another type of yam was grown.

With the growing of these staple crops, foods such as grass seeds and roots, that had previously been eaten in fairly small amounts, became the mainstay of the diet. Some people believe that this was a bad thing for human health because we were not adapted to eat large quantities of starch, but that is a debatable point. What may be more important is the fact that we are eating large quantities of the particular chemical 'armaments' found in these crops. Selection and plant breeding have reduced the amounts of these armaments substantially, of course, which is why our crop plants lack the bitterness of their wild equivalents, such as crab-apples or sloes. But it is possible that some chemicals with more insidious effects may remain, and that relying so heavily on a staple crop may expose us to excessive amounts of those chemicals.

ENZYMES

Enzymes are specialized molecules found only in living things (the ones in biological washing powders are extracted from living things). They are absolutely essential to life, because they make specific chemical reactions happen. For example, they join other molecules together to build up the cells that make up living bodies. They also break down food (digestive enzymes), so that the energy it contains can be utilized, and break down toxins (detoxification enzymes) to make them harmless. They transform surplus food into fat stores, or break down the fat to yield energy when food is short.

Although they cannot be seen, even under a microscope, there are hundreds of thousands of different enzymes in the human body. Each enzyme has a very specific job to do: most of them only control one reaction, although others are slightly more versatile. For example, some of the digestive enzymes can break down a variety of food molecules of the same general type. Enzymes themselves are controlled by smaller molecules which can turn a particular enzyme on or off.

Enzymes are just one type of **protein** molecule. Like all proteins, enzymes are made according to an inherited pattern which is passed on from parent to child. This pattern is stored in the genetic material, the DNA. In fact, DNA acts as a template, from which all enzymes and other protein molecules are made. If there is a change in the DNA – a **mutation** – then the enzyme which is coded for by that part of the DNA will be altered. Usually these changes are for the worse, and the enzyme does not work as well as the original version. What sort of effect this enzyme defect has will depend on how important the enzyme is, what sort of reaction it controls and how badly it has been affected. Defective enzymes may play a part in food intolerance – they will be considered in more detail in Chapter Twelve.

A possible suspect in this regard is wheat. Certain people, known as **coeliacs**, are made seriously ill by wheat (see p142). Coeliac disease is inherited, which suggests that there are genetic differences making some people better able to cope with a wheat-based diet than others. This was confirmed by experiments in which very large amounts of wheat protein were given to healthy volunteers. The relatives of coeliacs were made ill by these large amounts of wheat protein – so were 'normal' people, but the relatives of coeliacs suffered more.

It looks very much as if coeliacs are unfortunate casualties of the slow adaptation process between the human race and wheat. Wheat, after all, is a relatively new food – we have only had 10,000 years to get used to it, which is the blinking of an eye in evolutionary terms. Although natural selection should gradually eliminate any genes that make human beings susceptible to wheat (at least among wheat-eating populations) it seems to be a process that has not had time to run to completion. There is some evidence for this, in that wheat proteins reduce the absorption of starch in most people. (Starch, if unabsorbed, goes to feed bacteria in the gut, and could perhaps cause an overgrowth of unwanted bacteria.)

If this theory is correct, then it is possible that some non-coeliacs are adversely affected (though not as seriously) by defensive chemicals found in wheat. Not just affected by very large amounts, as in the experiment described above, but affected by a normal, everyday intake of wheat. Natural selection works more slowly on a gene that has mild ill-effects than on one with serious ill-effects, such as coeliac disease. So it is even more likely that *minor* problems with a new food would persist for thousands of years.

This could explain why wheat sensitivity is so common, although there are other equally plausible explanations. Wheat, along with milk, is the most commonly eaten food in Western countries, and may appear in every meal and snack of the day. There is little doubt that a food which is consumed frequently is far more likely to cause food intolerance (although no-one knows precisely why) and this alone could account for wheat's bad record.

Other foods, besides cereals, are a possible source of toxic or damaging chemicals. Some are known to cause **false food allergy** in susceptible individuals (p79) and a few can cause cancer. Others, such as coffee, have a drug-like (**pharmacological**) action on the body, which means that they produce marked physiological effects even though they are eaten in very small amounts. Some of these are looked at more closely on p83 and p165.

History lessons
Another of our cultural myths is that the past is a perfect guide to what we should eat. Hence the common criticism of ideas about food intolerance:

'Surely foods that have been eaten for thousands of years can't cause serious health problems – if they did it would have been noticed before.' In fact, experience shows that human beings are rather bad at identifying foods which cause non-acute, long-term illness. The rat, remember, only waits a day to see if a new food makes it ill. Like rats, we are programmed to notice short-term effects only.

The best illustration of this is the failure to identify wheat as a factor in coeliac disease until the 1940s. It took a famine in Holland at the end of World War II to remove wheat from the diet, and an observant doctor to recognize that his coeliac patients were miraculously cured. Similarly, the islanders of Guam have traditionally used the seeds of the false sago palm, a type of cycad, as food. Although they suffered from a high incidence of senile dementia, no-one made any connection between this and the cycad seeds. But in the 1950s an epidemic of dementia began, which continues to this day. Scientists have traced it back to the war years, when Guam was occupied by the Japanese, food was desperately scarce, and the islanders had to rely heavily on false sago palm as a result. A constituent of the seeds has proved to be responsible for degeneration of the nerves and brain.

A third example comes from China, where a cancer survey showed an unusually high level of oesophageal cancer in one province (the oesophagus is the tube that leads from the mouth to the stomach). The local tradition of making pickled vegetables in huge vats which were left to mature for months proved to be the cause. The thick layer of mould that grew on the pickles was producing **carcinogens** (cancer-producing compounds) which seeped into the pickles. Even though the mould was scraped off before the pickles were eaten, enough carcinogens were there to give susceptible people cancer.

The moral of these stories is *not* that food in general can cause fatal diseases – the cycad seeds and mouldy pickles are extreme in that respect. The important lesson to be learned here is that history is sometimes a poor guide to diet.

Digesting the facts

To add to the myths about food, there are some long-standing misconceptions about human digestion that fuel the arguments over food sensitivity. The most important one is that food is broken down into very small molecules before any of it is absorbed. Every school biology student is taught this: that the enzymes in the mouth, stomach and small intestine break down food into its basic constituents. **Starches** (**complex carbohydrates**) are broken down into **sugars**, and **proteins** are broken down into **amino acids**. These very small molecules are then absorbed and enter the bloodstream, but larger molecules are excluded by the gut wall – or so the story goes. If this were true, food could not cause allergic reactions in the skin or airways: the molecules that got through the gut wall would be too small to provoke any reaction by immune cells in the blood, which only respond to fairly large molecules, not to simple sugars or amino acids.

Research carried out in the last 10–20 years has shown that this picture of digestion is very simplistic and misleading, but the news has been a long time getting through. In one study, healthy adults were given potato starch dispersed in water to drink. After 15–30 minutes, blood samples contained up to 300 starch grains per millilitre of blood.

After a meal, a small number of undigested or partially digested food molecules are found in the bloodstream, so it is clear that the gut wall is not as impregnable as was once thought. In fact, specialized areas of the gut wall actually 'sample' the gut contents, actively taking up droplets of liquid that contain intact food molecules. The cells that do this are called **Peyer's patches** and they form part of the immune system. By sampling the gut contents they are able to prepare the body for the arrival of food molecules in the bloodstream. They ensure that the body makes a distinction between these food molecules and any disease organisms that may enter the blood. Under normal circumstances, this prevents the body from mounting unnecessary and damaging attacks against the food molecules. How this is achieved is explained on pp233–4.

Chapter Two

FOOD ALLERGY, MAST CELLS AND IgE

According to the most widely accepted definition, an allergy is *any* idiosyncratic reaction in which the immune system is clearly involved. However, the main agent of allergy is IgE, and allergists have traditionally concentrated on IgE reactions or **Type 1 hypersensitivity**. These form the subject of this chapter and the two that follow. Allergic reactions that have nothing to do with IgE or mast cells are described in Chapter Five, along with false food allergies.

The history of food allergy

Hippocrates, the Father of Medicine, was the first to record an allergic reaction to food. He observed that while cheese was a wholesome food for most people, some were made severely ill by eating it, even in very small amounts. Other Greek writers recorded violent reactions in certain individuals to eggs, honey, strawberries, nuts, oysters or other shellfish. While some of these cases may have been false food allergy (see p79) others were probably food allergy proper.

In 1921, two German scientists, Carl Prausnitz and Heinz Kustner, showed that something in the blood could reproduce such reactions. Kustner was sensitive to fish and developed urticaria, or nettle-rash, soon after eating it. A small amount of blood serum from Kustner was injected into Prausnitz's arm. The next day fish extract was injected into the skin at the same spot and produced a red, itchy bump. When tested previously, there had been no such reaction. The two scientists gave the name **reagin** to the unknown component in the blood that had caused the reaction in Prausnitz.

The test became known as the **Prausnitz-Kustner test**, or **passive transfer test**, and was at one time used in diagnosing allergies. (The only reason it is no longer used is that there is a risk of transferring viral infections such as hepatitis and AIDS.) Progress thereafter was slow, and it was over 40 years before scientists could say exactly what 'reagin' was. The breakthrough came in the 1960s, the result of painstaking research work by a Japanese husband-and-wife team, Kimishige and Teruko Ishizaka, working in the United States. They discovered that reagin is a type of **antibody**, now known as **IgE**.

PROTEINS

Proteins make up our skin, hair and bones. They are major components of the nerves, blood and all other cells in the body. Specialized proteins in the muscles produce contraction by sliding over each other. Another hard-working protein, called haemoglobin, carries oxygen around in the blood, while strong, elastic proteins make up our tendons and ligaments. Chemically adept proteins known as **enzymes** control all the chemical reactions in the body and regulate every living process (see p18). Antibodies, and many other crucial components of the immune system, are also proteins.

Proteins can do these many different jobs because they are made up of long chains of chemicals called **amino acids**. The types of amino acid present, and the order in which they occur, is different for each type of protein. Once the chains have been formed, they are folded up in a specific way to give a compact protein molecule, often spherical or sausage-shaped. In the case of enzymes, one small area on the surface of the molecule is the **active site**, where the crucial chemical reaction controlled by that enzyme occurs. Similarly, in antibodies, the particular combination and arrangement of amino acids at the **antigen-binding site** (see p24) decides which antigen it will bind.

There are 20 common types of amino acid each with its own distinctive chemical properties. Some are attracted to water, others repel it. Some can react with one type of molecule, others do not. It is the different combinations of amino acids that make proteins so different from one another. They give enzymes their impressive range of chemical abilities, and account for the versatility of antibodies.

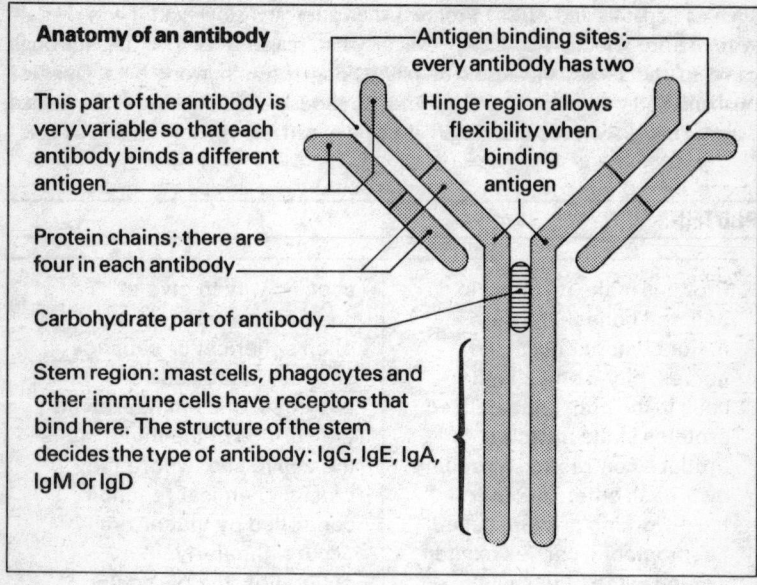

Anatomy of an antibody

Antigen binding sites; every antibody has two

This part of the antibody is very variable so that each antibody binds a different antigen

Hinge region allows flexibility when binding antigen

Protein chains; there are four in each antibody

Carbohydrate part of antibody

Stem region: mast cells, phagocytes and other immune cells have receptors that bind here. The structure of the stem decides the type of antibody: IgG, IgE, IgA, IgM or IgD

Fighting infections – the versatile antibody

Antibodies are special molecules produced by the body to fight off infections. They bind firmly to the bacteria or virus that causes the infection and, with luck, this stops the infection in its tracks. Antibodies can block infection in a variety of ways. With viruses, they may be able to prevent them from invading the body's cells simply by binding to them. With bacteria, however, antibodies alone are ineffectual. They need help to defeat the bacteria and their job is to act as signals to other cells and molecules in the body which have the power to kill. The antibodies form a coat on the surface of the bacterial cells and this stimulates the immune system's 'assassination teams' to go into action against the bacteria.

Antibodies are **protein** molecules, as are many of the important, hard-working components of the body (see p23). Proteins are infinitely variable molecules and this is what makes them so useful. In the case of the antibodies, their versatility is employed in making molecules that bind specifically to a particular target molecule, or **antigen**, and to no other. The measles virus, for example, is bound by antibodies that specifically recognize proteins in the outer coat of the virus – these being the measles antigens. They do not normally bind to anything else, apart from the measles virus.

The body produces a vast range of different antibodies – millions of them –

so that if it has to combat a new bacteria or virus it is certain to find an antibody 'in stock' that is just right for it. The antibodies are produced by special factory cells called **B cells**, and each B cell produces its own particular form of antibody. When faced with an invading microbe, the body selects a B cell with the right antibody to match that microbe, stimulates the cell to divide, and then instructs all the cells that are descended from it to produce their much-needed antibody. This continues until there is enough of the correct antibody to defeat the infection.

Different types of antibody

Antibodies are Y-shaped molecules, as the picture opposite shows. At the tip of each arm is an **antigen-binding site** where the antibody can bind to the particular feature of the antigen that it recognizes. These antigen-binding sites are the most changeable part of the antibody molecule – they vary enormously from one antibody to another. Their chemical structure determines which antigen is bound by that antibody.

The stem of an antibody can also vary, although nothing like as much. There are five basic types of stem, and they produce five different types of antibody, known as **isotypes**. The names of these isotypes (in order of abundance) are : IgG, IgA, IgM, IgD and IgE. In all cases the letters 'Ig' stand for **immunoglobulin** – another name for antibody. Imbalances between the different isotypes of antibody may play a role in food intolerance, and they will appear again in Chapter Twelve.

IgE and mast cells

IgE molecules are just as specific for their antigen as other antibody isotypes but they operate in a rather different way. Their main function is to defend the body against parasites such as ringworms and flukes – these are much larger than bacteria and viruses so the body has different strategies for killing them. In the tropics, where parasites are common, quite high levels of IgE may be found even in non-allergic people. Cooler conditions are not as favourable to parasites and they are far less of a health problem – in non-allergic people living in temperate climates, the level of IgE is usually very low.

Like other antibodies, IgE molecules are produced by B cells. But once they have been produced, the IgE molecules behave differently from most other antibodies in that they attach themselves to **mast cells** and **basophils.** These two types of cell look slightly different under the microscope, and whereas basophils are found floating in the blood, mast cells are embedded in the solid tissues of the body. Mast cells are better known and understood, so we will conveniently ignore the basophils from here onwards: the two types of cell probably work in much the same way.

Although the stem of the IgE molecule is attached to the mast cell, the antigen-binding sites are still free. So when the right antigen comes along, it will bind to the IgE molecules. This is the signal the mast cell has been waiting for. Packets of chemicals inside the cell are suddenly released to the outside, where they act as messengers, causing major changes in the cells and tissues around them. One of the main chemicals to be released is called **histamine** – hence the use of drugs that counteract its effects, **antihistamines**, in the treatment of allergies. The packets of chemicals inside the resting mast cell look like small granules under the microscope, so the process of releasing the chemicals is called **degranulation**.

Histamine and other chemicals released by mast cells are called **mediators**

THE UBIQUITOUS MAST CELL

Mast cells are found embedded in our tissues throughout the body. They are especially common around the tubes leading to the lung (the bronchi), in the nose and in the gut – in other words, they are well positioned to guard the body's vulnerable entrance points from parasites. Each mast cell can have as many as 100,000 IgE molecules on its surface. These will not all be from the same B cell – so they will respond to different antigens.

The chemical mediators that do so much damage to allergic individuals are stored in tiny membrane-bound packets inside the mast cell. These give the cell a granular appearance under the microscope. For the mast cell to release its mediators –

degranulate – an antigen must bind more than one IgE molecule on the cell surface. The crucial signal for degranulation is the cross-linking of two or more IgEs by an antigen.

Although this is the main way of making mast cells degranulate, there are other methods as well. Some foods contain substances that trigger mast cells directly causing **false food allergies** in certain people (see p79). Some bacteria produce toxins that can trigger mast cells directly. It may even be possible for the body to trigger mast cells itself, in response to an irritant substance in food, for example. These different methods of firing the mast cells make the diagnosis of allergy a complex business.

How a mast cell is triggered into action

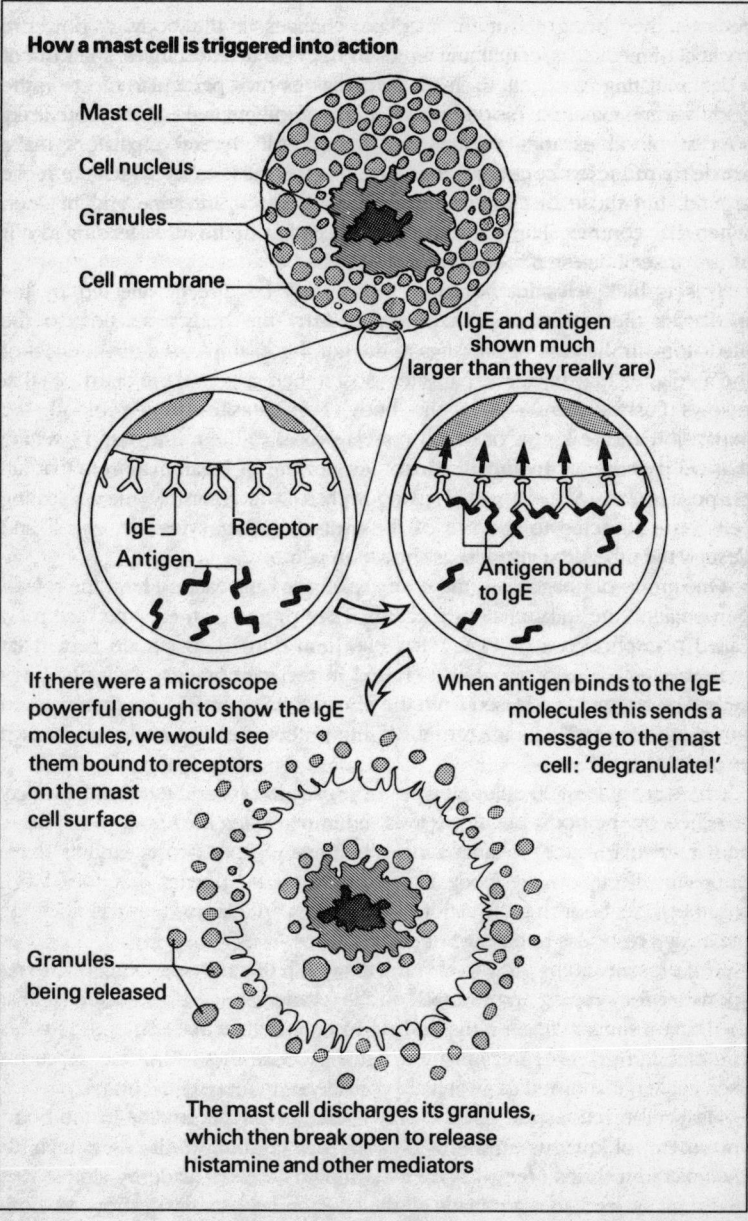

Mast cell

Cell nucleus

Granules

Cell membrane

(IgE and antigen
shown much
larger than they really are)

IgE ⌐ Receptor

Antigen

Antigen bound
to IgE

If there were a microscope
powerful enough to show the IgE
molecules, we would see
them bound to receptors
on the mast
cell surface

When antigen binds to the IgE
molecules this sends a
message to the mast
cell: 'degranulate!'

Granules
being released

The mast cell discharges its granules,
which then break open to release
histamine and other mediators

because they bring about or 'mediate' changes in the body. A powerful cocktail of mediators, containing ten or more separate substances, spills out of a degranulating mast cell. Each mediator has its own particular effect on the body – some make the blood vessels open out, others make them more leaky so that blood escapes through the vessel wall. Several mediators make **smooth muscles** contract – these are not the muscles by which we move around, but those that operate our lungs, stomach, intestine and bladder. When they contract sharply, air may be expelled from the tubes leading to our lungs, or semi-digested food from our bowels.

This is bad news for parasites, which may be directly affected by the mediators themselves, and then assaulted by the body's reaction to the mediators. In the case of parasites in the gut, for example, the direct effect of the mediators may make the parasites loosen their grip, and the diarrhoea that follows flushes them out of the body. For parasites in the blood, the expansion and leakiness of blood vessels produces the redness and swelling that we describe as **inflammation**. One feature of inflammation is that all-purpose defensive cells called **phagocytes** (which simply means 'eating cells') are attracted to the site of the invasion. Phagocytes can engulf and destroy the unwanted invaders as shown on p76.

One group of phagocytes, the **macrophages** ('big eaters') have the role of perpetuating the inflammation reaction. They produce an enzyme (see p18) called phospholipase or PLA. What PLA then does is to cut up certain fat molecules – the phospholipids – found in the membranes of all our body cells. The fragments released from the phospholipids by PLA are then worked on by other enzymes, which turn them into potent chemical mediators, known as **prostaglandins**.

There are at least 20 different types of prostaglandin, and they have a variety of effects on the body, but all are involved in regulating the immune response, and particularly the inflammation response. Some prostaglandins have opposite effects on the body from others, so it appears that they work together, one modifying the actions of the other. In this way they can fine-tune the body's response to damage or danger.

The prostaglandins produced in the aftermath of a mast-cell reaction are responsible for keeping up the attack on the invader. So it is no coincidence that they have a similar effect on the body to histamine: they make smooth muscles contract and promote inflammation. They produce the 'late phase' reactions seen in allergic individuals, which are considered in more detail on p42.

Mast-cell reactions are not the only source of prostaglandins in the body, and these ubiquitous messengers also play a role in diseases such as rheumatoid arthritis (see p124). Prostaglandins can be made by almost *any* body cell. Indeed, they are made all the time, and constantly destroyed before they can have any effect (a common type of control mechanism in living organisms). The effect of the macrophages, attracted by the mast cells, is simply to boost production of prostaglandins so that they are made faster than they are destroyed. Several other types of cell can boost prostaglandin manufacture in the same way.

How IgE produces allergies

Anyone who lives in a town or city will have been kept awake, at some time or another, by the sound of a burglar alarm ringing endlessly in an empty shop or house. The alarm is only meant to ring if someone breaks in, but it is triggered off by some other quite innocent event, such as a strong wind or the vibrations of a passing lorry. This is more or less what happens in the case of allergies. The mast cells, which are meant to respond to invasion by parasites, are triggered off by an innocuous substance such as eggs or cow's milk. But why should this happen?

The answer is that the body misguidedly makes IgE antibodies that fit the antigens in these substances. A very complex and intricate set of controls normally prevent the body from making IgE in response to such harmless materials, but in the allergic individual something goes awry and the control mechanisms break down.

In the case of Jane, her body had mistakenly made IgE antibodies to an antigen in peanuts, probably a protein. The strange symptoms that she experienced on eating peanuts were all produced by mediators released from her mast cells. Mast cells in the tissues of the mouth were triggered as soon as the food came into contact with them, producing symptoms almost immediately. Her lips and tongue swelled up because tiny blood vessels inside them became leaky, allowing fluid to seep out into the surrounding tissues.

The cause of Jane's collapse (anaphylactic shock) when she ate peanuts again was a sudden drop in blood pressure, likewise produced by the mediators. This time, it seems, more IgE was present and far more mediators released. By making the blood vessels all over her body expand, and at the same time become more leaky, the mediators left her without enough blood pressure to keep the vital organs functioning.

In the case of asthma, it is the effect of histamine on the smooth muscles of the **bronchi** that produces the symptoms. These vital tubes, which carry air to the lungs, go into a spasmodic contraction. How the allergens reach the airways, and the types of allergens involved, will be dealt with in Chapter Three. The way in which mast cells cause other allergic reactions, such as hay-fever and perennial rhinitis, will also be described there.

As one might expect, people with these allergic disorders tend to have a higher level of IgE in their blood than others. But there are a few whose IgE

SKIN-PRICK TESTS

The standard test for allergy is the skin-prick test, which looks at how the skin reacts to a range of common allergens – or to the suspect allergen where the likely cause of the trouble has been identified but confirmation is still needed. Allergen extracts are used, these being prepared from pure samples of foods, pollens, house dust etc. A drop of the extract is placed on the arm, and a prick or scratch made in the skin below the drop. A minute amount of the allergen enters the skin, and if the patient is sensitive to the allergen there will be a marked reaction, known as a **wheal-and-flare** response.

Skin-prick tests work well for some types of allergen, particularly inhalants. But where the allergen is found in food, they often do not produce a positive result, except in cases where the patient's reaction to the food is immediate and violent.

Skin-prick tests can be negative even though there is a genuine allergic reaction, simply because the reaction is localized – in the gut, nose or wherever. IgE antibodies can often be demonstrated in the part of the body that is affected, but they have clearly not entered the bloodstream, which is why they are not present in the skin.

levels are normal. Conversely, there are quite a large number of people who have high levels of IgE, *and* give positive skin-prick tests to common allergens (see box), but who display no symptoms. Perhaps these symptom-free individuals have fewer, or less accessible, mast cells than others, making them less susceptible to high IgE levels. Or perhaps the mechanisms behind allergy are more complex than they appear, and IgE is only part of the story.

Antigens and allergens

Are antigens and allergens fundamentally different from each other? This is a question that causes a lot of confusion and it is worth spending some time looking at what these two words actually mean.

An **antigen** is any molecule that can provoke the body into producing antibodies to it. To do this the molecule must be above a certain size, because the B cells and their colleagues in the immune system are programmed to ignore very small molecules. So simple chemical molecules such as water or salt cannot act as antigens. However, some quite small molecules, that are too small to act as antigens on their own, may combine with proteins in the body, thus producing molecules that *are* large enough to be recognized by the immune system. Small molecules of this sort are called **haptens**.

Living organisms are composed of a great variety of chemical compounds, and some make more effective antigens than others. The important point about an antigen is that it should have at least one distinctive chemical structure on its surface – a chemical 'handle' that the antibody can grab hold of. This structure, which the antibody recognizes, is called the **epitope.**

One major group of antigens are the **proteins**, which are widespread in all living things (see p23). The chemical variety of proteins makes them good antigens – there are plenty of distinctive 'handles' for an antibody (itself a protein) to seize on. Some other chemicals found in living things are less distinctive chemically and they do not readily act as antigens – fats and oils, for example. Complex carbohydrates – which are made up of chains of sugar molecules – can act as antigens, although the sort that we eat in quantity (such as the starch found in potatoes and bread) are very dull chemically and unlikely to be antigenic. These foods also contain proteins, however, and it is mainly these that act as antigens.

The other potential source of antigens in food, apart from the proteins, are small molecules such as phenols, amines and carotenoids. Some of these give the food its colour and flavour, others are there to deter animals from feeding on that food, or prevent it being attacked by bacteria and fungi. The majority of these small molecules are natural compounds, but artificial colours, flavours and preservatives greatly increase the number present in modern food.

Most of these molecules are too small to be antigens in their own right, but can act as haptens. To do this they must combine with proteins in the food itself, or with proteins in our bodies – something they may do quite easily as they tend to be very reactive. The extent to which these small molecules can act as haptens is somewhat controversial, and the issue is clouded by the fact that many of these compounds also have toxic or pharmacological (drug-like) effects on the body.

An **allergen** is essentially the same thing as an antigen, except that it happens to cause an allergic reaction in a particular person. The proteins in cow's milk, for example, are antigens to most of us, but for the child with cow's-milk allergy they are allergens. *The main difference between an antigen and an allergen is not in the molecule itself but in the way the individual's immune system reacts to it.*

Having said that, it does seem that some foods are more 'allergenic' – more likely to cause allergies – than others. Certain foods turn up again and again as the culprits in food allergy, while other commonly eaten foods are rarely encountered. Why this is so, no-one can say at present, but there are several possible explanations.

Perhaps these apparently more allergenic foods contain compounds with very unusual and distinctive chemical features that are 'easily recognized'. Such compounds might induce IgE antibodies more readily than others, although it is far from certain that the structure of antigens *can* exert such an influence over the immune system. The whole question of how the body scrutinizes incoming antigens and regulates its response to them is still very poorly understood. As yet no-one can say what role the chemical make-up of antigens plays.

An alternative explanation is that such foods contain substances which stimulate an immune response, known collectively as **adjuvants**. Adjuvants are used in the laboratory as a way of inducing immune responses for research purposes. These adjuvants are mostly derived from bacteria, but there are also adjuvants found in some plants. The extent to which these occur in foods, and their potential for stimulating IgE rather than other types of antibody, is unknown.

One group of compounds that *do* occur in foods, and may be important here, are the **lectins**, protein molecules that bind to human cells. These cling to cells in the gut, and they may also be able to pass through the gut wall into the bloodstream, thus reaching every part of the body. Some lectins are known to affect the immune response, and a few promote the formation of IgE at the expense of other antibodies, especially in people prone to allergies. Many of the foods that commonly feature in food allergy, such as peanuts, are particularly rich in lectins. Perhaps the peanut lectins make the body more inclined to form IgE – so producing allergies to the other constituents of peanut.

Finally, there are some foods that appear to be potent allergens but in fact are not. What happens is that they trigger mast cells directly, producing **false food allergy** (see p79). Strawberries, shellfish, eggs, tomatoes and fish all come in this category. Some people who react to such foods will be displaying true IgE-mediated allergy, while others will be suffering from false food allergy. Only laboratory tests can sort out one from the other.

The allergic family

Classical allergic disorders, such as hay-fever, perennial rhinitis, asthma and urticaria, tend to 'run in the family': parents who suffer from them are much more likely than others to produce children with allergies. And if *both* parents have allergic problems then the children have an even higher chance of being affected. Not that the child and the parent will necessarily suffer from the same disorder. The parent may have severe rhinitis while the child suffers from asthma and eczema – or vice versa. Indeed, the child may begin with eczema in babyhood, lose the symptoms when it is two or three years old, but then develop asthma instead. These facts all suggest an underlying predisposition to allergy that manifests itself in different ways.

Doctors describe this constellation of symptoms as **atopy**, a word whose derivation and meaning is difficult to pin down. It comes from the Greek and is variously defined as meaning 'no place', 'out of place' or 'another place'. It is generally understood to mean that there is a deep-rooted problem which may produce symptoms in various places on the body, not just in one place as with most diseases. Patients with any of these classical allergic symptoms tend to be described as **atopic**, especially if other members of their family have allergies. They almost always show a positive reaction to the skin-prick test (see p30) when tested with a variety of common allergens.

Although atopics have more IgE in their blood than the average person, if the offending allergen can be eliminated – by avoiding a particular food, for example – their IgE levels often return to normal. So it seems possible that the root-cause of the problem is a failure to suppress IgE production *to particular substances*.

Clearly the genes responsible for these control mechanisms are not operating normally, but why the controls are so specific for particular substances is not known. It is especially puzzling in individuals who are violently allergic to just one substance. Other, less fortunate, individuals are allergic to a wide range of substances and readily develop new allergic reactions – in such cases it would seem that there is a more generalized fault in the IgE control-mechanism.

All in the genes?

If atopy is inherited, then the genetic information that is passed on from parent to child must in some way be faulty. Studies of atopic families have led to some understanding of the genetic mechanisms involved, and they help to explain some puzzling features of the problem.

By looking at seven families with asthma and allergic rhinitis, researchers in Oxford have identified a single gene that they believe is largely responsible for allergies. This discovery, published in 1989, was a surprise to doctors and research workers, who had previously thought that several genes must be involved. (Some still suspect that this really is the case.)

Everyone carrying this gene shows some positive reactions to skin-prick tests, or to laboratory tests for IgE. However, 15 per cent of those carrying the gene have no symptoms. And among the other 85 per cent, the severity of the symptoms varies greatly. All this suggests that other factors are at work. They may be minor genes, that modify the effects of the main one, or they could simply be environmental factors, such as breathing polluted air, a damp or dusty home, infections or diet.

It is definitely the case that the environment affects the likelihood of developing allergic responses. Identical twins – who carry exactly the same genes – can differ in terms of allergy. One may be afflicted and the other not, showing that something in the environment, which only one has experienced (probably an infection) is also important. It is interesting that Scandinavian babies born in the spring, when birch pollen is in the air, are more likely to develop hay-fever later in life. And in the case of food, early exposure to potential allergens is risky for the children of atopic parents (see p252).

It is clear then, that the allergy gene creates a tendency to allergy, and environmental factors, especially early in life, may then push the individual into expressing that potential. The question remains whether these factors alone can explain why 15 per cent with the crucial gene have no symptoms, or whether minor genes might also be involved.

The fact that parents with no obvious symptoms, and no atopic relatives, can still produce an atopic child suggests the existence of minor genes. Either the mother or the father is probably carrying the main gene for allergy but its effects are masked by more beneficial genes. When all the parental genes are reshuffled to produce eggs and sperm, and then combined with genes from the other parent, a different genetic setting is produced. In this setting, the main allergy gene is no longer masked.

Allergy and age

If defective genes lead to allergy then one would expect most allergies to begin early in life, as indeed they do. Symptoms cannot be produced the first time a person is exposed to an allergen, however. Although the body already has the capacity to produce antibodies to the allergen concerned (in the form of as-yet-unactivated B cells), the antibody itself is not there. An initial exposure is required to enable the body to 'find' the right B cell from its extensive stock and multiply it up to useful levels. Once this has happened, a second exposure to the allergen can stimulate antibody (IgE) production. The allergen can then trigger off IgE-coated mast cells with devastating results.

Despite this, a baby may react to a food allergen the first time he eats it because molecules of the food may have reached him by other means. One such route is breast milk, which contains molecules from the foods the mother herself is eating – only a few, of course, but enough to sensitize a highly atopic baby. Some babies may even be sensitized before birth, by food molecules in the mother's blood that pass into the foetus's blood. So it is important for atopic mothers-to-be to think about their diet. Chapter Thirteen suggests practical steps that can be taken by parents to reduce the risk of sensitizing their children.

As children get older, their early symptoms often disappear or at least diminish. Allergies to milk, egg and soya are those most likely to disappear with age, while allergies to peanuts, nuts and fish tend to persist into adult life.

For some children, the initial symptoms of the allergy, such as eczema, may disappear, only to be replaced by other symptoms, such as asthma. Others apparently lose their allergic reaction entirely, but may succumb to other health problems in adult life, which turn out to be food-related. There has never been any systematic study of such patients, so it is difficult to know whether their childhood illness has in any way influenced their health later. But some doctors who specialize in treating food allergy believe that the child's allergic reaction to foods does not 'disappear' but is simply *suppressed* by the body, only to recur in adult life, often in a different form. Paediatricians say that children grow out of their allergies, but perhaps they only grow out of their paediatricians!

If this theory is correct, it might be better to investigate their allergic problems more closely in childhood, and, in the case of food allergens, to eliminate the incriminated foods from their diet, rather than simply waiting for them to 'grow out of it'. Experience shows that cutting out allergenic foods for a period of time – for a few months, a year, or sometimes longer – can often eliminate the sensitivity in the long term, as well as providing more immediate relief from the child's symptoms. But there are a variety of other factors to consider – some of which will be discussed in more detail later.

Although most allergies first appear in childhood, particularly the acute types of food allergy, there are a few adults who suddenly develop an allergy for no obvious reason. Dr A.W. Frankland, formerly of St Mary's Hospital in London, describes the case of a woman of 50 who suddenly became allergic to sesame seeds, which she had previously eaten without difficulty. One day while eating a biscuit containing sesame, her mouth and throat began to tingle, and urticaria (nettle-rash) developed on her skin. These symptoms disappeared after an hour. When she ate another such biscuit two weeks later the reaction was far more severe. Her lips and eyelids swelled, urticaria developed all over her body, and she collapsed unconscious on the floor. Only prompt medical attention saved her life. This is an unusual, but not an isolated case, and is difficult to explain in terms of what we now know about allergies as inherited disorders.

Chapter Three

THE CLASSICAL ALLERGIC DISEASES

The classical allergic diseases are hay-fever, perennial rhinitis, asthma, urticaria, atopic eczema and immediate-onset food allergy. The way in which IgE produces these problems, by stimulating mast cells and basophils to release damaging chemical mediators, is described in Chapter Two. This chapter looks at each disease in more detail, and considers the relative roles of different types of allergen.

Multiple causes

Allergens can be conveniently divided into four groups: those we eat, the **food allergens** or **ingestants**, those we breathe in, the **inhalants**, those that come into contact with our skin, the **contactants**, and those that are injected, such as insect stings or antibiotics, the **injectants**. **Airborne allergens**, such as pollen and dust, can act in two ways: as inhalants, when they are breathed in, and as contactants, when they land on the skin or eyes.

At one time, doctors thought that the type of allergic reaction depended solely on the sort of allergen involved – inhalants would only cause problems in the nose and lungs, contactants would only cause problems on the skin, and food would only cause problems in the mouth and gut. The demise of this simplistic view of allergies has been described on p11.

In any one allergic disease, there may be two or more allergens at work, some airborne, others ingested. Dr Harry Morrow-Brown of the Midlands Allergy and Asthma Research Association describes the case of a two-year-old boy whose eczema improved considerably after excluding milk and beef from his diet. However, he did not lose all his symptoms. Some months later, his parents took him on holiday, and to their surprise the child recovered completely while away. On the journey home, they picked up their pet dog from the boarding kennel and before they reached home the child was scratching as much as ever. It turned out that the particles of skin (danders) produced by the dog were a contributory cause of the eczema, aggravating the symptoms produced by milk and beef. With the dog banished and the house thoroughly cleaned, the boy's skin healed completely.

As this example shows, considerable detective work is often necessary to track down the many contributing causes of an allergic reaction. With problems such as asthma and rhinitis, particularly, it is essential to understand the part that airborne allergens play before trying to assess the role of food. Although this book is, strictly speaking, about food allergy, we must also consider the role of inhalants and contactants in these allergic diseases.

Hay-fever

Pollen, produced by plants and carried on the wind, is the most notorious of the airborne allergens – it causes the symptoms known to doctors as **seasonal allergic rhinitis and conjunctivitis** and to the rest of the world as **hay-fever**. Not all hay-fever sufferers respond to the same pollen, and the timing of the symptoms will depend on which pollen is the culprit (see p62).

Mast cells in the nose and eyes respond to the proteins in the outer coat of the pollen grain. The mediators that are released cause inflammation of the delicate membranes, which the hay-fever sufferer experiences as red, itchy, watery eyes, and a runny or congested nose. Some people also suffer from itching in the mouth or ears. Irritability and fatigue may accompany these physical symptoms, although whether these occur as a direct effect of the allergens on the nervous system, or simply as a secondary effect of the unpleasant physical symptoms, is debatable.

Food can probably contribute to hay-fever, though pollen is always the major allergen. Some people find that by avoiding particular foods they reduce their sensitivity to pollen, and a lucky few lose their hay-fever symptoms altogether. Sensitivity to foods can also *mimic* hay-fever, if the foods concerned cause rhinitis and are only eaten in the summer, or in much larger amounts then (see p63).

Perennial rhinitis – constant runny or congested nose

Hay-fever sufferers may feel sorry for themselves as the summer months approach, but they are envied by those afflicted with **perennial rhinitis**, who have to endure similar symptoms all year round. In their case it is usually airborne allergens, such as mould spores or house dust, which trigger mast cells in the nose. If the eyes are also affected this will cause conjunctivitis. It is almost always airborne allergens that affect the eyes, but the nose is also susceptible to allergens from other sources, including food. For the full range of allergens that can provoke rhinitis see pp61–7.

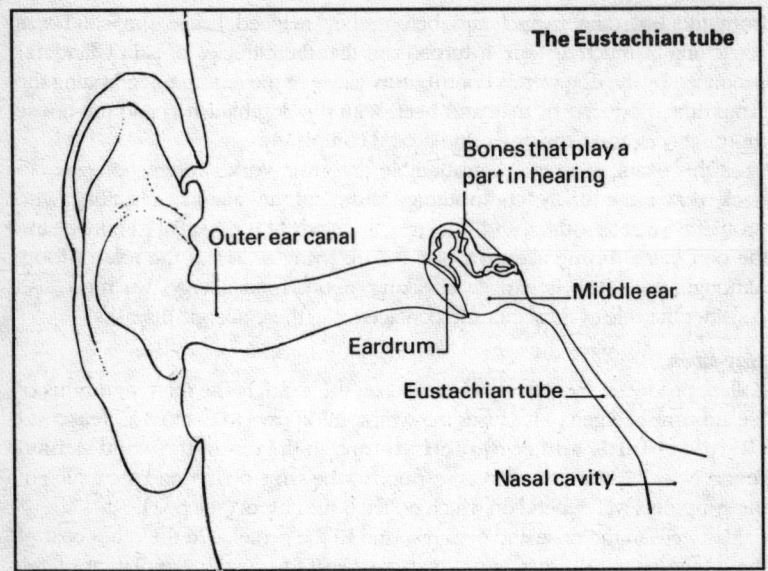

The Eustachian tube

Bones that play a part in hearing

Outer ear canal

Middle ear

Eardrum

Eustachian tube

Nasal cavity

Problems caused by rhinitis

The nose is intimately linked to several other organs and problems here are likely to have effects elsewhere. Because the nose is connected to the middle part of the ear by a tube (the **Eustachian tube**), perennial rhinitis can affect the ears as well. The Eustachian tube's function is to drain any fluid from the ear and allow air to get into the ear so that the pressure on either side of the eardrum is equalized. If the tube becomes blocked with mucus from the nose, air can no longer reach the middle ear and the air already there becomes replaced by a thick, sticky secretion produced by the ear itself. This mucus sticks to the delicate bones that play a vital role in our hearing, and thus causes deafness. The condition is known as **chronic secretory otitis media** (**CSOM**) or **glue ear**, and although it may be caused in other ways this is undoubtedly an important one. The problem is particularly common in children. Recently doctors have discovered that glue ear is related to 'passive smoking', that is, to a child living among cigarette smokers. It has long been known that tobacco smoke prevents the lungs from keeping themselves clear of particles, by paralysing the tiny hairs that sweep them clean, and it now seems that tobacco smoke has the same sort of effect inside the ear. House-dust mite is also said to be associated with glue ear.

Children suffering from glue ear are likely to complain of popping or itching in the ears, or say that their ears feel 'blocked up'. The first signs of deafness are sometimes mistaken for disobedience because they fail to do as they are told. In younger children there may be little outward sign of the problem, although some shake their head in a characteristic way or repeatedly scratch at their ears. Deafness may result in the child being slow to begin speaking – often the first indication that anything is wrong. Needless to say, there are a great many other reasons for delayed speech, and it would be a mistake to jump to conclusions on this basis alone.

CHRIS

Chris had been fascinated by aircraft since he was a small boy, and he loved his job as a pilot, flying helicopters out to oil-rigs. Unfortunately, he suffered badly with what he called hay-fever, although it affected him for most of the year. He had to take antihistamines to ease his streaming nose and eyes, but these made him drowsy, and now his job was at risk. His doctor tried a battery of skin-prick tests with common allergens such as pollen, house dust, feathers and cat fur, but there was no positive response to any of these. She then tried more direct forms of testing in which house-dust and other allergens were sprayed into the nose. These tests were also negative. Since so much depended on curing Chris's rhinitis, his doctor talked to him in detail about his lifestyle, in the hope of getting a clue to what might be the problem. Chris was sure that he lived a very healthy life – in fact he was something of a health fanatic who took lots of exercise and was keen on weight-training. He was also very careful about what he ate, and took yeast tablets every day for extra vitamins. The doctor asked him, as an experiment, to cut these tablets out for a while. She was aware of some people having allergic reactions to yeast, and while she though it unlikely that yeast could cause Chris's symptoms, anything was worth a try. To her surprise – and Chris's – his nose was completely clear within four days. When he tried taking the tablets again, his rhinitis promptly returned. Later he discovered that he would get a milder form of rhinitis from drinking large amounts of beer, or eating a lot of bread, but in general he has had no further problems.

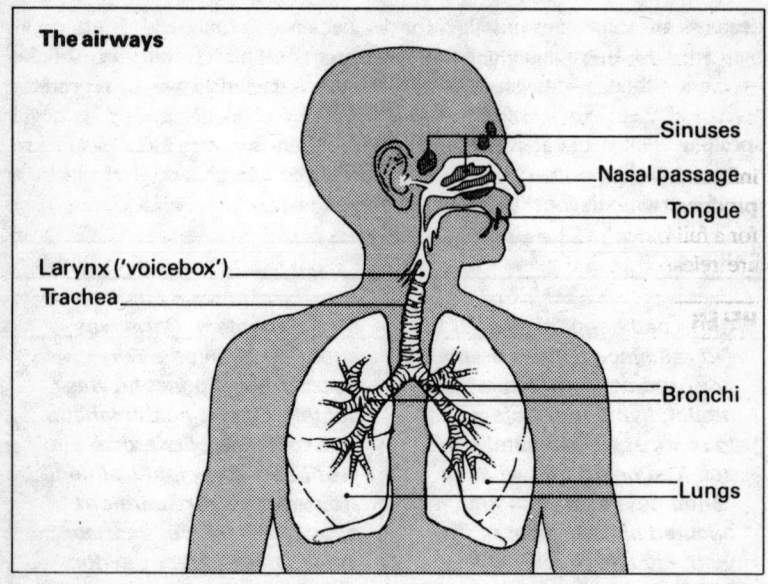

The airways

Sinuses

Nasal passage

Tongue

Larynx ('voicebox')

Trachea

Bronchi

Lungs

Other problems that can follow on from rhinitis are allergic sinusitis and nasal polyps. The sinuses are air-filled cavities in the skull which are lined with delicate membranes that link up with those lining the nose. Most cases of **sinusitis** – inflammation of these membranes – result from an infection in the nose that spreads outwards. But allergic reactions can also occur here. The main symptoms of sinusitis are a severely blocked nose, with a headache over the eyes, if the frontal sinuses are affected, or an ache in the cheeks if the maxillary sinuses are inflamed.

Prolonged irritation to the membranes of the nose and sinuses can result in swelling, and this may eventually produce **nasal polyps** in some people – small grape-like protrusions of the membrane. The polyps are usually harmless but they may obstruct the nasal passage making breathing difficult. The sense of smell can also be lost, and there may be symptoms similar to sinusitis if the opening between a sinus cavity and the nose becomes blocked. The polyps can be removed surgically if they do cause discomfort. For some inexplicable reason, many cases of nasal polyps are seen in people who are sensitive to aspirin (see p57).

One final problem that should be mentioned in connection with rhinitis is **post-nasal drip** (sometimes known by the general name 'catarrh'). Excess mucus from the nose trickles down the back of the throat and thus into the trachea – the main tube leading to the lungs – to be coughed up later. Post-nasal drip can follow various infections, but it is sometimes allergic in origin.

Asthma

The inhalants that cause rhinitis can also cause asthma, the 'target organs' in this case being the tubes leading from the trachea to the lungs, known as the **bronchi**. A variety of airborne allergens may be responsible, see pp61–7.

When these allergens trigger mast cells in the bronchi, they cause inflammation of the membranes lining the tubes which become thicker and produce more mucus. This restricts the free passage of air and sets the stage for a full-blown asthma attack. Such an attack occurs when sufficient mediators are released by the mast cells to make the smooth muscles of the bronchi

HELEN

Helen had eczema as a baby and began to have asthma attacks when she was about six. These got a great deal worse when she was eight years old, and on close questioning the doctor discovered that her parents had recently built an aviary inside the conservatory that was attached to their house. Skin-prick tests showed that Helen had a strong reaction to feathers, and when the birds were removed from the house her asthma settled down to its previous level. In the hope of getting rid of it completely, her parents replaced all feather pillows and cushions with foam-filled ones. Although this seemed to help a little, Helen still had asthma attacks once or twice a month. These frequently came on after parties or outings, and the doctor suggested that it might just be excitement triggering off the attacks. Then her asthma started to become more frequent again, and as the attacks often took place at school, it was interfering with her studies. Helen's mother began to wonder if foods that Helen only had at parties or at school, during breaks, were responsible. Crisps, squash and other food containing additives were obvious suspects as Helen was not given this sort of food at home. She agreed to go without these foods for a month to see if this had any effect. Within a few days her attacks virtually disappeared and tests with different types of additives showed that artificial colourings and sulphites could bring on an attack within a few hours. As long as she avoids 'junk food' Helen is now free from asthma.

contract. The bronchi suddenly become much narrower. Stale air inside the lung cannot easily escape, so the lungs have difficulty in drawing in fresh air with its life-giving oxygen. The air whistling through the constricted openings makes the characteristic wheezing sound.

While most asthmatics conform to the general pattern described above, there are also milder forms of the disease in which there is no wheezing and no asthma 'attack' as such. In such cases the predominant symptom is a persistent cough combined with some breathlessness.

The only way of telling if such symptoms might be due to asthma is to try out an anti-asthma treatment (see pp322–4) and see if there is any improvement. If there is, further tests should be made to confirm the diagnosis and try to identify the allergens involved.

Although inhalants are the major culprits in asthma, foods can also play a part. Often there is more than one allergen involved (see p62).

LATE-PHASE REACTIONS

If an allergic patient is given a skin-prick test (see p30) there will be a strong response – known as a **wheal-and-flare reaction** – almost immediately. This redness and itching subsides after some time, but then a different sort of reaction can set in, producing a larger, less itchy, but more painful lump. This is known as the **late-phase reaction**, and it is produced by the messenger substances called **prostaglandins** (see p28).

When a person encounters allergens in everyday life, late-phase reactions are more difficult to discern, especially if there is frequent exposure to the allergen. But such a reaction can sometimes be observed in asthmatic patients, for example. Brief exposure to their allergen will produce an acute reaction almost immediately, followed by recovery, followed by a more insidious return of the asthma between four and 12 hours after the exposure. The late-phase reaction has usually exhausted itself by the next day.

Late-phase reactions are important, because they probably contribute substantially to the development of 'chronic' allergic reactions – a long-term condition in which the patient is scarcely ever free

Asthma without allergens

Asthmatics who are constantly exposed to their allergen – as is the case with house-dust sensitivity – are likely to have bronchi that are highly 'irritable', because of the inflammation in the membranous linings. The late-phase reaction, described in the box below, plays a large part in producing this state of chronic sensitivity. Once it has developed, all sorts of irritating stimuli can then spark off an asthma attack. Common irritants include smoke (cigarettes, bonfires etc), factory fumes, infections, very cold air and sulphur dioxide (given off by various foods and drinks, see p301).

Becoming emotional or afraid can have the same effect as these airborne irritants, as can strenuous exercise. It was the ability of the emotions to bring on an asthmatic attack that led to the idea of asthma being largely 'psychosomatic'.

Eating large amounts of the food additive monosodium glutamate, can also provoke an asthma attack, according to Dr David Allen, a respiratory specialist

of symptoms, although the severity of the symptoms may fluctuate. During late-phase reactions, the affected organ (eg the bronchi or the skin) tends to be more sensitive to non-specific irritants, so the symptoms may be sparked off again very easily, even if the allergen has been removed. A succession of late-phase reactions can easily lead to a situation where the organ is constantly over-reacting to minor irritants.

Certain drugs block late-phase reactions by preventing cell membranes from releasing the phospholipid molecules that would normally be used to make prostaglandins. The drugs that do this are **corticosteroids** (eg prednisolone) which mimic the action of hormones produced by the body. The fact that corticosteroids are so useful in controlling asthmatic symptoms shows what an important role late-phase reactions can have in allergic illness.

Corticosteroids are not simply used for allergy treatment – they suppress inflammation generally because prostaglandins are widespread messengers, produced in a variety of ways. They therefore find a use in diseases such as rheumatoid arthritis where inflammation needs to be controlled.

from Royal North Shore Hospital in Sydney, Australia. He believes that MSG – common in Chinese cooking, packet soups and other convenience foods – has an effect on the central nervous system which triggers off the attack. Similar claims have been made for diets that are high in salt, although how salt in food might contribute to asthma is unknown.

Nettle-rash and oedema

There can be several different causes for urticaria (also called nettle-rash or hives) of which allergic reactions are just one. Where allergy *is* at the root of urticaria, it is probably the mast cells found in the lower layers of the skin that cause the problem. When they degranulate, the mediators released have a powerful effect on the tiny blood vessels, or **capillaries**, that lie all around them in the skin. These capillaries become more leaky, allowing **serum** (the watery part of the blood) to seep out into the skin itself. This produces the characteristic swellings and itchiness of urticaria.

Where there is a great deal of seepage from the blood vessels, the tissues below the skin may also become filled with watery fluid. This produces a puffiness that doctors describe as **localized angioedema** (or **oedema**). About 50 per cent of people who are afflicted with urticaria also get angioedema, and some people have angioedema *without* any urticaria. However, there are a large number of other disorders that can produce angioedema, some of them very serious – they should all be eliminated by a full medical examination, before the possible role of allergy is investigated. (See also pp75–7.)

There are two forms of urticaria which differ mainly in their timing. The type which troubled Kustner (see p22) is acute urticaria, which comes on very rapidly and usually clears within 24 hours. It is usually accompanied by other symptoms, such as feverishness, faintness or nausea. Chronic urticaria, the other form, is a persistent rash, or one which comes and goes over a much longer period of time.

The blame for acute urticaria can usually be pinned on a food that was eaten just before the attack began, although there are other causes of acute urticaria, including insect stings, drugs (notably penicillin), and, more rarely, something that was applied to the skin. Whatever the cause, the reaction is usually so prompt and unequivocal that the patient easily makes the correct diagnosis.

With chronic urticaria, things are not so simple. Only about 20 or 30 per cent of people with this distressing problem are likely to discover the underlying cause. Two-thirds of those afflicted do not have high IgE levels, nor any other allergic illness, and it is not at all certain what causes their symptoms. However, those that *can* identify the source of their problem very often find that there are several triggers, including food or food additives. Whether they are acting as allergens, or have a drug-like effect, is an open question.

Something that is worth trying for chronic urticaria is a diet low in histamine. Research has shown that many patients with chronic urticaria cannot break histamine down as well as they should, and histamine absorbed from food could be causing their illness. The foods to avoid are given on p83.

Histamine is also produced by the bacteria of the gut, and the amount can be excessive if a lot of starchy foods, or a lot of fruit and vegetables, are eaten. If someone suffers from chronic urticaria, and it gets worse shortly after every meal, bacterially generated histamine is a possibility that should be considered. Reducing starch intake, or fruit and vegetable intake (or both) may help. Eating live yoghurt may also be useful in improving the balance of different kinds of bacteria in the gut.

The subject of urticaria will come up again in Chapter Five, because even when the rash is truly allergic it can be caused in more than one way.

Atopic eczema

Eczema is a term that is often used rather loosely for a variety of skin conditions. Strictly speaking it means a red, itchy 'rash', which tends to flake and then ooze or 'weep' as it progresses. The disease is far more common in children, who usually compound the damage by constant scratching. Bacteria may infect the oozing skin and make matters still worse, while prolonged scratching will cause bleeding.

In adults, oozing does not generally occur, and the skin tends to become thickened instead. Some doctors feel that these symptoms should not be

RICHARD

Richard had suffered from eczema since he was just two months old, and when he was eight he still needed twice-daily applications of cream to keep the itching under control. Since he did not seem to be growing out of his eczema, his mother asked the doctor if she could try changing his diet, to see what effect that had. She was told to avoid eggs, milk and all milk products as a first step, which she did. Within a week Richard's eczema had cleared up, and even when the cream was stopped it did not return. When milk was reintroduced into his diet, Richard was fine, but 24 hours after eating egg he began to scratch furiously. By avoiding eggs he has remained free of eczema.

described as eczema, although they are undoubtedly the counterpart of childhood eczema. They therefore use the term **atopic dermatitis** as a general description of both types of disease. In this book we will use **eczema** for both children and adults, since this is the most widely understood term.

There are several different kinds of eczema, but what concerns us here is the variety known as **atopic eczema**, which is seen mainly in atopic individuals. What distinguishes it from other forms of eczema is the pattern of distribution over the body. The red itchy patches usually start on the face, particularly on convex areas such as the cheeks and chin. In time the skin on the face heals and for some children this will be the end of their eczema. But for others the rash appears on the body, eventually settling in the folds of skin at the buttocks, knees, ankles, elbows and wrists. In severely affected cases, the rash may cover the whole body.

Atopic eczema is mainly a disease of childhood although there are rare instances of it first appearing in adult life. About three-quarters of children affected develop the disease before they are a year old, and most in the first six months of life. The disease tends to come and go thereafter, and usually disappears by the age of 15. Because this type of eczema is so common in the children of atopic parents, and because it is usually followed (or accompanied) by hay-fever or asthma, it is considered to be an allergic disease. However, there is no clear evidence that IgE antibodies (see pp25–6) actually play a role in producing atopic eczema, and it is not obvious how they might produce the characteristic symptoms.

If IgE is at the root of eczema, then the question of how the allergens reach the skin arises. This is a matter of great medical controversy, but there is growing evidence that what goes into the mouth can produce a reaction in the skin, and that food is an important factor. Allergens which are inhaled and absorbed into the bloodstream may also play a part, and airborne allergens that land on the skin could contribute to the problem, along with contactants in clothing, creams and cosmetics.

However, allergens are often only part of the problem. General irritants, such as detergents, are also thought to be important, and these can bring on eczema in the sensitive individual.

Allergies to food

The medical profession's original, rather limited concept of food allergy, as described on p11, was of an immediate, violent reaction to food. Jane's reaction to peanuts was a textbook example of such an allergy. General advice on how to cope with such food allergies is given on pp50–4.

Not all allergic reactions to food occur immediately after eating it, however.

There is a rare form of food allergy in which the allergen is not an intact food molecule but one of the products of partial digestion. Eating the food produces no ill-effects at first, but violent symptoms begin several hours afterwards, as the food begins to break down in the stomach (see p52).

Delayed reactions are also seen when food contributes to allergic symptoms such as asthma, rhinitis, eczema or chronic urticaria. It may be several hours or even days between the food being eaten and the symptoms appearing. With symptoms of this sort, it may also be necessary to eat quite large amounts of the food, or to eat it for several days in succession. If the food is one that is eaten regularly – as is often the case – the link between cause and effect is likely to be obscure, and food allergies of this type often go unrecognized. An elimination diet, of the kind described in Chapter Fourteen, may be necessary to work out what is causing the problem.

The idea of food producing symptoms in distant parts of the body, such as the nose or bronchi, may at first sight seem implausible, but research shows that allergens can be absorbed into the bloodstream intact (see p21) and these must then be carried to all parts of the body. It is thought that these blood-borne allergens can react with mast cells in any susceptible organ. If the allergen were to interact with mast cells in blood vessels around the bronchi, for example, the mediators released by the mast cells would affect the nearby bronchial linings and the bronchial muscles – exactly the same effect as for airborne allergens. Not surprisingly, if a food produces asthma it usually produces other symptoms as well, because the allergen is being carried throughout the body.

In the case of rhinitis, the allergen can be carried to the nasal membranes in the bloodstream, producing symptoms 6–10 hours after the meal, or even later – up to 24 hours in some patients. Alternatively, the action of chewing food in the mouth may transmit allergens into the nasal cavity, thus provoking a response in the nose directly. Similarly, asthmatics can react to minute food particles that are inhaled while eating. Children with an exceptional sensitivity to peanuts have even been affected by *someone else* eating peanut butter nearby, but this is extremely rare.

Without doubt, most sufferers from rhinitis, asthma and associated problems are responding to airborne allergens alone. But a significant proportion suffer from food sensitivities that contribute to their symptoms, *and food may be the sole cause of the problem in some cases.* Until fairly recently, most doctors did not appreciate the importance of food in producing such symptoms and many children were diagnosed as having 'intrinsic asthma' – that is, asthma with no obvious external cause – when their wheezing may have been due to food. Similarly, atopic eczema has usually been treated with corticosteroid creams, which are successful for some but not the most severely affected. Trying to identify potential food triggers may be a better approach for such children.

Food allergy in babies

Food allergy usually shows itself in childhood, and the most common problem is a reaction to cow's milk among babies and young children. Babies who are bottle-fed are obviously at greater risk of developing a sensitivity to cow's milk, but atopic babies who are breast-fed can react badly to foods that the mother is eating, because minute quantities get into the breast milk. Again, cow's milk is a common problem, but it is certainly not the only one – any food that the mother eats may act as an allergen for the breast-fed baby, especially if eaten in large quantities.

Babies may react immediately to their allergen, with symptoms such as vomiting, urticaria, and swelling of the lips, face and eyes. In such cases there is usually a positive skin-prick test. Once the allergen has been identified it must be avoided, for a while at least (see p225). Some babies grow out of the allergic reaction in time.

Not all babies react to their allergen immediately. Some have a delayed reaction with symptoms such as eczema, diarrhoea, asthma or rhinitis. Irritability, restlessness and crying are also reported, although most doctors would not accept these as allergic symptoms. Infants with delayed symptoms often fail to give a positive skin-prick test, and the link with food may not be at all obvious, either to the mother or the doctor. Diarrhoea in babies is dealt with more fully on pp210–11. General guidelines for dealing with food sensitivity in babies and young children are described on pp221–9.

A few babies suffer recurrent pneumonia as a result of allergy to cow's milk. They will also have diarrhoea or vomiting, show little appetite, and may have asthma or a runny nose as well. It seems likely that some milk is inhaled during feeding, and this causes an allergic reaction in the lungs.

If a baby is anaemic, then allergy to cow's milk should be suspected, because this can cause bleeding from the digestive tract, which in turn leads to a shortage of iron. Sometimes the bleeding goes unrecognized so that anaemia is the first noticeable sign of the baby's food allergy.

Chapter Four

TREATING CLASSICAL ALLERGIES AND IDENTIFYING FOOD ALLERGENS

Allergies are well-recognized conditions, and those suffering from true food allergy are far more likely to receive adequate medical treatment than those with food intolerance. Even so, well-informed patients can make a significant contribution to their own treatment. This is particularly true if, as so often happens, there is no allergy specialist (**allergist**) overseeing the treatment. There are still very few allergists, and most allergic symptoms are treated by other specialists. A patient with multiple symptoms may see an ear-nose-and-throat specialist for rhinitis, a chest specialist for asthma, a dermatologist for eczema and a gastroenterologist for bowel disorders due to food. The net result is that there is no one doctor considering the whole allergic picture in that patient.

The patient who understands something about allergies is at less of a disadvantage in such circumstances, and may be able to help the doctor in unravelling the complexities of cause and effect. But it is important to stress that self-help should only be an adjunct to proper medical treatment, never a substitute. Some allergic conditions can be life-threatening, others can deteriorate to the point where they produce irreversible damage to health. No-one should attempt to treat them without medical supervision.

OPTIONS IN ALLERGY TREATMENT

Because the mechanism behind true or 'classical' allergies is well understood, the potential for treating them with drugs is very good. The preparations used include **corticosteroids** (sometimes referred to simply as **steroids**, although they are not the same as the steroid drugs used by athletes), which have a general suppressive effect on inflammation, **antihistamines**, which counteract the effect of the mediator histamine, and **bronchodilators** for use in asthma. (For more details on these drugs and how they work see pp320–6.) Although at one time there were serious side-effects associated with many anti-allergy drugs, the modern formulations have overcome most of these problems. The drug treatments now available are both safe and effective.

Before embarking on any other form of treatment, such as an elimination diet, it is important to weigh up the costs and benefits of that treatment as compared with using drugs to combat the symptoms. In cases where the symptoms are relatively mild, it may be better to rely on drugs alone. The decision involves a great many personal considerations, including, for example, the relative importance of food to the person concerned, their perseverance and will-power, and the number of meals that have to be eaten away from home. Nutritional needs also have to be taken into account. It is a decision that can only be made by the individual patient (or by the parents in the case of a small child) in consultation with the doctor concerned.

What to do about immediate allergic reactions to food

This is the one area where tracking down the source of the problem is unlikely to be difficult, except in the case of babies and small children, where some detective work may be necessary (see pp221–7).

What *is* hard is living with such an allergy. In the vast majority of cases, a food allergy of this type is lifelong and irreversible, and for highly sensitive individuals it can be life-threatening. Assuming that you know which food or foods you are allergic to, the best policy is to avoid them scrupulously. It is probably wise to keep the food out of the house entirely, so that there is no risk of a small amount contaminating the food of the allergic person. You must also be very cautious about eating in restaurants and cafes and religiously read the labels on packeted food. Labels can be deceptive, however, because they often use unfamiliar words to describe a potentially allergenic food component – such as 'lactalbumin' for one of the proteins found in cow's milk. For a full list of such synonyms, see p302.

Peanut-sensitive individuals should watch out for a new product, about to be launched in America, which could be exported to other countries. These are peanuts that have been stripped of their original flavour by chemical treatment, reflavoured as almonds or other more expensive nuts, and moulded to the appropriate shape. The packets will have to declare their ingredients of course, but the bowl of nuts on a bar or party table may not be quite what it seems. There are also now available pretzels with a peanut paste filling which is quite unexpected, and therefore potentially dangerous.

Never try to pick out the offending food from a dish that has already been prepared, and then eat what is left. There will be some unseen molecules of the food that have seeped into the mixture, and you may be sufficiently sensitive to react to them.

The biggest problem is eating out. In a recent American study, researchers looked into seven deaths from violent allergic reactions to foods and found that six of these occurred when eating away from home. One of these unfortunate victims ate chilli in a restaurant, quite reasonably expecting it to contain meat, beans, chillies and vegetables. It turned out that the cook had used peanut butter to thicken the sauce, and the man was highly allergic to peanuts. Peanuts or peanut butter may also be used inconspicuously in cakes, biscuits and sweets. Some Chinese restaurants use peanut butter to stick down the ends of egg rolls.

One obvious strategy when eating in a restaurant is to choose plain food, such as grilled fish or meat, where 'what you get is what you see'. This is not always possible and, if such foods are not available, you will have to make sure you know what is in the food you are eating. Try to speak to the chef directly if you can, but accept that this may not always be possible (in many restaurants now there *is* no chef, the food being prepared in a factory and delivered in pre-packed portions). Waiters and waitresses are often too busy to really take the trouble to find out what is in the food, and if they don't understand the seriousness of food allergy they may not bother. Most of the cautionary tales about allergic reactions in restaurants have as their villain the waiter or waitress who *said* they'd checked with the chef but hadn't.

One way around this problem is to telephone the restaurant in advance and discuss the problem with them – say that you need to know exactly what is in the food you are eating. You should be able to judge how helpful they are prepared to be from this initial contact. For the person who is sensitive to milk, Chinese or Japanese food is a good bet because there is no tradition of using milk in Oriental cuisine.

Anyone who has had a severe reaction to food in the past should be aware that a further exposure can sometimes precipitate a worse reaction. If you have ever experienced swelling of the tongue and lips, difficulty in breathing, or generalized urticaria, then you should be very cautious indeed about trying the food again. If you have ever collapsed after eating a food (anaphylactic shock) then under no circumstances should you eat it again, however small the amount. Even a relatively mild reaction, such as vomiting and nettle rash in response to a food, can be the foretaste of something much more serious, and it is vital that such warnings are heeded.

Asthmatics are at particular risk because a general anaphylactic reaction will induce a severe asthma attack at the same time and this in itself can be fatal. Anyone with a true allergy to food who is also taking the drugs known as beta-blockers (used for a variety of heart conditions) should be aware that they increase the risk of a severe anaphylactic reaction.

An initial test that can be done at home, is to apply a small amount of the food to the face, making sure that none of it goes anywhere near the mouth. If this produces a rash, then the food should certainly not be eaten. If it does not, then it is worth approaching your doctor to see about skin-prick testing, which should show if the food is now safe to eat.

For those who have had a severe reaction of this type, it may be advisable to carry a syringe containing emergency medication, in case the food is inadvertently eaten again. The syringe can be used only once, and contains adrenaline, which counteracts the effects of the mast-cell mediators by causing the blood vessels to contract. It is still necessary to avoid the food, of course – the contents of the syringe will only be effective if a very small amount has been eaten. Do not delay in using the syringe if you begin to experience a severe reaction to the food. In this situation, a 'wait-and-see' attitude could be disastrous. The sooner you use the adrenaline, the more effective it will be, and you will avoid the possibility of lasting, irreversible damage to sensitive parts of the body. Having used the syringe, contact your doctor or go to a hospital quickly, because you may need further doses of adrenaline. The dose should be repeated every 15–20 minutes until you are fully recovered. Tell the doctor if you have been taking corticosteroids as these may suppress your body's normal ability to produce its own corticosteroids, which are needed in this crisis situation. You may require a dose of corticosteroid, as well as adrenaline, to counteract the effect.

Not all anaphylactic reactions come on immediately. They can sometimes take an hour or even two hours to develop. There are usually some initial signs that things are amiss, such as itching or swelling in the mouth, nausea and stomach pains. If the food is affecting the throat, hoarseness or a 'lump in the throat' sensation may be the first signs.

Should these be followed by more generalized feelings, such as itching all over, sneezing, runny nose, diarrhoea and weakness, then a serious anaphylactic reaction may be developing. Other odd sensations that may accompany this stage are a feeling of warmth and a sense of dread or apprehension. Incontinence, disorientation and abdominal pains may also be experienced.

If there are any signs such as these **do not delay getting medical help**. Go to a casualty department if you can, and make sure you are seen quickly – don't sit quietly waiting your turn. Tell the doctor if you have been taking corticosteroid drugs.

Anyone who has had a severe reaction in the past should consider wearing a medical information bracelet with the relevant information on it. If you were to eat your culprit food by mistake while away from home, and were found unconscious, it could save your life. Without it, you might not get the correct medical help.

If you have had an immediate, violent reaction to food, but are not sure which food component is responsible, then you are in a more difficult position. It is important to identify your allergen, so that you can eat safely with the minimum of dietary restrictions. A little intelligent detective work may help you to guess the identity of the culprit, and your doctor should be able to arrange for a skin-prick test to check your conclusions.

One possibility you should consider is that you are reacting to an additive rather than a food. If you consistently react to commercial ice-cream, for example, but not to milk, cream or home-made ice-cream, then you may be allergic to polysorbates, which are used as stabilizers in ice-cream manufacture. Careful reading of labels and some cautious experimentation with suspect additives should help you to identify the source of the problem. Appendix VI gives more details on food additives, and identifies 'families' of additives which are chemically similar to each other – if you are allergic to one, you may also react to others with a related chemical structure.

Another rather remote possibility is that you are allergic to a digestion product of the food rather than the food itself (see p47). Vomiting and diarrhoea begin some hours after eating, and anaphylactic shock is a possibility. This sort of allergy is thought to be very rare.

Immediate, violent reactions are particularly common with shellfish, but are often inconsistent – a person will react severely on one occasion but not at all on another. One reason for this is that shellfish actually comprise two separate animal groups (see p304). Another is that the shellfish themselves vary, depending on what they have been eating. They tend to accumulate various chemical compounds, including toxins, from the creatures that they eat. These are passed on intact to the human consumer. The adverse reaction that follows may be an allergic one, or it may be a false food allergy (see p79) or simply a straightforward case of poisoning by toxins that the shellfish have accumulated. With increasing pollution of coastal waters by raw sewage, there is also the very real possibility of infection by bacteria or viruses, which may further confuse the picture.

To add to the complexities, shellfish are often treated with preservatives, known as benzoates, after they are caught. A few people are allergic to these widely used additives, and while they will certainly react to various other foods as well, the reaction to shellfish is likely to be more marked because of the prodigious quantities of benzoate used. The amount will vary tremendously from one batch of shellfish to another, and this may explain the variable reactions seen in a small proportion of those sensitive to shellfish.

Another possibility which should be considered, in puzzling cases of food allergy, is sensitivity to antibiotics. Because these are added to animal feeds, they can turn up in trace amounts in meat, eggs and milk. Someone who is

CATHERINE

Catherine had suffered from asthma since childhood – she could not remember a time when these attacks of breathlessness and wheezing did not set in once or twice a week. Skin testing had always been negative and she had simply learned to live with the problem, controlling her symptoms with drugs. Then, in her forties, Catherine began to suffer from frequent headaches and felt very tired. Her doctor could find nothing wrong and suggested that she might like to try an elimination diet to see if this was of any help. Catherine cut out milk, eggs, wheat and citrus fruits, and found that she felt a great deal better. When she retested milk, this brought on a headache within an hour, followed by a severe attack of asthma. On a diet with no milk or milk products her headaches are few and far between. To her great surprise, she is also free from asthma attacks for the first time in her adult life.

extremely sensitive to a particular antibiotic may react to the tiny amounts found in such foods.

Other foods can also be present as contaminants if processing machinery has not been cleaned thoroughly when switching from one product to another. Once again, peanuts cause more trouble than any other food. A factory producing both peanut butter and almond butter caused a serious allergic response in a peanut-sensitive individual by contaminating the almond butter with peanuts. Sweets can suffer the same problem. With growing awareness of the potential hazards, manufacturers may now be taking more care. If you are ever doubtful about a food, proceed cautiously, taking a very small amount at first. You can also apply some to your face first, as described above.

Finally, there are some food-allergic individuals who only produce symptoms if they take strenuous exercise after eating the food. Exactly why this should occur is unknown, but changes in the state of the blood vessels that occur naturally during exercise must somehow trigger off adverse reactions in the mast cells. This type of reaction can lead to collapse (**exercise-induced anaphylaxis**), which can sometimes be fatal. (Some people react in this way, not as a reaction to specific foods, but to *any* food. This is not an allergic reaction.)

What to do about asthma

A balanced approach is advisable in the case of asthma. Firstly, medicinal drugs may be necessary to control the immediate symptoms and make life bearable for the patient. The drugs currently in use are described on pp320–6. Secondly, an effort should be made to identify airborne allergens. Some careful detective work, using the list of allergens on pp61–7, may help to pinpoint the culprits. Skin-prick tests can also be useful here, although they are not always accurate. Once airborne antigens have been identified they can be eliminated as far as possible from the home, using the methods described on pp69–70. If something in the workplace is responsible for the asthma, either as an allergen or an irritant, every effort should be made to change to a different working environment. The asthma may get worse as the years go by, and as the bronchi become more sensitive they react to lower and lower levels of irritant – and they may begin to react to other, milder irritants as well.

After 6–8 weeks, the effect of eliminating airborne allergens and irritants can be assessed, and if there are still serious symptoms then it may be worth trying an elimination diet. Continue with the basic measures for avoiding airborne allergens while the diet is in progress. Where foods provoke asthma, it seems that skin-prick tests are not all that useful in identifying the problem food. So a diet – such as that described in Chapter Fourteen – is the only reliable means

---

Coping with an asthma attack

The most important thing to remember during an asthma attack is to stay calm. Sitting upright with your elbows resting on the back of a chair can be helpful. If the back of the chair is not high enough, add a pillow or two. Sitting in this position lifts your ribcage and reduces the amount of muscular effort needed to breathe. Fresh air is valuable, so open a window as long as it is not too cold. A large group of anxious onlookers tend to increase the asthmatic's anxiety and thus make matters worse.

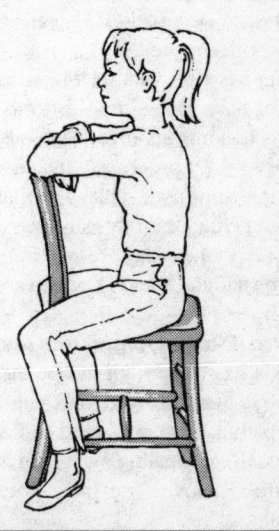

of diagnosis. In the case of babies and young children, see pp221–7. Remember that children should not be put on an elimination diet without medical supervision. *This is particularly important for anyone who has ever had a very severe attack of asthma, because there is a risk of death if a serious reaction occurs when a food is reintroduced.* If you are testing foods at home, your doctor should be able to give you a supply of suitable medicine for use in a severe asthma attack.

Where asthma is brought on by food, the reaction is sometimes dependent on some other factor being present at the same time, such as alcohol, aspirin, cold drinks, or exercise just after the meal. In such cases it can be quite difficult to pinpoint the exact causes of asthma attacks.

If foods do turn out to be instrumental in the asthmatic attacks, then avoiding those foods entirely is the simplest solution. Where this proves too difficult or dull, then the drug sodium cromoglycate, taken by mouth, may be of benefit – see pp320–1.

Asthma is a complex disease which may not be entirely due to allergy. For this reason, not all asthmatics will be able to track down the source of their problems using the methods described, and some will have to rely mainly on drugs to control their symptoms. For this group, and indeed for all asthmatics, avoiding exposure to irritants such as smoke and fumes will help greatly. Certain jobs carry a very high risk of asthma because they involve exposure to particular chemicals – these are described on p66. Anyone with a history of asthma, *even if they have been free of symptoms for many years,* should try to avoid such occupations, because of the likelihood of precipitating asthmatic attacks once more.

There is one way in which food might actually help to *combat* asthma. Studies have shown that fish oils can help to reduce the number of asthma attacks in some sufferers. Fish oils are thought to have a beneficial effect on all sorts of bodily processes, and seem to exert a calming influence on over-active immune responses. This is probably due to constituents known as fatty acids. You can either eat oily fish once or twice a week, or take cod liver oil. One or two teaspoons a day are recommended – do not take too much, as the oil is rich in vitamins A and D, which are toxic in excess.

What to do about rhinitis and associated problems

Rhinitis has quite a lot in common with asthma – indeed the two conditions often go hand in hand, and patients who can avoid the allergens that trigger their asthmatic attacks tend to find that their rhinitis clears up as well. So the approach to dealing with rhinitis is much the same as that for asthma, described above. The same goes for associated conditions such as allergic sinusitis.

The first step should be an attempt to identify airborne allergens, using the list on pp61–7. Skin-prick tests are useful in pinpointing the inhalants that trigger rhinitis, but of little use for foods. Efforts to eliminate airborne allergens should continue for some months to allow a fair assessment of the effects. It is best to begin in the winter, because pollen and outdoor mould spores are at their lowest levels then – their presence may mask any good effects achieved by eliminating house dust or pets, and this can be very discouraging. If such clean-up measures *do* produce an improvement, continue them through the summer months to see if the symptoms recur.

At the end of this process, it should be clear if any airborne allergens are involved, and which ones they are. Where it is difficult to avoid such allergens, desensitization treatments may be worth considering – see pp296–300.

If the symptoms persist despite all these measures, then an elimination diet could be used to assess the role of food – see Chapter Fourteen for the detailed procedure. For babies and young children, see pp221–7. Where the rhinitis is fairly mild, using drugs to control it may be a more practical solution. The drugs that can be prescribed are detailed on pp320–2 and 324–5.

One particular set of symptoms calls for a special mention here. In the case of **nasal polyps**, especially if accompanied by urticaria (nettle-rash), sensitivity to aspirin should be a prime suspect. How aspirin might produce this cluster of symptoms is unknown: the aspirin may be acting as an allergen, but it is more likely to be having some direct pharmacological ('drug-like') effect on the nasal membranes and skin.

Avoiding aspirin and aspirin-containing painkillers is simple enough as long as you remember that the following synonyms may be used: salicylate, salicylic acid and acetylsalicylic acid. Most brand-name painkillers contain some aspirin, and it is important to read the contents list carefully. Plain paracetamol tablets are aspirin-free.

For most people, simply avoiding aspirin drugs should be sufficient. However, some people also react to related drugs (see p327).

If avoiding aspirin and related drugs proves ineffective, then some doctors suggest that restricting the diet may be worthwhile. Aspirin-like compounds (salicylates) occur in various plants, the drug originally being extracted from the bark of willow trees. Certain fruits, nuts, vegetables and spices are rich in salicylates: a complete list is given on p301. If you are sure aspirin aggravates your symptoms, but are still not well despite avoiding aspirin drugs, then you could consider trying a low-salicylate diet to see if you improve.

There are unconfirmed reports that sensitivity to aspirin is linked with an inability to tolerate benzoate preservatives (p314), azo-dyes (p315) and metabisulphites, used to preserve wines and some foods (p301).

What to do about eczema

In general, atopic eczema is a mild disease that disappears in time, and most cases are probably best treated with creams or other medication (see pp325–7). It is certainly not fair on an eczematous child to deny the relief that these medications can bring, while attempting to sort out the problem with dietary investigations. A balanced approach using drugs, diet and other investigations is required. Where there is a secondary bacterial infection then a course of antibiotics may be necessary. With dry, uninfected eczema, there is a promising new form of drug treatment based on traditional Chinese herbal remedies. The herbs are made into a tea, which is drunk once a day. The taste is not at all pleasant, but the beneficial effects are usually worth it – about two thirds of patients are substantially better, and these are people whose eczema has resisted all the usual forms of treatment. Generally speaking, the herbal treatment works better in adults than in children. At present this treatment is not widely known, but it may soon be available on prescription through your family doctor.

Another new form of treatment for eczema is to give the bacterium *Lactobacillus acidophilus*, which is a natural inhabitant of the gut, but can become depleted. This can be taken in capsule form, although there are doubts about how many live bacteria are found in these capsules. A more reliable method is to eat live yoghurt (see pp199–200).

For the child (or adult) with severe eczema, life can be misery and it is certainly worth investigating the possible role of food in the illness. The best response is usually seen in babies less than a year old, and guidelines for investigating their reactions to food are given on p221. In older children, the difficulties of sticking to a diet may outweigh the benefits, although some children are very good at sticking to a diet, once they see the benefits.

The diagnosis of food sensitivities in children with eczema can sometimes be made by a skin-prick test (see p30). Although it is not foolproof, this test can give an indication of which foods may be responsible, and this may be a useful first step. The diagnosis should be confirmed by eliminating all the suspect foods from the diet and then reintroducing them one at a time. Check that your doctor approves of this procedure before you start. Creams and other medication can be used during this procedure, to alleviate the itching. The strength of medication used should be carefully chosen to damp down the symptoms without eradicating them entirely, so that the response to foods can be assessed.

If skin-prick tests do not indicate any particular foods, then a simple form of elimination diet, avoiding the foods that are most often a problem in eczema, may be tried (see p226).

Before any dietary investigation is started, however, the possible role of airborne and contact allergens should be considered. This involves a certain amount of detective work, thinking over times when the child is better, or much worse, and looking for clues as to what is causing these changes. Bear in mind that eczema is likely to fluctuate considerably anyway, and not every change will be in response to a change in the allergen load. What you should be looking for are major changes that occur regularly in response to a particular event – a marked improvement during holidays for example, or a deterioration when staying in a particular house. The list of allergens on pp67–9 can be used as a starting point for your investigations.

If you feel that some airborne or contact allergen might be contributing to the eczema, then take whatever steps you can to eliminate it before embarking on dietary investigations. Reducing dust, damp and moulds in the house (see pp69–71), keeping wool off the skin, avoiding low-temperature washing powders (see pp67–8) and rinsing clothes thoroughly after washing are basic measures that anyone with an eczematous child should try. If there are pets, then removing them temporarily, or keeping them away from the child, should be added to this list.

Non-specific irritants may be even more important than allergens, and these too should be eliminated. Simple measures include putting pure cotton clothing next to the skin, not using too much soap, and avoiding contact with chemical preparations as much as possible. Keeping a child's fingernails short reduces the damage done by scratching, and not allowing the house to get too hot is also helpful – heat aggravates the itchiness in the skin. Special cotton clothing, and mitten-pyjamas, which alleviate the effects of scratching, can be bought by mail-order (see p337).

All these measures may take a little while to have any effect and you should allow several months to elapse before coming to any conclusions. If the eczema is still troublesome, it may be worth trying an elimination diet.

Anyone who has suffered from eczema as a child would be well advised to avoid exposure to irritants in later life, even if their eczema appears to have cleared up. Surveys have shown that such people are far more likely to suffer from irritation to the skin on their hands. Occupational dermatitis – a common complaint of cleaners, beauticians, hairdressers, motor mechanics, nurses and laundry-workers – is roughly ten times more likely among those who once suffered from eczema. Such jobs should be avoided, and so should the use of cosmetics – sparing use and a regular change of brands is the best policy. 'Hypoallergenic' cosmetics are useful, in that they lack perfumes and other potential irritants, but the name is somewhat misleading, because they too can provoke allergies if used often enough.

Housework, of course, is a necessary evil, which only the lucky few can avoid. The obvious way to prevent trouble is to wear rubber gloves.

Unfortunately, rubber itself can be an irritant, especially in the warm, humid conditions that prevail within such gloves. Wear cotton gloves inside the rubber ones to prevent direct contact with the skin, and avoid using very hot water because the cooler the hands are within the gloves the better. Alternatively, wear PVC gloves – see pp338–9.

What to do about chronic urticaria

Sensitivity to aspirin is a fairly frequent cause of urticaria, and one that is easily tracked down. If you take aspirin regularly, cut them out for a few weeks and see if the urticaria improves. To check that it really was the aspirin, take a normal dose and see what effect this has. (You should not try this test if you have ever had a severe asthma attack.) Other drugs similar to aspirin (**non-steroidal anti-inflammatory drugs**) can also produce urticaria. These drugs (see pp327–8) are used to treat rheumatoid arthritis, osteoarthritis, period pains and headaches. Some are available without prescription.

ELIZABETH

As a schoolgirl, Elizabeth suffered from a rather odd type of nettle-rash that only came on when she was cold. It made her very miserable in winter, with an unbearably itchy rash on any exposed part of her body. She found this difficult to live with because she was very keen on sport, and could not play hockey, netball or other outdoor games in winter. Cold-induced urticaria, as her problem is known, can indicate more serious underlying problems, but medical tests showed that this was not the cause of the symptoms in her case. The standard test for cold-induced urticaria is to place an ice cube on the patient's arm for three minutes. When the doctor tried this on Elizabeth she reacted with nettle-rash on the arm. Purely as an experiment, the doctor decided to try Elizabeth on an elimination diet. After five days excluding all commonly eaten foods, she did not react to the ice-cube test. But when she reintroduced milk, and later eggs, she reacted in the same way as before. By avoiding these foods in winter, or only eating them occasionally, she is free from the nettle-rash. This has allowed her to do something she never thought possible before – to go on a skiing holiday!

Another approach to treating urticaria is to try a no-sugar, no-yeast diet, as described in Chapter 10. Some doctors use this diet, often in combination with anti-fungal drugs, as a treatment for supposed 'candidiasis'. Although the treatment is often very helpful, it is not known exactly why it should work, but there may be some imbalance in the gut flora (see pp186–7).

If a no-sugar, no-yeast diet is not effective, and other possible causes have been ruled out by your doctor, then you should consider the possibility of food sensitivity. Food additives are often the source of trouble, and the Stage 1 diet described in Chapter Fourteen should identify such sensitivities. If it does not, progress to the Stage 2 diet. Alternatively, skin-prick tests may be able to show which foods or additives are the source of the problem. However, skin-prick tests are not foolproof in urticaria, and for some people an elimination diet will be the only way of getting to the root of their problem.

It is rarely a single food or food additive that is implicated in chronic urticaria. As with acute urticaria, antibiotics and other medicinal drugs can play a part. So too can contactants, such as the nickel found in cheap jewellery, although this is unusual.

Identifying your allergens

The lists that follow (pp61–9) can be used as a starting point in tracking down your allergens. Careful detective work will be needed to identify allergens with any certainty – beware of jumping to conclusions, or you may be burdening yourself and your family with unnecessary avoidance measures. There is one list for asthma and rhinitis, and a second for eczema.

ALLERGENS THAT SHOULD BE SUSPECTED IN ASTHMA AND RHINITIS

GENERAL POINTS

- **Infections**
  Infections can trigger asthmatic attacks, so attacks that are worse in the winter do not necessarily point to a particular allergen. In some children, wheezing only occurs during infections and there is probably no allergen involvement. The viruses involved appear to produce substances that directly trigger mast cells in the bronchi.

- **Salt and MSG**
  Too much salt in the diet may make asthma more likely – try reducing the amount of salt eaten to see what effect this has. Monosodium glutamate (MSG) may have similar effects. The most common sources are tinned and packet soups, convenience foods and Chinese food.

● *Irritants*

Various airborne irritants can provoke both rhinitis and asthma, *eg:*

Smoke from cigarettes, bonfires, incinerators etc

Perfume and even strongly scented flowers

Industrial fumes, especially those containing sulphur dioxide

Sulphur dioxide is also given off by some foods and drinks (p301). Chewing and swallowing quickly can help to reduce the amount of sulphur dioxide released, but avoidance is probably a better solution.

If possible, reduce exposure to these irritants before trying to work out which allergens may be involved. In particular, eliminate cigarette smoke from the environment, as it is bound to make these conditions worse. Once allergens are identified and dealt with, the asthmatic may be able to cope with certain irritants again because the bronchi are less sensitive, but no asthmatic should be expected to tolerate someone else's cigarette smoke in their own home.

● *Other non-specific triggers*

Cold air, exercise, fear, anger and other emotions can also trigger attacks, so you should consider the possible involvement of these factors. However, there is likely to be some other factor that is the primary cause of the asthma. It is only when the bronchi are already sensitized that they respond to triggers such as these.

● *Multiple triggers*

Remember that there may be more than one allergen producing the same symptom – food may be one cause and inhalants or contactants another. Where foods are involved they may make the bronchi more sensitive, so that an airborne allergen then triggers an attack. *In such cases, the food alone may not bring on an asthmatic attack.*

POTENTIAL ALLERGENS

● *Pollen*

Mostly causes seasonal allergic rhinitis (hay-fever). The timing of the symptoms will depend on the type of pollen at fault: in Britain this is February-May, with the peak in April, for tree pollen, June-July for grass pollen and July-August for weeds such as nettles, plantains and mugwort. Pollen can also cause asthma. Where there is sensitivity to perennial allergens as well, the rhinitis may persist all

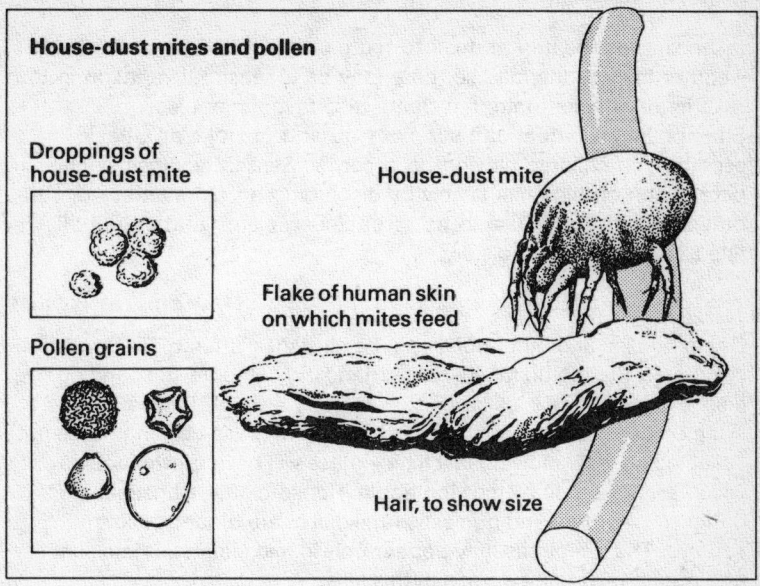

House-dust mites and pollen

Droppings of
house-dust mite

House-dust mite

Flake of human skin
on which mites feed

Pollen grains

Hair, to show size

all year, but get worse in spring or summer. 'Hay-fever' that begins in
late July or August and continues into the autumn is more likely to be
mould allergy.

In some people, certain foods can heighten sensitivity to pollen.
Foods eaten only in summer (or in greater quantities then) can
produce symptoms that may resemble hay-fever – suspect summer
fruits, orange squash and ice-cream.

● *House dust*
Sheep's wool or other components of dust may be the problem, but
more often it is the **house-dust mite**, *Dermatophagoides* ('the skin-
eater'). This minute animal lives on flakes of human skin shed by all
of us in great quantities. It is not an insect, as is often stated, but a
mite – a distant relative of the spiders. Although it is not an insect, it
is killed by some insecticides. Some people react to the mites
themselves but most are allergic to the **faecal pellets** (droppings).
These are covered with a thin layer of protein produced by the mite,
and it is the protein that acts as an allergen. House-dust mites thrive
in old sofas and armchairs, mattresses and carpets. Sunshine and
dry air are the mite's greatest enemies, so it prefers fitted carpets
cleaned with a vacuum cleaner, to loose rugs or carpets that are

taken outside, beaten and left to hang in the sun for a while. Damp weather favours the mite so there may be a seasonal variation in the severity of attacks (note that damp also favours moulds).

Shampooing a carpet can stir mites up and provoke an attack – especially in children playing on a carpet. Sensitivity varies: some people can obtain relief simply by discarding an old mattress or sofa, others require the house to be scrupulously clean, and free of all fitted carpets and upholstery.

● Moulds

Damp houses and other buildings (*eg* churches, church halls) provoke symptoms. Raking up fallen leaves, handling compost, or spending time in a greenhouse, cellar or conservatory also tend to make symptoms worse. So does mowing the lawn, if grass-clippings were not collected up after mowing last time – these will have grown moulds which are stirred up by mowing again. House-plants, Christmas trees, damp straw or hay and domestic humidifiers are other possible sources. The symptoms may appear only in midsummer or late summer and autumn – or may worsen at this time.

● Pet dogs, cats, rabbits, horses, hamsters, mice etc

Symptoms may not appear until many months after the pet is acquired – sometimes as much as a year. In very sensitive individuals, clothing that has been in contact with an animal can trigger an attack. Traces of animal allergens can linger in a house where pets have lived previously, even if carpets are removed. Old horsehair sofas or mattresses can affect someone who is sensitive to horses.

A brief exposure to an animal can cause symptoms that persist for up to a week. The symptoms may be mild and transient when the animal is actually there, with a more severe, delayed reaction that sets in later.

● Feathers

Pet birds, feather-filled pillows, eiderdowns, duvets and cushions can all cause symptoms. However, some people who appear to react to feather pillows are actually sensitive to house-dust mite.

● Wool, cotton, other textiles

Fibres are common in the air in most homes. People working in textile or clothing factories may become sensitized at work.

● *Barn mites in stored grain*
These can cause allergy in farmers and farmworkers.

● *Flour, grain dust, sawdust and other inhaled particles*
Workers in flour mills, sawmills etc, are most likely to become
sensitized. With allergies to wheat flour, eating bread may also provoke
symptoms. The dust from castor beans is particularly troublesome,
mainly because it contains lectins (see p32) that act as general irritants
– but it can also produce true allergies.

● *Airborne food particles or droplets*
Examples include egg applied by a spraying machine to glaze pies.
Once sensitized, an individual may also react when they eat the same
food.

● *Animal urine*
Those working with laboratory animals are the most likely to be
affected.

● *Vaccines*
The use of eggs for culturing certain vaccines (*eg* influenza, measles-
mumps-rubella) can lead to problems for those who are highly
sensitive to eggs, because a minute amount of egg protein persists in
the purified vaccine.

● *Foods*
Any food could, in theory, cause asthma. Other symptoms, such as
pain in the abdomen, diarrhoea, eczema or rhinitis are likely if food is
the cause. The reaction may occur rapidly in response to a small
amount of the food, or may be delayed by several hours or even days,
and require a large portion of the food. Some individuals have to eat
the food for several days in succession before there is a response.
    Foods can also cause rhinitis. In addition, hay-fever sufferers,
especially those sensitive to birch pollen, may experience an itching
mouth and swollen tongue after eating certain fruits or nuts. This is
due to a cross-reaction between pollens and certain foods – see p305.
Such symptoms may occur rapidly, but more often the rhinitis begins
many hours after the food is eaten.

● *Yeasts*
Alcoholic drinks, over-ripe fruits, breweries and bakeries are common

sources, but see p198 for a full list. Mould and yeast sensitivity may sometimes be helped by a no-sugar, no-yeast diet – see pp193–6.

● *Food additives*
As for foods, although the response time is usually shorter. Colourings used in food may also be present in medicinal drugs.

● *Drugs*
Antibiotics and aspirin are the common culprits, but any drug, in theory, could provoke an allergic response. The highly sensitive individual may respond to trace amounts of antibiotic found in meat, eggs or milk.

Aspirin (salicylate) can trigger off asthma, and is sometimes the cause of nasal polyps, especially where these are accompanied by urticaria.

● *Paints, air-fresheners, aerosols, natural gas, fumes from cavity-wall insulation*
Many household chemicals produce vapour that may act either as an allergen (when combined with a protein) or as an irritant. They can contribute to both asthma and rhinitis. Air-fresheners are actually *designed* to fill the air with vapour – keeping the house clean and well-ventilated is a much better way of combating household smells.

● *Industrial fumes, dust or other airborne particles in the workplace*
Dust in factories manufacturing antibiotics is often implicated, and may lead to sensitivity to the same antibiotic taken by mouth, whether as a drug or in food. Similar problems affect insulin production.

Fumes released during the manufacture of plastics, polyurethane foam, varnishes, paints, adhesives and synthetic fabrics may act either as allergens (when combined with a protein in the body) or as irritants. Isocyanates and phthalic anhydride are common offenders. Fumes released when plastics are heated or burned are also potential triggers. Phenylene diamine, used in the fur industry, and piperazine, a drug used to kill parasites, are other common causes of asthma. Enzyme manufacture, soldering (especially of electronic components), textile dyeing, beauty care and hairdressing are other high-risk occupations. The disease may begin soon after the first exposure, or it may take several months or years to appear – over a decade in some cases. The attacks may be delayed and not occur until the evening, when the patient is at home. Symptoms may clear up at weekends, but not in everyone. Once someone has become sensitized, very small

amounts – carried on the clothing of another person for example –
may be sufficient to trigger an attack.

ALLERGENS THAT SHOULD BE SUSPECTED IN ECZEMA

GENERAL POINTS

- *Irritants*
  Remember that in eczema, irritants may be more important than
  allergens in causing the symptoms. Common irritants include:
  Detergents
  Soap
  Shampoo, hair-dye etc
  Household chemicals of all kinds
  Rough clothing, including wool and synthetic fibres (pure cotton is
    the least irritating)
  Hard (calcium-rich) water
  Solvents and other chemicals used in the workplace
  Heat
  Scratching

POTENTIAL ALLERGENS

- *House dust*
  See pp63–4.

- *Moulds*
  See p64.

- *Pets*
  See p64.

- *Wool*
  Woollen jumpers or wool-mixture clothing are the usual sources. Wool
  may act as a general irritant rather than an allergen.

- *Enzymes*
  The enzymes used in 'biological' washing powders are the usual
  source. The use of enzymes is so widespread now, that the term
  'biological' is not always used. In general, any powder designed for use
  at low temperatures will contain enzymes. For enzyme-free detergents

that contain a minimum of potential irritants see p338.

● *Foods*
Any food can act as an allergen in eczema, but those most often
implicated in children are milk, egg and citrus fruits (mostly oranges).
Chicken, nuts, fish, wheat, peanuts, tomatoes, lamb and soya are also
common offenders. See pp260–75 for details of how to investigate the
role of food, or pp221–6 if the patient is a baby or small child.

● *Food additives*
Colouring and preservatives are frequent culprits, particularly the azo-
dyes (see p315) and benzoate preservatives. They may be acting as
non-specific irritants rather than allergens. Colourings used in food
may also be present in medicinal drugs, including antihistamine
preparations. See pp313–15 for details of food containing additives.

● *Drugs*
Eczema is seen in some patients who are sensitive to aspirin
(salicylate), although this is not thought to be an allergic reaction to
the drug.

● *Pollen*
Pollen grains landing on the skin may contribute to eczema in some
children, but they are unlikely to be the sole cause.

● *Grass and other plants*
Direct contact with some plants may provoke eczema in the sensitive
individual.

● *Metals*
Nickel, chromium and cobalt are the most frequent offenders. Women
are more likely to be nickel-sensitive than men because inexpensive
jewellery frequently have a high nickel content. So do the metal studs
in jeans

● *Cement*
The chromate in cement causes skin irritation in many construction
workers.

● *Chemicals in the home and workplace*
Various chemicals can cause skin irritation and eczema, particularly
rubber chemicals and plastics. High temperature and humidity makes

the skin even more sensitive, so wearing rubber gloves can readily produce sensitivity to rubber – see p60 for suggestions on how to overcome this problem.

ELIMINATING COMMON AIRBORNE ALLERGENS

● *House-dust mite*

Many allergy-sufferers are primarily affected by the house-dust mite allergens in their mattresses. It was once thought that interior-sprung mattresses were more troublesome than foam mattresses, but research has shown that any mattress can harbour large numbers of mites. Getting into bed, or turning over in bed, forces out a blast of air from within the mattress, air that carries a heavy load of allergens. This can be prevented by a mattress cover that holds in the mite allergens. The best covers are made of a microporous material which allows water vapour through (suppliers are listed on p337). Alternatively, the cover can be made of ordinary (impermeable) plastic, such as builder's plastic, but this tends to make the sleeper hot and sweaty.

Before the mattress cover is put on, it is preferable to treat the mattress with a spray that kills mites (acaricide spray) or a special liquid nitrogen treatment. Suppliers for both are listed on p339. If not killed, the mites will flourish inside the covered mattress, and when the cover is removed, or if a hole develops, allergens will leak out. The sprays are considered extremely safe, but very occasionally asthmatics experience symptoms in response to them. Anyone with chemical sensitivity should avoid using them. Liquid nitrogen is absolutely innocuous (the air around us is mostly nitrogen), and kills mites by reducing the temperature below freezing.

Covering the mattress is all that some patients need, while others are more sensitive to house-dust mite, and must therefore take other precautions. If symptoms still occur in bed, or first thing in the morning, try buying new pillows and covering them with microporous covers. Duvets can also be covered; they should be washed or dry-cleaned first, then thoroughly dried. Blankets should be regularly washed (a temperature of 60°C is needed to kill the mites) or dry-cleaned. Air the bed every day, and air the room by opening the window, to reduce moisture levels – humidity favours the mites. The allergy sufferer should stay out of the bedroom for some time after bed-making to allow the allergens in the air to settle.

You may also have to treat the bedroom carpet, if it is harbouring a lot of mite allergens. Thorough vacuum cleaning may help, but most people also need mite-killing sprays or liquid nitrogen treatment.

Some highly sensitive people must remove fitted carpets from the bedroom, along with any unnecessary fabrics, soft toys, clothes, etc. Rugs, if hung up outside in the sun regularly, and beaten to remove dust, harbour far fewer mites. Curtains should be washed regularly.

If symptoms are experienced in other parts of the house, improving the ventilation may be helpful as this will reduce mite numbers. Should this alone prove ineffective, consider replacing any very elderly armchairs or settees, since these can often be full of mites. Other upholstered furniture can be treated with mite-killing sprays or liquid nitrogen. Vacuum clean the upholstery afterwards.

If symptoms occur within a few hours of vacuum-cleaning, mite allergens dispersed into the air by the vacuum cleaner are probably at fault. Special vacuum cleaners that keep in the allergenic particles are now available. Filters that can be fitted to existing vacuum cleaners also reduce the number of particles becoming airborne. See p338 for suppliers of both these products. Dusting should be done with a damp cloth.

It may be difficult to part a child from its favourite teddy, even if this *is* harbouring millions of house-dust mites. Should you be faced with this problem, wash the soft toy as thoroughly as possible, dry it quickly (*eg* in a tumble-dryer) and hang it out in the sun for a day or two. Thereafter, the house-dust mites can be kept at bay by placing the teddy in a plastic bag and leaving it in a deep-freeze for one day each week.

● *Moulds*

Take all necessary measures to eliminate damp and condensation from the house. Ventilate all rooms, cupboards etc. Electric space-heaters are cheap to run and can help to keep a troublesome damp spot dry – do not use fan heaters as these churn up the spores.

Cover pans when cooking to reduce the amount of steam generated. Fitting an extractor fan in the kitchen can also reduce the amount of moisture in the air, which in turn reduces condensation.

Avoid having vinyl wallpapers, metal window-frames and other household fittings that favour condensation. Have baths rather than showers as these create less steam.

Check for signs of dampness and mould growth behind furniture and in cupboards, refrigerators and deep-freezes regularly. The rubber door-seals often harbour black moulds.

Throw away any furniture, curtains, carpets or cushions that have been damp and smell of mildew – even if they are now dry they will still contain mould spores.

Do not leave vegetables and fruit lying around for too long before eating them.

Do not have too many plants in the house. Remove dead leaves and flowers, and do not overwater them. Take off the top layer of soil and replace it from time to time.

Do not use humidifiers.

Heat the whole house well – do not leave some rooms permanently cold and unventilated.

Make sure clothes and shoes are thoroughly dry before putting them away in drawers or cupboards.

● *Animal skin (danders) and feathers*

Don't keep furry or feathered pets. If you already have pets which you cannot bear to get rid of, consider housing them outside or in part of the house that the affected person can easily avoid. Do not allow pets into the bedroom of the person affected. If they sleep on furniture or carpets, clean up after them with a vacuum cleaner.

For very sensitive individuals it may be necessary to avoid people and clothing that have been in contact with animals.

For those sensitive to feathers, eliminate all bedding stuffed with feathers, also cushions, armchairs and sofas. If you are also sensitive to synthetics, then duvets filled with wool or silk are available (p337).

For those sensitive to horses, check that you do not have any old items of furniture stuffed with horsehair.

● *Pollen*

This is the most difficult allergen to avoid. Keeping windows closed on warm, sunny days can be helpful. They should remain closed in the evening and during the night in large cities. When driving or travelling by train, avoid opening the window.

Keep away from meadows, parks and other grassy areas when it is warm and dry. Wearing sunglasses may help to reduce symptoms in the eye.

For very sensitive individuals, a stay at the seaside during the height of the pollen season is recommended – the sea breeze brings in pollen-free air. Alternatively, air filters can be used (p338) and are usually effective – as long as the patient stays indoors with the windows closed.

Chapter Five

OTHER FORMS OF FOOD ALLERGY

The first part of this chapter covers allergies to food that are not due to IgE. The second part deals with reactions that, strictly speaking, are not allergies at all: false food allergies, and problems caused by histamine in foods. This last section is relevant to all types of food sensitivity. Histamine-rich foods can be a problem for people with either food allergy *or* food intolerance, because both may have gut walls that are abnormally leaky.

NON-IgE FOOD ALLERGY

Doctors recognize four types of reaction in which the immune system responds to an antigen so strongly that unpleasant symptoms are caused. These are called **hypersensitivity** reactions. The reaction caused by mast cells and IgE is the most common and troublesome of the four, and is known as Type I hypersensitivity. The other three reactions involve different parts of the immune system. Type II hypersensitivity is not relevant here, while Type IV hypersensitivity is a very slow immune response produced by a particular group of immune cells. It may be involved in some reactions in the gut, such as Crohn's disease (see pp118–20) but it is not generally relevant to food allergy. This section is therefore confined to Type III reactions. These occur when there is a substantial production of antibodies in response to an antigen in the blood. It is the sheer weight of numbers that causes the problem – the antigens and antibodies, bound together in **immune complexes**, are like so much litter going round in the bloodstream.

In the case of food, undigested molecules get into the blood through the gut wall, after a meal (see p21). This is a normal process that occurs in the healthiest of individuals, although in the food-sensitive person it is likely to be more pronounced because the gut wall is more leaky. Once the food

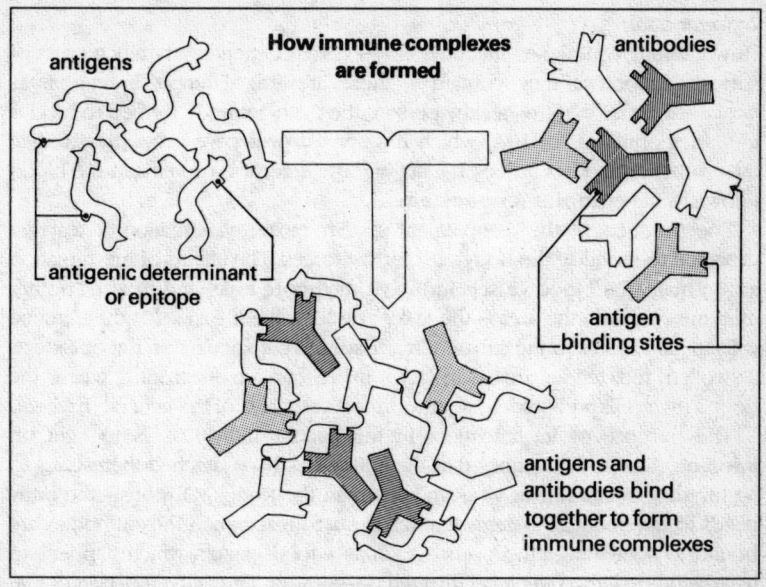

molecules enter the bloodstream they encounter antibodies – again a natural, healthy process which leads to the formation of immune complexes when the antibodies and antigens bind together. Immune complexes attract the attention of phagocytes or 'eating cells', the vultures of the immune system that clear up any debris, dead cells and invading bacteria they come across.

Immune complexes form all the time, whenever antibodies encounter their antigen. Normally they are cleared from the blood by the phagocytes within a few hours. But if the immune complexes are both large and numerous, the phagocytes may not be equal to the task. Then the immune complexes accumulate in the blood, and eventually they are deposited in the blood vessels. This is the condition known as **Type III hypersensitivity** or **serum sickness.**

Serum sickness happens in autoimmune diseases, such as **SLE** (systemic lupus erythematosus, or **lupus**; see pp140–1), where there are a great many antibodies to the patient's own proteins circulating in the blood. It is also believed to happen, to a lesser degree, in rare cases of food allergy – in some types of kidney disease, for example, where the disease seems to be induced by food. Although there is no definite proof for this, the circumstantial evidence is quite strong (see pp75–6).

Inflammation

How immune complexes affect the blood vessels depends very much on what sort of antibodies they contain – there are five different **isotypes**, as explained on p25. In the healthy person, the main antibody formed to food is immunoglobulin A, or **IgA**, which has special protective properties. Unlike most other antibodies it does not activate the defensive proteins in the blood known as the **complement system**.

The products of the complement system cause inflammation, a reaction designed to mobilize the body's protective forces. The effects of inflammation are to make the blood vessels in the vicinity more leaky and to attract other immune cells into the area – the leaky vessels make it easier for the immune cells to gain access to the surrounding tissues. What appears on the outside as a swollen, red, tender area is in fact a microscopic battleground, where the body's own cells and tissues are unfortunate casualties of the general mayhem.

The purpose of inflammation, in the healthy individual, is to fight off infection. The body assumes that the antibodies have attached themselves to an invading bacterium or virus and sends in the troops. Obviously the body needs to have control systems that tell it *not* to react when the antibodies are bound to something innocuous – such as a food protein which happens to have wandered into the blood through the gut wall. This is the function of IgA. Because it does not activate the complement system it can quietly mop up non-harmful antigens for disposal by the phagocytes, without setting off a damaging episode of inflammation.

For this system to work, the body must somehow distinguish food from other sorts of antigen. And it must make sure that IgA – rather than IgG, another more inflammatory type of antibody – is manufactured to fit the food molecules. The details of how the body does this are still far from clear, but a general picture is emerging from current research, and this is described in Chapter Twelve. The process is known as 'the induction of oral tolerance'.

What, if anything, goes wrong with this system? There is only a limited amount of evidence available, but it does seem that the system for producing IgA rather than IgG to food molecules breaks down in some people. Where this occurs, the immune complexes circulating in the blood after a meal will be potentially inflammatory. If they are deposited in a blood vessel, damage to the walls of the vessel will follow.

Such people may also have IgE in their food-molecule immune complexes, so mast cells could be triggered to add to the inflammation. Whether this actually happens is not clear. But if it does, then there are important implications for the way we think about allergies: the dividing line between Type I (IgE) food allergy and Type III food allergy may not be as sharp as is often assumed.

Symptoms produced by immune complex deposits
Patients with the autoimmune disease SLE (see p73) illustrate the sort of symptoms that can be produced when immune complexes are deposited in the blood vessels. Among other things, they suffer from skin rashes, painful joints and damage to the kidneys and lungs.

All these symptoms are produced by the deposited immune complexes causing inflammation in tiny blood vessels known as capillaries. In the case of the joints, the capillaries supplying blood to the joints become inflamed and this causes pain.

In the kidneys, immune complexes can become deposited around the delicate membranes that do the important job of filtering the blood. Their task is to remove excess salts and certain toxic compounds from the blood so that they can be flushed out of the body in the urine. Proteins in the blood are not normally allowed to escape into the urine, but when there is damage to the structure of the kidney, then this can occur. Because the body's much-needed proteins are being lost in the urine the general state of health will eventually deteriorate, especially in children, who need protein for growth. The failure of the kidneys also means that excess water is retained, so there is puffiness in various parts of the body (oedema).

Food and kidney disease
The question of whether *foods* might produce excess immune complexes in the blood, and thus cause the same sort of damage to the kidneys, is a highly controversial one. Two groups of doctors, one working in Japan, the other in Miami, Florida, have made a special study of children with kidney disorders, and they believe that food is the source of the problem for *some* of these children. When put on an elemental diet (a synthetic food mixture that contains a minimum of antigens, see p263), children with certain types of kidney disease may improve. Those who do recover are then challenged with various foods and some reproduce their original symptoms – protein loss in the urine, and retention of water leading to puffiness in various parts of the body.

The food most often implicated is cow's milk – the most common allergen of childhood. But the majority of these children appear to be sensitive to several foods, and to various airborne allergens, such as pollen. Some of them also show sensitivity to environmental chemicals, a subject that is dealt with more fully in Chapter Nine. By putting these children on restricted diets, their symptoms have been fully or partially controlled. There are reports that neutralization treatments (see pp297–9) are also useful, where the food or foods concerned are difficult to avoid.

It must be emphasized that children such as these are rare, and the vast majority of cases of kidney disease are due to other causes. Nevertheless it does seem that food allergy can cause kidney damage in some children. Whether it can affect adults in this way is an open question.

Almost all the children affected in this way are atopic – that is, they show one of the classical allergic disorders, such as asthma or eczema. This raises the possibility that IgE and mast cells are somehow involved in the damaging reactions in their kidneys. While this is possible, it does not seem that IgE has a central role. Neither is it entirely certain that deposition of immune complexes is to blame. Some of the available evidence suggests that it is, but other studies point to different forms of immune reaction producing the damage.

Finally, Type-I allergic reactions to *airborne allergens*, such as pollen, may sometimes be linked with kidney disorders. Reactions of this type are thought to be extremely rare. It is not known whether IgE and mast cells are responsible for the damage in the kidney, or whether some other mechanism is at work.

Inflammation of the blood vessels and spontaneous bruising

If inflammation occurs in the walls of the blood vessels, the vessels become more permeable as we have already seen. When the inflammation is not too serious, and mainly affects the tiny blood vessels (capillaries) in the skin, the

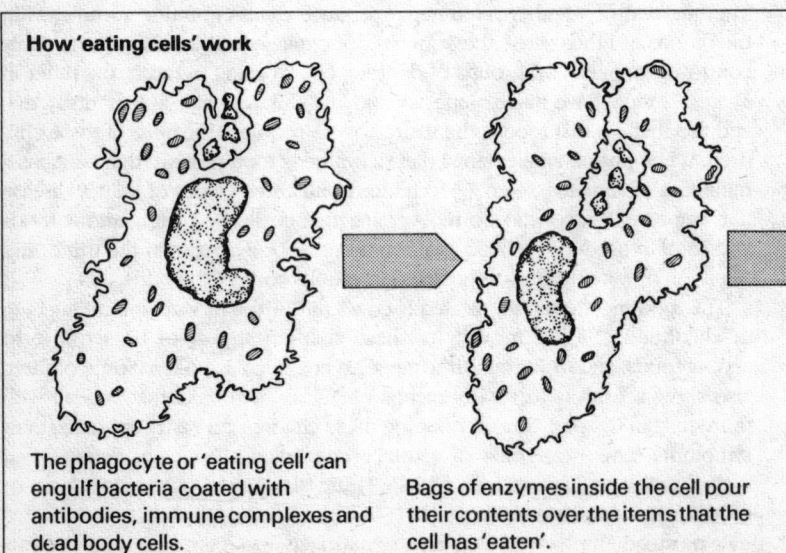

How 'eating cells' work

The phagocyte or 'eating cell' can engulf bacteria coated with antibodies, immune complexes and dead body cells.

Bags of enzymes inside the cell pour their contents over the items that the cell has 'eaten'.

result is likely to be urticaria or nettle-rash (see p44). In such circumstances it is mainly fluid that leaks from the blood vessels, with few cells making an escape. (The approach to dealing with this form of urticaria is much the same as that described on pp60–1, although the possibility of chemical sensitivity should also be investigated.)

If the inflammation is more serious, then the blood vessels can become much more leaky and even break open, so that red and white blood cells escape into the surrounding tissue, as well as fluid. This condition is known as **vasculitis** and it may affect larger blood vessels as well as capillaries.

The first noticeable sign of vasculitis is usually swelling, or **oedema**, due to water leaking from the blood into the surrounding tissues. If there is generalized oedema – a reaction that affects the whole body – there will be a marked gain in weight, as much as 5 kg (over 11 lb) in 24 hours. There may also be aches and pains, especially in the legs, that tend to come and go.

As the condition gets worse, the blood vessels become more leaky and eventually rupture. Red blood cells start to seep into the tissues and are noticeable externally as tiny reddish spots, which then turn purple or black, and finally yellowish before disappearing – the same sort of colour changes as are seen in a bruise. The condition is known as **purpura**. Larger escapes of blood produce **spontaneous bruising.**

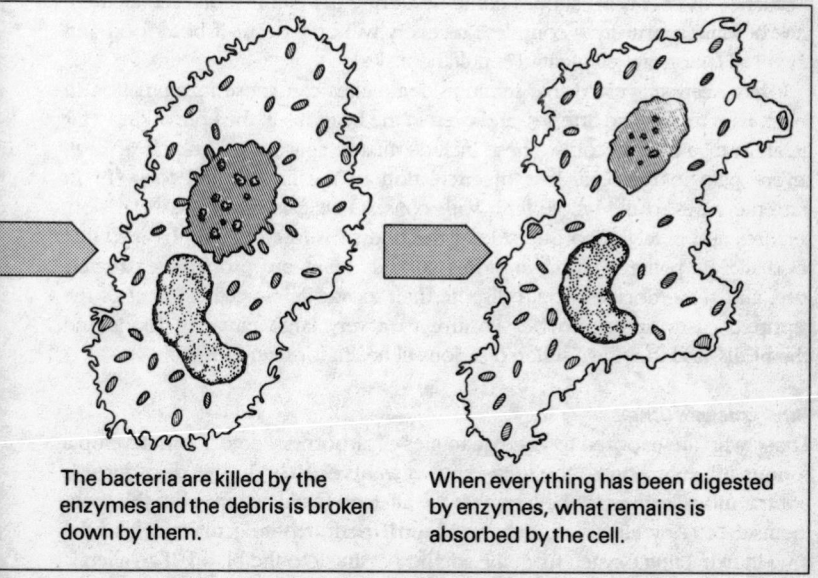

The bacteria are killed by the enzymes and the debris is broken down by them.

When everything has been digested by enzymes, what remains is absorbed by the cell.

If vasculitis is allowed to continue unchecked, more serious damage to the vessel wall may occur, and this can eventually lead to a vein becoming permanently inflamed or even completely blocked. Such damage is serious and often irreversible, so it is important to treat vasculitis at an early stage.

A role for food?

There are various causes for vasculitis and purpura. Infections can precipitate an attack, as can certain drugs. A shortage of **platelets**, the tiny particles in the blood that promote clotting, can also lead to purpura – such a shortage occurs in some autoimmune diseases, where the body attacks its own tissues. If all these possibilities have been eliminated, then it is worth considering allergy as a potential cause. In rare cases, food allergens circulating in the blood can be responsible – these can be identified by an elimination diet of the kind described in Chapter Fourteen. There may also be instances of IgE-mediated allergy producing vasculitis. An acute attack of vasculitis and purpura can accompany the sudden collapse (anaphylactic shock) that sometimes occurs on eating a food allergen.

Many of those suffering from allergic vasculitis show sensitivity to various chemicals, so it is important to eradicate these from the immediate environment before trying an elimination diet. This may be sufficient to clear the symptoms or at least reduce their severity. Even if it has no apparent effect, avoidance of chemicals should continue during the elimination diet, as there may be dual sensitivity – complete recovery will only occur if both food and chemical factors are eliminated simultaneously.

It has been suggested that immune complexes can cause inflammation in much larger veins and arteries, and even in the heart itself, thus provoking a far greater range of symptoms. These include muscle spasms, irregular heartbeat, severe pain in the legs, loss of circulation to the fingers and toes (or in extreme cases to the whole limb with consequent gangrene), loss of vision, seizures and paralysis on one side of the body. It should be emphasized that food-allergic patients with symptoms such as these are probably extremely rare, and some doctors would dispute their existence altogether. Most of the reported cases appear to be sensitive to a very large range of foods and chemicals, and they have suffered serious ill-health for many years.

Bird-fancier's lung

Those who are exposed to large quantities of airborne allergens can develop a serious inflammation of the lungs known as **alveolitis**. In this disorder it is not the tubes leading to the lung that are affected (as in asthma) but the lungs themselves. Tiny air-sacs known as **alveoli** perform the actual work of the lung in extracting oxygen from the air and passing it to the blood. If an allergic reaction to airborne allergens occurs in the alveoli, the large number of immune complexes produced can be deposited there and cause highly damaging inflammation. The structure of the alveoli begins to break down, causing shortness of breath, tightness in the chest, fever and a dry cough.

There are several forms of alveolitis, including farmer's lung and mushroom-worker's lung, but the only one likely to have any relevance to food allergy is bird-fancier's lung. In this disorder, it is tiny particles from the birds' droppings that initiate the allergic reaction in the alveoli. The connection with food allergy is a tenuous one, but some doctors claim that eating eggs can exacerbate the symptoms in a few patients. This might occur if the antibodies produced to the antigens in the droppings also bind to antigens from egg proteins carried in the bloodstream. This dual binding – known as **cross-reactivity** – can occur where antigens are chemically similar. Laboratory experiments suggest that there *is* cross-reactivity between the antigens of chicken's eggs and the antigens found in the droppings of budgerigars and pigeons.

FALSE FOOD ALLERGY

False food allergy, as used in this book, means unusual reactions to food that are caused by the foods *triggering mast cells directly*. In other words, these reactions involve mast cells, but they do not depend on IgE antibodies being formed to the food in question. Because the reaction is produced by mast cells releasing mediators, the symptoms are indistinguishable from true IgE-mediated food allergy.

When food bites back

Food, as we have already seen in Chapter One, is not necessarily the nice, passive, innocuous stuff that we have traditionally believed it to be: neither plants nor animals want to be eaten, and they have ways of fighting back. In plants, particularly, there are many chemical weapons to deter would-be diners, and some of these chemicals persist, even in modern crop plants. That we are not made ill by them more often is a tribute to our own abilities in breaking down such chemicals – abilities that have been acquired in the course of evolution.

One particularly cunning type of chemical weapon turns the body's most potent defence force on itself: it fools the mast cells into degranulating. There are dozens of different substances found in food that can perform this trick. Some bind to IgE molecules, effectively bridging two adjacent molecules, in much the same way as an antigen might bridge them. Others bind to the receptors on the mast cell that normally attach themselves to IgE, thus bridging the receptors. Because bridging of the IgEs (and thus bridging the receptors) is the signal for the mast cell to degranulate, both types of substance cause the release of damaging mediators such as histamine. Other substances may produce the same effect simply by binding to the mast cell membrane and changing its structure so that it becomes more permeable.

One group of compounds that can have this effect on mast cells are the **lectins**. They are produced in particularly high concentrations by peanuts, beans, peas and lentils, all of which are members of the legume family of plants. Lectins are also found in edible snails, and in wheat.

The main characteristic of lectins is that they bind to carbohydrate molecules carried on the surface of all cells. As a result, they make red blood cells clump together, and this is how they are recognized in the laboratory. The deadly poison, ricin, used in the KGB's infamous umbrella-tip murder of Georgi Markov, is a type of lectin. Fortunately not all lectins are as potent as this, but many can cause rather more subtle damage. Apart from triggering mast cells, they can also bind to the lining of the gut wall and make it more leaky, so that more undigested food molecules get into the blood stream. These molecules can act as allergens, causing further damage as they travel around the body in the blood. There is also some evidence that, in atopic individuals, certain lectins can stimulate the body to produce IgE in preference to other antibodies. All these different effects could contribute to adverse reactions to food, but the major factor in false food allergy is the direct effect of lectins on mast cells.

Many lectins are inactivated by cooking, but they need to be heated for a long time and at fairly high temperatures to destroy all their activity. The powerful lectin found in kidney beans or haricot beans (*Phaseolus vulgaris*) can cause serious diarrhoea and abdominal pain if the beans are not soaked and cooked properly. Using low-temperature 'slow-cookers' to prepare casseroles containing beans has caused many outbreaks of such illness.

Whereas the lectin found in raw or badly cooked kidney beans is damaging to almost everyone, other lectins are more selective – indeed, the word lectin comes from a Latin word meaning 'choosing'. Each of us is slightly different in our chemical make-up, and one important way in which people vary is in the short carbohydrate molecules that sit on the surface of our body cells. It is mainly these carbohydrates to which the lectins bind, and they are highly specific for the individual sugars that make up the carbohydrate. Each type of lectin is specific for a particular sugar. (There is also a short carbohydrate chain in every antibody molecule, and it may well be that lectins trigger mast cells by binding to the carbohydrate component of IgE.)

It seems likely that individual differences in the carbohydrate chains (either on the cell surface, or in IgE molecules) could make some people susceptible to a particular lectin which has no adverse effect on the majority of the population.

But if susceptibility to particular lectins causes false food allergy, why is this problem so rare? The answer must be that natural selection has weeded it out, because it would have been a serious disadvantage among our distant ancestors if an important element in the diet could not be eaten. Any individual who suffered such an affliction would probably have died early, without leaving any offspring. In this way, the genes that could make a person susceptible to false food allergy would have remained very rare. But even such damaging genes can survive if they are capable of being masked by other 'healthy' genes – this means that some people can carry the gene, without suffering any ill-effects, and pass it on to their children.

Other foods that can trigger mast cells

Although lectins are probably the best-studied, they are certainly not the *only* food components that can trigger mast cells directly. Several foods contain **peptides** (small protein-like molecules) which also bind to mast cells and make them degranulate. Among the foods known to contain such peptides are egg-white, strawberries, crustacean shellfish (prawns, shrimps, crabs, lobsters), tomatoes, fish, pork, alcohol and chocolate.

Pineapple and papaya both contain very powerful protein-breaking enzymes that can attack the membranes of any body cell, including mast cells. This again may cause the mast cells to degranulate. It is not certain whether some individuals are more susceptible than others, but it is not advisable for anyone to eat raw pineapple or papaya on an empty stomach because of the damage done to the stomach lining by these enzymes. Tinned pineapple is safe because the heat used in canning inactivates the enzyme.

Yet another group of foods contain substances that appear to trigger mast cells but whose chemical identity is unknown. The foods in question are buckwheat, sunflower seeds, mango and mustard. The offending ingredient – which is assumed to be a peptide or protein – binds to the IgE of susceptible individuals.

Diagnosing false food allergy

Sorting out false food allergy from the real thing is far from easy. A skin-prick test (see p30) will not distinguish someone with false food allergy from someone who has true IgE-mediated food allergy – both can produce a positive result. The radioallergosorbent test or RAST (see p82) is usually positive as well, because the lectins or other offending food components bind IgE – in a true case of allergy, the IgE will bind the food antigen, but the results of the test look just the same. A simple modification of the RAST reveals the truth however; if extra food extract is added to the mixture, false food allergy will still give a positive test, but true food allergy will not.

Distinguishing between these two distinct types of food reaction is important to researchers, seeking to understand food allergy and establish its prevalence. As far as the patient is concerned, the distinction is less important, because the consequences and treatment are much the same. In most cases avoidance will be necessary. If drugs are used they will be ones that prevent

THE RADIOALLERGOSORBENT TEST (RAST)

The radioallergosorbent test, or RAST, measures the level of IgE antibodies that a person has to a specific substance, such as a food protein or a pollen. There are four stages to the test:

1. An extract of the food (or other potential allergen) is applied to beads made of a substance called sepharose. This is an inert substance that simply acts as a surface on which reactions between the allergen and the antibody can take place. The food molecules remain attached to the sepharose beads throughout the test.

2. A sample of the patient's serum (the liquid part of the blood) is allowed to flow over the beads. If the blood contains IgE antibodies to that food, these will bind to the food antigens on the beads. The beads are later rinsed to remove everything that is not bound – only the IgE molecules should remain.

3. Another liquid is poured over the beads. This contains a special type of antibody called anti-IgE, which binds specifically to the stem of IgE molecules. If there is IgE stuck to the beads, these anti-IgE antibodies will bind to them. If no IgE is present, then all the anti-IgE will be washed away.

4. The anti-IgE was previously marked with a radioactive marker or a coloured marker. This means that the amount of IgE present can be worked out by measuring the radioactivity or colour given off by the beads. The amount of anti-IgE present is a measure of how much IgE (specific for that food) there is in the patient's blood.

Of course, the test will also give a positive result if the food contains something that specifically binds to IgE (as long as there is *some* IgE in the blood). This does indeed happen in some patients with false food allergy, and is discussed on p81.

mast cells from degranulating or counteract the effect of the mediators – in either case, it does not matter how the mast cells are being triggered.

It is possible, however, that those with false food allergy have some underlying deficiency that may make them more susceptible. It has been found that 50 per cent of patients with false food allergy are deficient in the element magnesium. A shortage of magnesium is known to affect histamine release and increase sensitivity to histamine. A nutritional assessment (see pp270–2) might be advisable for anyone known to have false food allergy.

Surprisingly enough, it is possible to 'grow out of' false food allergy. Children who have such a reaction to a particular food sometimes lose it, usually by the time they are eight years old. Exactly why this should happen is far from clear. There could be a change in the structure of the tissues that surround the mast cells in the gut, making them less accessible to food molecules.

HISTAMINE IN FOODS

Some foods contain large amounts of histamine, and this can cause unpleasant symptoms when they are eaten. The histamine has a drug-like (pharmacological) effect on the body. Although this is not false food allergy (according to the definition we are using), it is appropriate to discuss it here – since histamine is also the main mediator produced by mast cells, the effects are similar.

Histamine is formed in foods by the action of certain bacteria. These are not disease-causing bacteria, and their presence is normally harmless, but if they are too numerous the histamine they generate can cause problems. The principal foods concerned are well-ripened cheeses and Continental sausages, especially those that are kept for a long time. Some types of fish, principally mackerel and tuna, may cause similar problems if they are not kept at low temperatures before being eaten or canned. Bacteria in the fish produce a cocktail of toxins that includes generous quantities of histamine. Fish affected in this way have a sharp, peppery or metallic taste. Tinned fish of any kind, sauerkraut, and many alcoholic drinks can also be rich in histamine.

The symptoms of histamine poisoning are nausea, diarrhoea, skin rashes, flushing and headaches. The liver is well-equipped to detoxify histamine, and these unpleasant symptoms are relatively short-lived, usually clearing up within 12 hours. However, the drug isoniazid, used for the treatment of tuberculosis, reduces the liver's ability to break down histamine, and anyone taking this drug should avoid histamine-rich foods. Viral hepatitis and cirrhosis of the liver also make the body less able to detoxify histamine. Some people with chronic urticaria seem to be unusually susceptible to histamine and it is worth avoiding it for a while to see if the urticaria clears up.

Any increase in the leakiness of the gut wall increases susceptibility to histamine in foods, simply because more histamine gets through. It seems likely that greater permeability of the gut is a common feature of both food allergy and food intolerance, so avoiding histamine-rich cheeses and sausages may be generally advisable.

Chapter Six

THE GREAT CONTROVERSY

No-one writing about food intolerance can claim to be reflecting 'majority opinion', because there are such widely differing views on the subject. By looking at those differences in opinion first, before considering food intolerance in detail, we hope to give the reader a better understanding of our own viewpoint on the subject.

Why is there so much disagreement over food intolerance? And why do so many doctors regard it as a 'media illness', the outcome of ill-informed publicity? There is no simple answer to this question, but it is an important one nonetheless. The disagreement is not over whether food intolerance exists – few doctors would dispute that it does. What is at issue is the *prevalence* of the problem, and the *sort of symptoms* it can cause.

The question of *prevalence* is problematic because there are no reliable data available. Estimates of how many people suffer from food intolerance range from a very conservative 0.3 per cent to a rather implausible 90 per cent. Most of the doctors who study food intolerance in the UK would put the figure at somewhere between 10 and 25 per cent.

Controversy over the *sort of symptoms* caused by food intolerance is equally fierce. The orthodox view is that foods are unlikely to cause symptoms such as rheumatoid arthritis or Crohn's disease (a severe inflammation of the bowel), and that only certain sorts of foods might trigger off migraine. The idea of foods causing mental problems, such as depression, anxiety, hyperactivity or even psychosis is considered quite outrageous by most orthodox doctors and psychiatrists. The list of complaints attributed to food intolerance, given on pp109–42, contains many other controversial items.

A related issue is the type of symptoms caused by food *allergy*. Although most allergists have now come round to the idea that allergic reactions to foods may cause asthma and eczema, not all have. And few are willing to accept that other problems, such as hyperactivity in children, might be linked to food allergy. For historical reasons, these debates are linked to those over food intolerance (see p11), so they too form part of this chapter.

In the course of this chapter, we will look at these bones of contention in some detail, assess the scientific evidence, and try to discover why the question of food sensitivity generates so much heated debate.

Cause-and-effect thinking

In the eighteenth and early nineteenth centuries, doctors tried to explain why they saw certain patterns of diseases. Epidemics broke out in the crowded urban slums created by the Industrial Revolution, due to a lack of sanitation and clean water supplies. Knowing nothing of bacteria and viruses, doctors constructed the theory of 'miasmas' to explain them.

Miasmas were elusive, unidentified atmospheric conditions that could somehow cause disease. To explain the great variety of diseases that appeared in the same crowded areas, the miasmas were assumed to be non-specific – they might cause cholera in some people, yellow fever in others, and so on. As an extension of this idea, other factors in the environment were assumed to cause disease. Cold was an obvious one, and it too was seen as being non-specific – different people suffered different symptoms when they lived in cold houses or breathed cold air.

In the 1860s and 1870s, a revolution occurred in medical thinking. Dr Robert Koch in Germany and Louis Pasteur in France discovered that micro-organisms caused a great many diseases. More importantly, they found that *specific* bacteria caused *specific* illnesses. This is a fact that we now take for granted, but in its time it was a remarkable and novel idea. The **germ theory**, as it was known, quickly replaced the old way of thinking, where a miasma or other environmental factor could cause a great variety of different ills.

The change in medical thinking brought about by the germ theory was a radical one. In a reaction to the vagueness of the old ways of thought, a dogmatic insistence on cause-and-effect thinking took over. From then on, each disease had to have a specific set of symptoms and a specific cause. This way of thinking, with its obvious scientific merits, has dominated medical education for the past century.

Food intolerance, as it is presently understood, is anathema to this way of thinking. The range of symptoms claimed for it is vast. No two patients are alike, and there is no single symptom that is common to all. Different foods are at fault in different patients – and they cause different symptoms. Some patients are apparently sensitive to other things as well, such as house-dust mite or synthetic chemicals. There are no tests for food intolerance and no obvious physical signs – indeed, the patients often look well. To cap it all, there is no obvious mechanism.

As Dr William Bynum, a medical historian at the Wellcome Institute observes: 'There is a general reluctance among the medical establishment to accept things that are non-specific and don't always cause the same symptoms. It smacks too much of the old ideas of causation in medicine – cold weather was supposed to cause head-colds in some people and rheumatism in other people and so on. Causal thinking before the germ theory was extremely loose and it did not satisfy the usual canons of scientific explanation about cause and effect. There has been a strong reaction to that, and the problem with so-called food intolerance is that it goes against the grain of present-day thinking.'

Two other factors help to make food intolerance seem dubious. Many of the symptoms that are claimed for it are symptoms of a general type that can be caused in all sorts of different ways. Headache, for example, can be due to a bump on the head, anxiety, overwork, a brain tumour or a wild party the night before. What is more, many of the symptoms are those that can be produced by psychosomatic illness, in which emotional or mental distress evokes physical symptoms in the body (see pp150–2). Both these factors make the phenomenon of food intolerance seem even less credible.

Doctors come to food intolerance with a set of preconceived ideas that automatically prejudice them against the whole concept. And unlike the general public, they are not readily swayed by stories of miracle cures, however numerous those stories might be. This sort of evidence is referred to in medical science as 'anecdotal', and is quite rightly treated with great caution. The human body and mind interact in mysterious ways, and a person may recover from an illness spontaneously, or in response to an entirely ineffective treatment. This is known as the **placebo effect**, and is described on pp153–5. These and other factors make individual case-histories a doubtful item of evidence. Even if diets *are* helpful in clearing up the symptoms, it may be for some other reason entirely – perhaps the person's previous diet was unsound nutritionally, or contained an unhealthy amount of caffeine or some other drug-like substance that was causing the symptoms.

The history of medicine is littered with bogus 'miracle cures' that apparently worked wonders in their day. Hydropathy, popular in the nineteenth century, was said to be a cure for all sorts of nervous complaints and long-term illnesses. The treatments consisted of alternate hot and cold baths, wrapping the patient in wet blankets, and requiring him to drink huge quantities of water. These measures were supposed to 'strengthen the fibres' of the body and rid it of poisons. 'Direct Faradism' (named after Faraday, who helped to discover electricity) involved giving mild electric shocks to the arms and legs. It was recommended to anyone who was tired, run down or had other nervous afflictions. The electric shocks supposedly 'stimulated the constitution'. Both these therapies were highly regarded in their day, and thousands felt they had benefited from them. Mass enthusiasm is a strange thing – simply feeling caught up in some wonderful new discovery may be a powerful form of treatment.

There are various other preconceived ideas that work against food intolerance – the belief that food is essentially passive and innocuous for example (p15), the notion that what we have eaten for thousands of years must be good for us (p20) and the simplistic model of digestion which assumes that no complex molecules reach the bloodstream (pp20–1). These mistaken ideas all contribute to the understandable scepticism of the medical world.

Seeing the light

A combination of factors such as these make it very difficult for doctors, however open-minded they may be, to accept many of the effects now being claimed for food sensitivity. Dr Doris Rapp describes in her book *Allergies and the Hyperactive Child*, how she became a 'convert' to the idea that foods and inhalants could cause hyperkinetic syndrome: 'I am ashamed to admit that from 1960 to 1975 while in practice as a paediatric-allergist, I seldom recognized or diagnosed this problem. Then, as often happens in medicine, my patients taught me.'

One of the patients involved was a five-year-old girl whose nose, eye and chest allergies, for which Dr Rapp was consulted. The parents mentioned that she was also irritable, over-active, depressed and weepy, and suffered from stomach aches, headaches and diarrhoea. Dr Rapp suspected brain damage as the cause of the behavioural problems, which of course would be incurable. Her main concerns were the allergies, and these she attempted to treat with an elimination diet, plus suggestions for the removal of major allergens from the home. 'In three days, her mother called to say she was extremely pleased. I assumed Paula's hay-fever and asthma had improved, but her mother said no, Paula's disposition and her activity were better. I was amazed and perplexed. The mother said Paula's teacher had called to find out which "drug" the child was taking . . .'

A succession of similar experiences were enough to change Dr Rapp's outlook. 'How could I have missed it for so long?' she goes on to ask. 'The answer is that a doctor often sees what he wants to see and is trained to see. If parents noticed their child had a better disposition, stopped wetting the bed, or seemed less tired or less over-active after a diet, I always believed that it was because the nose and chest allergies were better . . .'

Many other doctors who work in the field of food sensitivity have similar tales to tell. Some have come to the idea because they themselves, or members of their families, were plagued by mysterious illnesses. In desperation, they tried an elimination diet and found that symptoms which had troubled them for years cleared up within a week or two. This encouraged them to look again at some of their long-term patients with unidentified illnesses, and when they began to try elimination diets on such patients they found that many of them responded very well.

Belief and disbelief

So far, we have only looked at attitudes to food intolerance in terms of beliefs and preconceived ideas, which will undoubtedly seem odd to anyone with a scientific turn of mind. In theory, medical beliefs should be secondary to the scientific evidence, for or against, although in reality they rarely are. Dr David Atherton of the Institute of Child Health in London, who specializes in treating eczema, writes: 'I am often asked by sceptical colleagues whether I "believe in all this food business". It is a sad reflection on current medical practice that such an important question as the relationship between a patient's diet and their disease should be relegated to one of belief or disbelief.'

In the next section we will consider the scientific evidence, but as we do so the importance of prejudice will again become evident. Even in the most scientific studies of this subject, it seems that the beliefs of the experimenters can influence the outcome. In general, those who 'believe' in food intolerance tend to get positive results, while the disbelievers usually get negative results. *The conclusions you draw from this will, of course, be influenced by what you believe!* But, as we hope to show, there are simple explanations for these apparently contradictory findings.

THE SCIENTIFIC EVIDENCE
Safety in numbers

Medical science is never exact, for a variety of reasons. For a start everyone is different, both in the genes that make them what they are, and in the environmental conditions that shape them from birth. Those environmental conditions include childhood and adult illnesses, standard of nutrition, type of work, nature of relationships with other people, past medical treatments and present living conditions. A collection of patients also differ in their age and sex, two very important factors in health and illness. Their response to treatment is bound to differ for these reasons alone.

A second major factor is the imprecise nature of diagnosis. Names may be given to diseases – 'rheumatoid arthritis', for example, or 'migraine' – but this does not mean that they are single, clearly defined conditions, in the way that infectious diseases such as measles or cholera are. Doctors suspect that, although the symptoms look similar, there are a multitude of different disorders sheltering under such umbrella terms. One of the ways in which medicine advances is by recognizing different subgroups within such diseases, and giving new names to the symptoms shown by those subgroups – 'classical migraine' and 'common migraine', for example. But in many diseases, there are no obvious subgroups, even though it is clear that the patients are not all the same. This is particularly true in food intolerance.

To overcome these problems in medical trials, it is important to study as large a group of patients as possible. Because the patients suffering from a disease can be so diverse, a new treatment may only be effective for, say, 10 per cent of them. A study that only includes 20 patients should, in a perfect world, include two patients who will respond. But when numbers are this small, the laws of chance dictate that there could easily be no patients of this type in the group. So a group of 100 patients may be needed to give a convincing result – but such large-scale trials are costly and difficult to organize.

Different doctors, different patients

A third factor that influences medical trials is the type of patients a particular doctor sees. To take one example, a consultant gastroenterologist working in a large hospital will see a wide range of patients with persistent diarrhoea, who have been referred by their family doctor. These patients will vary in all sorts of ways, including their own ideas about their illness. Some may think that particular foods cause their symptoms, but most will have no clue at all why they are ill. An allergist, on the other hand, will not see many patients with diarrhoea, but those he *does* see will probably have been referred by their family doctor because they believe their symptoms are caused by 'allergies' to food. Experience shows that such patients have often tried some form of self-diagnosis, or alternative therapy, without success.

A proportion of the allergist's patients may be people with psychosomatic problems, who have latched on to diet as an explanation for their symptoms because they find the label 'psychosomatic' unacceptable (see p156). Despite their lack of success in identifying dietary triggers for their symptoms, they are unwilling to give up. Of course, the first group of patients – those seen by the gastroenterologist – may well include some with psychosomatic problems, but they are probably fewer than in the group seen by the allergist.

When referring patients, family doctors take account of the consultant's views, and, it must be said, their own personal preferences. A 'difficult' patient whose diarrhoea is accompanied by a patently neurotic personality is likely to be referred to a consultant whose main interest lies in psychosomatic causes. Another patient with much the same bowel symptoms, whom the family doctor believes to be mentally well-balanced, will probably be referred to a consultant who is more interested in physical causes. This again biases the 'sample' of patients that a particular consultant sees, and tends to reinforce medical prejudices.

Neither of these two groups of patients is a representative sample of *everyone* in the country with persistent diarrhoea. A survey which showed that a third of 'apparently healthy' people suffered some form of bowel disorder (see p114) also discovered that the majority had not sought medical treatment. So the statistics produced by any medical study are not necessarily applicable to the population at large.

Studies of food intolerance

In the face of all these difficulties, it is reasonable to ask why anyone bothers with such studies. But they do, in the interests of establishing scientifically valid forms of diagnosis and treatment. Attempts to do this in relation to food intolerance are many and varied, and we will not try to cover them all. What matters in such studies is the *care* with which they are designed and the *details* of how they are carried out. To assess a trial properly, one must look carefully at the details and we will therefore concentrate on five trials – two dealing with rheumatoid arthritis, two dealing with irritable bowel syndrome, and one dealing with migraine. These trials are the main ones carried out in Britain within the last eight years, and they are among the most scientific attempts to evaluate the food-intolerance concept.

Trials dealing with rheumatoid arthritis

Rheumatoid arthritis is a disease in which the joints become painful, swollen and warm, due to internal inflammation. There are characteristic changes in the level of certain factors in the blood that help to confirm the diagnosis. Contradictory results from different trials are often due to a failure to diagnose rheumatoid arthritis properly. This disease should not be confused with other forms of joint pain, which are more transient and do not produce the same sort of changes in the blood, or damage to the joint – it is well known that joint pains of this type can be due to allergic reactions to food. What is at issue is whether foods can ever be a factor in *true* rheumatoid arthritis. In the two studies described here, all the patients involved were diagnosed as cases of rheumatoid arthritis by a standard set of tests.

Dr Gail Darlington, a consultant rheumatologist at Epsom District Hospital in Surrey, carried out one such trial, with the help of Dr John Mansfield, a private practitioner with many years' experience of elimination diets. Dr Norman Ramsey, an experienced medical physicist, helped with the assessment of changes in the patients' symptoms.

This was a reasonably large-scale study with 53 rheumatoid arthritis patients involved, and 44 actually completing the trial. They all underwent a two week 'wash-out' period, when the medicines they had been taking were withdrawn, and they all received paracetamol instead, plus a dummy tablet that they were told was a 'new drug'. This sort of treatment is known as a **placebo**. Placebos play an important part in scientific trials as explained on p156.

After two weeks, the patients were split into two groups, one of which began an elimination diet. For the first week, this diet consisted of twelve rarely eaten foods. All milk products, eggs, cereals, beverages and additives were excluded, along with most meats and all commonly eaten fruits and vegetables.

After the first week, these excluded foods were reintroduced, one at a time. Any foods that caused a flare-up of symptoms were not eaten again. The assessment of the patients continued for six weeks – long enough for them to have tested most foods and established a workable diet that excluded all 'incriminated' foods.

While the first group of patients was undergoing the elimination diet, the other group kept on taking their dummy tablets. After six weeks they were told that a different form of treatment would be tried – and they were then put on to the elimination diet. The objective here was to use the second group to assess the **placebo effect** – the improvement that is produced by *any* new form of treatment. Their response during the first six weeks on the dummy tablets was a measure of the placebo response that might be expected in the other group during the elimination diet.

The joint symptoms of all the patients were assessed using various standard measurements of pain and stiffness, plus routine blood tests that help evaluate the severity of rheumatoid arthritis. Dr Ramsey, who was unaware of which patients belonged to which group, and was therefore unbiased, made the assessments. The patients who received the dummy tablets first did show some improvement – so there *was* a placebo effect – but the group that undertook the elimination diet did far better. When the placebo group later went on to the diet, they too showed a much more striking improvement.

Notice that these measurements are a rather crude assessment of improvement in the group as a whole: when considered individually, some showed little change, while others seemed to respond dramatically to the treatment. (The reasons for assessing patients as a 'job lot', rather than individually, will become clear when we look at the next trial.) At the end of the diet, three-quarters of the patients claimed to feel 'better' or 'much better' than at the outset.

Elimination diets often act as weight-reducing diets, and on average, Dr Darlington's patients lost about 4.5 kg (10 lbs) during the trial. Being overweight has a bad effect on diseased joints, especially those in the knees and ankles. So one might argue that the loss of weight could have contributed significantly to the improvement seen. To check this, Dr Darlington compared weight losses in those that had responded well and in those that had responded poorly. There was no difference, so this seemed unlikely to have been an important factor.

In spite of these striking results, Gail Darlington is in no way a propagandist for the food-intolerance idea: 'I'm a very routine, orthodox physician and rheumatologist. If I spend the next ten years of my life helping to prove that the whole thing is a nonsense, or a placebo effect, or a non-specific manipulation of the immune system, I won't be at all concerned – I simply feel it's an area that needs to be investigated in just as scientific a way as we look at Drug A versus Drug B. Before 1981, most people in the UK thought that food intolerance was rubbish in a rheumatological context, as indeed I did at that time – one is fairly definitely trained to believe it's rubbish. But I was impressed by the results I saw in my patients who had gone to other people to have their diets manipulated. After seven years working in this field, I've gradually come to believe that it *is* relevant to some patients. To take one example, I have a patient of 33 who has changed from being a limping acute arthritic to being a perfectly fit, normal young man – and that is an improvement he has maintained for two and a half years.'

Rheumatologists tend to attribute such results to natural remissions, because rheumatoid arthritis is a disease that comes and goes for no apparent reason. It is also notoriously susceptible to placebo effects. Gail Darlington understands these doubts, but feels they are misplaced: 'Yes, obviously, it could be purely coincidental, but I do have quite a few patients in this bracket now, and it does seem unlikely that they *all* just happened to go into natural remission at the moment they began their diet. As for placebo effect, our trial was carefully designed to measure this in the control group. We showed that there was a placebo effect, but that it certainly couldn't account for all the improvement seen in the patients on the diet. What is more, when the control group were later put on elimination diets, they responded just as well as the first group – *far* better than they had done on the placebo.'

If Dr Darlington is right, then why did a similar trial, carried out three years earlier, produce such different results? This trial was conducted at Northwick Park Hospital in Middlesex, by Dr Michael Denman, Dr Bruce Mitchell and Dr Barbara Ansell. They studied 18 patients with rheumatoid arthritis, putting them on diets which excluded various foods for periods up to six months. In their opinion, the effects of eliminating foods cannot be assessed over shorter time intervals, because rheumatoid arthritis is such a variable disease. (Dr

Darlington's study overcame this problem by using a large group of patients and measuring their symptoms as a whole – in this way, the week-to-week variations in individual patients should cancel each other out.)

Only three of Dr Denman's patients stuck the course for the full six months. Thirteen dropped out before two months, and the report does not say how long they were on the diet. None of the patients showed any improvement.

One problem with this study was that the diet *did not eliminate wheat*, which other studies of food intolerance have identified as one of the most common offending foods. The diet also allowed chicken, tea, coffee, and all kinds of vegetables – including commonly eaten ones such as potatoes that are often incriminated by elimination diets. This failure to exclude several suspect foods, combined with the small number of patients involved, could well explain the poor results.

Trials involving IBS

Irritable bowel syndrome or IBS is a disorder characterized by chronic diarrhoea or constipation, or a mixture of the two. (**Chronic** in medical parlance means 'long-term'.) In most patients, there is also abdominal pain.

A major trial of IBS patients was carried out at Addenbrooke's Hospital, in Cambridge, by Dr John Hunter and Dr Virginia Alun-Jones. Twenty-one patients were involved, and they were placed on a diet of nothing but lamb, pears and water for the first week. Other foods were then reintroduced one at a time. Fourteen of the patients – 66 per cent – improved considerably on the diet and were then able to identify culprit foods. Eleven of these patients were later tested **double-blind** (see p147) to check that the effects were not purely psychological. Normal-sized portions of the food were eaten, disguised in a strong-tasting lentil purée that effectively concealed the identity of the food. All the patients responded in much the same way as they had done when they could taste the food being tested.

One obvious criticism of this trial is that the numbers involved were small. However, Dr Hunter and Dr Alun-Jones followed it up with another trial involving 122 patients. The percentage who responded to the diet was slightly higher – about 70 per cent. When a follow-up questionnaire was sent out, two to three years later, 86 per cent of patients replied, and 87 per cent of those who replied were still following the diet and benefiting from it.

In another trial of IBS, although there was a response to an elimination diet, the percentage who benefited was much smaller. This study was carried out by Dr David Pearson and Dr Stephen Bentley of the University Hospital of South Manchester, and Dr Keith Rix, a psychiatrist at the University of Manchester. The patients had all been referred to an allergy clinic at the hospital, because they suspected that their bowel symptoms were caused by food.

Nineteen patients completed the diet, and 14 of these showed an improvement in their symptoms. When tested with foods, ten produced consistent reactions to foods, while four did not.

At this stage, two patients with consistent reactions dropped out of the study, so only eight were left. They were tested double-blind with food in capsules, and five of them failed to react to foods that they had previously identified as causing problems when they could taste the food. This left just three whose bowel symptoms could definitely be related to food – only 15 per cent of the number who took part. Some of the patients were diagnosed as having mild psychiatric disorders, and this led the doctors involved to conclude that psychosomatic problems were an important factor in causing the symptoms for the remaining 85 per cent. This aspect of the study is discussed on p157.

Unfortunately, there are several major drawbacks to this study. Firstly, the number of patients involved was very small, and they were probably what doctors call 'a highly selected group': that is to say, they were not representative of IBS patients as a whole, for reasons that have already been discussed (see p90). Secondly, 59 per cent of the patients studied refused to undertake a full elimination diet, and according to the authors 'wheat was not excluded in all these patients'. Thirdly, the methods used for double-blind testing were questionable. Some patients were given the food disguised in soya milk, which will inevitably give false results if patients are sensitive to soya. (Reactions to soya are increasingly common.) Other patients were given the food in powder form, contained in gelatine capsules. The amount contained in the capsules was probably too small to identify food *intolerance* (rather than allergy), as was pointed out in a joint report by the Royal College of Physicians and the Nutrition Foundation, entitled *Food Intolerance and Food Aversion*. It is widely accepted, by orthodox and unorthodox doctors alike, that food *intolerance* reactions do not occur with such small amounts of food. Food *allergy* reactions can, of course, and the test procedure was probably designed with these sort of reactions in mind. It is significant that the three patients who showed consistent positive reactions also had a range of atopic symptoms – asthma, eczema, urticaria or hay-fever. In other words, the double-blind test was probably detecting those with IgE-mediated allergic reactions to food and missing others with food intolerance. As the authors themselves admit '. . . even patients with clear evidence of immunologically mediated sensitivity may not react every time they are exposed, particularly if the dose is limited.'

Another trial of IBS patients, carried out two years later by a different group of doctors, produced similar results. In this study, only three out of 49 patients were found to be food intolerant. Unfortunately, this study followed a similar procedure to that of the Manchester group – wheat and citrus fruits were not excluded, and capsules were used for double-blind testing.

Trials involving migraine

Migraine is generally defined as a severe headache, usually one-sided, that may be accompanied by nausea, vomiting, and visual or perceptual changes. The symptoms vary greatly from one person to another, and there is considerable disagreement among doctors about what should or should not be described as migraine. This makes the design and interpretation of trials involving migraine especially difficult.

The most comprehensive and frequently quoted trial of migraine patients was carried out at Great Ormond Street Hospital for Sick Children in 1982–3. It involved 88 children with severe and frequent migraine, most of whom had other symptoms as well. Over two-thirds suffered from abdominal pain, diarrhoea and flatulence, and almost half showed disturbed behaviour, the majority being hyperkinetic (see pp212–16). Aching limbs and runny or congested noses were also common, and some children also suffered epileptic fits, recurrent mouth ulcers, vaginal discharge, asthma or eczema. A few showed signs of permanent damage to the nervous system.

The majority of children with migraine do not show such a huge range of other symptoms, and in this sense the children studied were a 'highly selected group'. Because Great Ormond Street is the major specialist centre for children's diseases, their patients tend to be the most severely affected. This is the major criticism made of this study – that it is not generally applicable. Even so, it is of great interest, because of the high degree of response obtained.

The children were initially placed on a low-risk diet, consisting of one meat, one fruit, one vegetable and either rice or potatoes. Vitamin and calcium supplements were taken to compensate for any deficiencies in this diet. The children stayed on this diet for three to four weeks, and those that showed an improvement then began reintroducing other foods, one per week. Those who did not improve after four weeks were put on to another very simple diet, with a different selection of foods, to check whether they were sensitive to one of the components of the first diet.

If foods caused symptoms when they were reintroduced, they were withdrawn again, and the children continued until they had tested all commonly eaten foods. They were then tested again with *one* of the foods that seemed to cause a bad reaction, but this time the tests were done double-blind – neither the child, the parents nor the experimenter knew which foods were being eaten. To this end, the foods were disguised in a strongly-flavoured purée and supplied in tins to be given to the children at home. The tins were identified by a code number, and it was only when the code was broken at the end of the experiment that it became clear which tin contained the suspect food, and which tin was the placebo – unadulterated purée, that should have caused no symptoms.

For various reasons, some children could not be tested double-blind, but 40 were tested in this way.

The results of this trial were a surprise to many doctors, not least to those involved. Of the 88 children who completed the diet, 78 recovered completely on one or other of the simple diets that were tried during the first stage of the experiment. Another four children 'improved greatly', and only six showed no improvement whatever. The response, in other words, was 93 per cent, a staggeringly high figure by any standards. Of the children who improved, eight remained well even when foods were reintroduced, and they continued to be healthy on a normal diet. That left 74 children for whom particular foods could be identified as a cause of migraine in open trial. Of the 40 who were then retested double-blind, 35 were made ill by the tin containing the suspect food, but not by the placebo tin. Three reacted to neither tin, and two were made ill by the placebo. Given the vagaries of food reactions generally, 35 out of 40 is an impressive response. The results would have been more convincing if the children could have been tested for *all* the foods to which they reacted on open trial, and if they could have been tested more than once, but the practical difficulties of doing this in such a large-scale trial are obvious.

One of the most unexpected features of this trial was the extent to which other symptoms cleared up during the diet. These symptoms – such as epileptic fits, hyperactivity and aching limbs – were generally assumed to be unconnected with the migraine. Yet in the majority of children, they disappeared during the initial stages of the diet, and reappeared when incriminated foods were eaten. So too did symptoms such as abdominal pain, diarrhoea, flatulence, mouth ulcers and vaginal discharge. The atopic symptoms – rhinitis (runny nose), asthma and eczema – only cleared up in about half the children, suggesting that unidentified airborne allergens were playing a part. The only major symptoms not to clear up in any of the children were those due to permanent nervous-system damage.

One interesting feature of this trial is that four of the five researchers involved were highly sceptical about the importance of food at the outset. The exception was Professor John Soothill, who wished to set up the trial and persuaded the others to assist him. Their report of the experiment records that they 'embarked on this study believing that any favourable response, such as that claimed to substantiate the dietary hypothesis, could be explained as a placebo reponse. The positive double-blind controlled trial . . . provides clear evidence that a placebo response was not the explanation.'

Two American research teams have carried out similar studies with adult migraine-sufferers. Professor Lyndon Mansfield of the University of Texas looked at 43 migraine patients. The patients were given skin-prick tests for allergy, and if the tests were positive these foods were eliminated from the diet. Patients with no positive skin tests were put on a diet eliminating wheat, corn, milk and egg. There are several problems with this approach. Skin-prick tests rarely pinpoint problem foods in migraine, as Professor Mansfield now acknowledges. And the elimination diet used for the other patients was not really strict enough. Despite these defects, the research team still found that 30 per cent of the patients had far fewer migraines. Of those tested with double-blind challenges, 70 per cent responded to the food that had already been incriminated by 'open' challenges (those where the patient knew what food was being eaten).

Another study, by Dr T. Ray Vaughan of Fitzsimons Army Medical Center in Colorado, looked at 104 patients, asking them to eliminate wheat, corn, milk and eggs, as well as any food that gave a positive skin-prick test, and any foods suspected of causing migraine. This approach produced an improvement in 66 per cent of the patients, and 38 per cent had less than half as many migraines. Not all patients could identify a food that caused migraine when they tested them openly, but 75 per cent could. More than half of these identified the same food on double-blind challenges.

In both these studies, the double-blind challenge was carried out with capsules, and these contained only 8 g of freeze-dried food – about a third of an ounce. This was taken three times a day, for each 'challenge', so an ounce was eaten in all, but it is still a very small quantity. This capsule test probably failed to identify some genuine reactions simply because so little food was given.

Other tests in adult migraine sufferers, using a full elimination diet, have produced a very good response (total or almost total relief from migraines) in over 60–70 per cent of sufferers. (Unfortunately, these trials did not use double-blind challenges to check the subsequent food reaction.) If the trials by Vaughan and Mansfield had used a more extensive elimination diet they would almost certainly have got a higher recovery rate among their patients. As it is, they found that about a third of patients were significantly better, and up to 10 per cent lost their migraines altogether. Their studies are useful because of the double-blind challenges, which showed convincingly that common foods, such as wheat, milk, egg and corn, can cause migraine.

Migraine – the arguments against

With rheumatoid arthritis and irritable bowel syndrome, we were able to present another scientific trial that failed to find any response to elimination diet. As far as we know, there has been no such trial with migraine.

Paradoxically, the fact that foodstuffs already have an accepted role in the orthodox view of migraine is partly reponsible for this. Certain foods, such as chocolate, cheese, red wine and citrus fruits are well-known migraine triggers. They are thought to spark off migraine attacks because they contain chemicals known as 'vasoactive amines' that can have a drug-like effect on the blood vessels. For more about these amines, see pp128–9.

A great many migraine sufferers have benefited by avoiding these 'trigger' foods, but few find that their migraines clear up altogether when they avoid them. Other trigger factors, such as bright lights, television screens, or emotional scenes, still have to be avoided, and some migraines are experienced regardless of all these precautions. This is an important difference between the chocolate/cheese/red wine sort of food response and the intolerance of commonly eaten foods, such as wheat and milk, diagnosed by elimination diet. When foods are identified by elimination diet and then avoided, it is common for migraines to *disappear altogether* – non-specific triggers, such as bright lights, no longer seem to be a problem. This was noticed in the Great Ormond Street study, and is commonly reported by other doctors treating migraine with elimination diets.

In the orthodox approach to migraine, getting patients to avoid specific high-risk foods such as chocolate, and then record any reduction in their attacks is a standard part of treatment. Unfortunately, as ideas about intolerance of everyday foods has filtered through, this same method has been extended to those foods. So patients who enquire if commonly eaten foods might cause their symptoms are told to omit wheat for a couple of weeks, then milk for a couple of weeks, and so on. *The collective experience of all those treating food intolerance is that this approach simply does not work.* The majority of people, if they are sensitive to any foods, are sensitive to more than one, and it is only if *all* are withdrawn *at the same time* that any improvement is noticed. This is why a proper elimination diet is necessary to detect this sort of food sensitivity. Yet the majority of migraine specialists dismiss the idea of food intolerance as a major, fundamental cause of migraine – and they do so on the basis of having asked patients to exclude foods from their diet one at a time.

Assessing the evidence
Sceptics might suggest that we have deliberately chosen to describe trials that support our 'case' – ignoring trials with negative results unless they had some obvious flaw, for example. In fact, the studies described here are not a carefully chosen selection – they represent the major scientific trials of food intolerance carried out during the last 15 years.

We believe that the studies which produced no evidence for food intolerance in rheumatoid arthritis and irritable bowel syndrome are both seriously flawed. The doctors carrying out these studies are sceptical of the whole idea, and this has led them to disregard some important aspects of food intolerance – that it is vital to exclude all the likely foods at once, that wheat and citrus fruits are common culprits, and that normal-sized portions are usually needed to provoke a reaction during testing. The number of patients studied in these trials was small, and in the case of the IBS trial, they may not have been representative.

No medical trial is ever perfect, and various criticisms can be made of the three trials that showed a good response to an elimination diet. But they are all fairly minor criticisms, and they do not invalidate the overall findings. The doctors who carried out these trials were well aware of the controversial nature of their approach, and all took special care to design their trials very carefully. Moreover, some of the doctors who planned these trials believed that they would not see any response, or that it would be a placebo effect if they did. *Their own results changed their minds.*

FOOD AND THE MEDICAL FRINGE
Thus far, it might seem that the controversy over food intolerance is a two-cornered fight: orthodox medical opinion on the one hand, versus various 'unconventional' doctors (called **clinical ecologists** in the USA) on the other. Life would be a great deal easier if this were true, but it is not.

To complicate matters, a great many unqualified practitioners have moved into the food-intolerance 'market'. Doctors will, of course, be shocked to hear any medical field described as a market, and that, perhaps, is part of the problem. The medical world may feel it is above such things, but in fact it is just as much subject to the laws of supply and demand as any other profession. The news about food intolerance, and what it might do for those with migraine, irritable bowel syndrome, and other long-term illnesses has filtered through to the general public, despite medical disapproval. People suffering from such illnesses are understandably interested to know more, since most have been told by their doctors: 'There's nothing much I can do, you'll just have to learn to live with it.' These patients represent a large segment of the population whose need for treatment is not being met by conventional medicine.

Not surprisingly, many people have turned to alternative therapies, such as acupuncture or homeopathy, for treatment of this sort of illness. Some such treatments may have some benefits, perhaps through their effects on the autonomic nervous system (see p150) and most do no harm. But the more recent involvement of alternative therapists in dietary treatments is far more worrying. Many of these therapists have little understanding of nutrition – or of food sensitivity for that matter. Some have endangered the health of their patients by putting them on such restricted diets that they are short of essential vitamins, minerals or protein. A case of scurvy (a serious deficiency of Vitamin C) has been reported. Young patients are especially vulnerable, since children need food to fuel their growth and development. Over the past few years, paediatricians have begun to see children with severe malnutrition as a result of ill-advised diets.

This has caused great concern among the medical professon, and led some doctors to mount what can only be described as a crusade against the whole idea of food intolerance as a commonplace illness. Qualified and reputable private practitioners working in this area have found themselves as much under attack as the unqualified practitioners – everyone has been 'tarred with the same brush'. These vociferous critics have been very influential, and the air of controversy and doubt that surrounds food intolerance owes a lot to their activities.

While their anger at cases of malnutrition is entirely understandable, in a sense these doctors are helping to perpetuate the very situation they deplore. The reluctance of most family doctors and consultants to take food intolerance seriously undoubtedly springs from its disreputable image, rather than from a careful weighing of the scientific evidence. Unable to get help from their doctors, patients who think that food might be at the root of their problems turn to alternative practitioners, and so the situation is perpetuated.

Of course, doctors should not go along with every fashionable therapy, simply because there is a demand for it from their patients. And of course there are some ailments that really *are* incurable, and for which 'you'll just have to learn to live with it' is the best advice. But we believe that the scientific evidence is now strong enough to merit a major medical rethink on food intolerance. That same evidence suggests that common illnesses such as migraine, irritable bowel syndrome and rheumatoid arthritis should not be regarded as 'incurable' in all patients. For a significant number of people, eliminating certain foods can bring relief from such symptoms.

Dubious tests for food allergy and intolerance

An elimination diet is not an easy method of diagnosis, and unless the patient fully understands the procedure it may not work at all. Doctors have been searching for a simpler method of diagnosing food intolerance for many years, but so far without success.

As alternative practitioners have moved into this field, they have found the elimination diet too difficult and time-consuming, and have sought easier diagnostic tests. Some, such as the pulse test and the cytotoxic test, are based on methods that were originally devised by conventional doctors but found to be too inaccurate. Others are frankly unscientific. All have helped their practitioners to earn a very comfortable living, without necessarily doing the patients a great deal of good. We will only consider the most common tests.

The cytotoxic test

This involves taking a blood sample, extracting the white blood cells (immune cells), and then exposing them to food extracts. The theory behind the test is that if a patient is sensitive to a particular food it will affect the white blood cells, causing changes that are visible under a microscope. In severe reactions, the white blood cells are said to swell up and break open.

Scientific appraisals of the cytotoxic test show that food extracts do sometimes affect the white blood cells in this way, and a recent study under carefully controlled conditions produced 70–80 per cent accuracy. If this could be achieved consistently, and, perhaps, improved upon, the test might be of some value, but the commercial tests presently available give so many wrong answers that they are of very little value. Tests sometimes show a reaction to foods which the patient can eat without getting any symptoms (a **false positive**) or they may fail to pick up a known food sensitivity (a **false negative**). In one investigation, commercial laboratories offering cytotoxic tests were sent duplicate samples of the same blood. Unaware that these were from the same person, the laboratories gave a different list of food sensitivity reactions for each sample.

There may well be *some* value in the cytotoxic test, but not as currently practised. Scientific attempts to improve it are going on at present – in particular, the assessment of the reaction by the blood cells needs to be automated rather than assessed by someone looking down a microscope. Such assessment is highly subjective, and the results are known to vary from one observer to another. A more accurate version of the test may be available in a few years time, but at present it is not worth the money.

Hair analysis

Hair is mainly made up of a protein called keratin. Analysing it involves breaking it down to determine the mineral content of the hair, which can be useful in showing if the body is deficient in certain minerals. This is the main use of hair analysis.

It is very difficult to see how the composition of hair could possibly indicate anything about the body's response to foods, but hair analysis is advertised as a method of diagnosing food intolerance. Objective trials have shown that the test has no value in the context of food sensitivity.

Pulse rate changes

This is a diagnostic method that was devised by an American allergist, Dr Arthur Coca, in the 1940s. According to Coca, the pulse would increase markedly after a food-sensitive patient ate an offending food, and this could be used in diagnosis. Most doctors who have tried it say that although there *is* sometimes a rise, it is not dependable enough to be of diagnostic value – there are plenty of false negatives. The pulse can also quicken for many other reasons – so that there are also many false positives.

Other diagnostic tests

The other diagnostic tests on offer include those that use pendulums or dowsing rods to test patients, those using radionic boxes, 'energy boxes', Vegatest electrical devices or other instruments. There are also tests derived from applied kinesiology, which mostly measure muscle strength. Most of these tests are based on ideas about energy fields or energy flows in the human body that are 'disturbed' by illness. There is little evidence to support these ideas about energy fields, and even their proponents claim that they are untestable in a scientific sense.

Even if such energy fields or flows *do* exist, the logic behind the tests does not stand up to scrutiny. Every therapist has his or her own version of the tests and it is therefore difficult to generalize. However, many therapists claim to identify problem foods simply by applying their chosen method of testing to the patient's body, or to a hair sample or blood sample. In other words, they claim that the energy 'disturbance' is so specific that it can reveal precisely which foods cause the illness – this is surely stretching credibility to its breaking point, especially when there are several foods involved.

Furthermore, the practitioners of these tests believe that it is the disturbed energy fields that produce the physical symptoms. But it is a common observation in food intolerance that there is, by and large, no relationship between the type of physical symptoms that a patient suffers and the type of foods that he or she is sensitive to. If the physical symptoms do not relate to the type of food responsible, then how can the changes in the 'energy fields' (that are supposed to produce those symptoms) be so food-specific?

The implausible nature of the reasoning behind these tests becomes evident when one looks more closely at what some practitioners actually do. Some claim that they do not need to have the patient present at all to perform the diagnosis – they can get to the root of the problem by swinging a pendulum over a list of foods, while thinking about the patient. And it does not matter if the practitioner and patient have never met, apparently.

No amount of logic will dissuade those who firmly believe in this type of medicine, of course. But there are a great many others who turn to such therapists simply because they are ill, and desperate to find out the source of their illness. Such methods can seem attractive short-cuts to a cure, but in reality they are most unlikely to work, and none have been evaluated scientifically. Anyone who thinks they may have food sensitivity would be much better advised to put their time and energy into an elimination diet – it is far more likely to help, and it will be a great deal cheaper.

'But it worked for my friend . . .'

The therapists practising these techniques would not stay in business if they had no successes of course, and you may well meet people who claim to have been cured by such methods. This proves very little, however. Given that the most common sources of food intolerance are wheat and milk, such therapists can achieve a reasonable success rate by diagnosing sensitivity to these two foods in all their patients. If eggs, oranges, chocolate, tea and coffee are added to the list, they may well achieve success with 50 per cent or more, and some patients will benefit from the placebo effect alone (see pp153–5). But there will be other patients who are not helped at all, or who are only partially better when they could be fully well if they had identified all their culprit foods. And even those who *are* better are not getting a very good deal – they are almost certainly avoiding some foods unnecessarily.

Quite apart from the inconvenience and social disruption that this causes, such people may not be eating an adequate diet. Indeed, anyone who cuts out certain foods without medical advice runs this risk, which is why we urge you to consult your doctor before embarking on an elimination diet, and to check with the doctor subsequently to ensure that the diet you are eating is adequate.

Chapter Seven

FOOD INTOLERANCE

There is a disease that is well known to doctors, although it does not feature much in medical textbooks. It is called 'thick note syndrome'. Those who suffer from it are waiting-room regulars, and they have been referred to innumerable consultants for further examination – which is why their medical notes are so voluminous. Their symptoms are usually minor ones, but very varied, and they affect many different parts of the body – they may have headaches, indigestion, diarrhoea, aches and pains, rashes and a host of other problems. In most cases, no physical disorder can be found to explain them.

It is generally assumed that patients with 'thick note syndrome' are suffering from psychosomatic illness (which is discussed in the next chapter). But as food intolerance has become more widely recognized, doctors have begun to realize that many of these people may be sensitive to food. Multiple symptoms, affecting any and every body system, are a key feature of this disorder.

The second part of this chapter looks at each of those symptoms in turn, while the first considers the general features of food intolerance. Because so little scientific research has been done on food intolerance, much of what follows is based upon general impressions gained by many different doctors treating large numbers of people. This is not hard evidence, from a scientific point of view, but it is all we have to go on at present.

Given the controversial nature of food intolerance, many of the statements in this chapter might be disputed by some doctors. Ideally, we should qualify each contentious statement, but this would make the chapter very long and ponderous. We have therefore summarized the arguments over food intolerance in the previous chapter. On the basis of the evidence presented there, we believe that the case for food intolerance is very strong, and the present chapter is written from that viewpoint.

GENERAL FEATURES OF FOOD INTOLERANCE

Everyday foods

In food intolerance, it is almost always commonly eaten foods that are the source of the problem. In Britain and other western countries, this means wheat and milk, which are usually consumed several times a day. In America, wheat and milk are just as important, but sensitivity to maize (corn) is also widespread – this finds its way into many prepared foods, in the form of cornflour, cornstarch and corn syrup. These maize products are also used in the UK, but less corn is eaten overall, and sensitivity to corn is not quite as common here. In the same way, peanuts are a frequent problem in America, because so much peanut butter is eaten, but they are less important in Britain at present. As eating habits change, so too do sensitivities. Now that soya beans and soya flour are more widely used in processed foods, cases of intolerance to soya are being seen for the first time. Where wheat and milk are not staple foods, other sensitivities prevail – a doctor practising in Taiwan found that the most common culprit foods there were rice and soya beans.

The impression gained from patients' case-histories is that a large intake of one food, regardless of what it is, can trigger off intolerance of that food. For the breast-feeding mother, large amounts of a food can have a sensitizing effect on her baby.

Any food can produce intolerance, but it does seem that some foods are more likely to be a problem than others. Oranges, for example, are regularly identified as culprit foods, whereas apples are incriminated much less frequently. Yet apples and oranges are probably eaten in roughly equivalent quantities. Similarly, wheat appears to be a more potent cause of intolerance than other cereals. However, the idea that some foods are completely 'safe' and can never produce food intolerance is wrong – this claim is sometimes made by alternative therapists, particularly those 'dietary therapists' who emphasize the supposedly magical qualities of rice.

The general pattern of food intolerance seems to be as follows. The patient begins with sensitivity to milk, wheat, maize, eggs or some other commonly eaten food. At this stage, they probably have just one or two minor symptoms. As time goes by, new sensitivities appear, to foods that are eaten less often. With new sensitivities come new symptoms and the person's health deteriorates. In those who have had food intolerance for many years, a large number of foods may be at fault – sometimes as many as 20 or 30. Such people tend to be quite severely affected by their symptoms, to the extent that they cannot lead a normal life. However, these cases are a minority. Most people who need treatment for food intolerance are sensitive to between one and five foods, and they are able to function quite well, despite their illness.

The amount of food needed to provoke symptoms is generally much larger in intolerance than in allergy. Someone with true food allergy may react to a single drop of milk, or a trace of food left in a cooking utensil. One young man who was allergic to fish even fell victim to his girlfriend's kiss – she had eaten fish half an hour beforehand. The food-intolerant individual never shows this sort of 'exquisite' sensitivity. They usually need normal-sized portions to provoke a reaction, although some will react to just a few mouthfuls of the food.

Slow reactions

Unlike food allergy, where the reaction to a food can happen within minutes, food intolerance generally produces very slow responses to food. The symptoms may appear several hours after the food is eaten, or the following day, or even 48 hours later in the case of bowel symptoms. Because the food (or foods) in question are being eaten so frequently, there is no obvious link between the food and the symptoms. This effect was referred to as 'masking' by the early clinical ecologists, and the name 'masked food allergy' is still sometimes used for food intolerance.

For many of those with food intolerance, it is difficult to pinpoint a moment when the illness started. The symptoms can begin with mild problems that most of us take for granted, such as headaches or excessive tiredness or frequent bouts of indigestion. Over the years, there is a slow decline into ill-health, but it is often so gradual that the person does not really notice how bad things are getting. For some patients, however, food intolerance has a more definite beginning. It may follow on from a bad bout of influenza or other viral infection. Or it may stem from a course of antibiotics, such as those given before some operations eg hysterectomy. Where people have been exposed to toxic amounts of pesticides, or other synthetic chemicals, food intolerance sometimes sets in immediately afterwards.

Most people with food intolerance have symptoms that fluctuate from day to day, and there may be periods when they are worse for a while, or better. Changeable factors, such as stress, probably play a part in these fluctuations, by making the patient more or less susceptible to the foods they are eating.

Following an elimination diet, during which the offending foods are withdrawn for a week or more, the reaction time may speed up considerably. If a culprit food is eaten again after this period of avoidance, the reaction is likely to be both more prompt and more severe. In some people there is an almost immediate reaction, such as vomiting, flushing, itching or a sudden flow of mucus from the nose. (However, sudden severe swelling of the lips and tongue – the characteristic symptom of immediate reactions in food allergy – is not seen.)

More puzzling still, the symptoms that appear on testing are not necessarily the same ones that the patient had before. To orthodox doctors, this is a very dubious aspect of food intolerance, and one that puts the whole phenomenon in doubt – it is a fundamental part of the scientific approach to medicine that the same cause should always produce the same effect. However, the common observation with food-intolerant patients is that the symptoms really do vary in some people, especially after abstinence from the food. How this might be explained is not known at present. But given the fact that food intolerance is probably a result of many interacting factors (see Chapter Twelve) then changing symptoms may not be so implausible as they seem at first sight. If changes occur, following exclusion of the food, it may be because one cause of sensitivity is more easily 'cured' by avoidance than another. Not eating the food could alter the balance of causative factors, and thus produce a different type of symptom.

Getting over food intolerance

Food allergy, especially the immediate-reaction type, is usually lifelong. Food intolerance, on the other hand, tends to diminish if the food is avoided for a while. After a period of months, or sometimes a year, the same food can be eaten without ill-effects. But the potential for a reaction remains: if the food is eaten on a daily basis again, the intolerance is likely to reappear within a month or so. A viral infection can also spark off food intolerance again.

Sometimes intolerance reactions disappear very quickly after avoidance of the food, and do not reappear even though the person returns to their previous diet. This seems to happen more often in children than in adults.

In general, the longer offending foods are avoided, the better the patient becomes (as long as other foods are not eaten too regularly or in too great a quantity). With improving health, the person is better able to cope with both their diet and other environmental factors – airborne allergens, for example, or synthetic chemicals. Just as there was a gradual decline into ill-health, so there is now a steady recovery, with the body becoming stronger and less sensitive at each step.

Food addiction

Craving the culprit food is the most bizarre aspect of food intolerance – it affects about 50 per cent of patients, at a very rough estimate. These patients tend to crave the particular food or foods that cause their problems. They may be aware of the craving, and just regard it as a personal quirk, or they may be unaware of it, but unconsciously select foods containing their culprit food. With wheat and milk, it is quite easy to do this unawares – the person who has to have biscuits and a milky drink before bed, eats wheat cereal and milk for breakfast and always has a cheese sandwich for lunch, may well be a 'food addict' of this sort.

If the food is avoided for a while, the cravings eventually disappear. But unfortunately, they reappear all too easily. Eating the same food (or a related food – see p265) on a regular basis again can quickly reestablish the 'addiction', and the downward spiral is particularly difficult to combat. Because eating the food initially gives great satisfaction and well-being to a person in this 'addicted' state, self-control is all the more difficult.

One would not want to take the analogy with drug addiction too far, but 'food-junkies' seem to suffer withdrawal symptoms when they give up their favourite food, just as heroin addicts and alcoholics do when forced to kick their habit. One of the problems of doing an elimination diet is that the first few days are often very unpleasant due to these withdrawal symptoms.

Although this aspect of food intolerance sounds very peculiar and unlikely to anyone new to the subject, none of the doctors working in this area are in any doubt about it – they have seen too many people with this same curious pattern of eating behaviour. There is now a tentative explanation for this strange phenomenon (see pp240–1).

THE SYMPTOMS OF FOOD INTOLERANCE

Every illness dealt with here can be caused in some other way as well, and it is important to remember this when thinking about your own problems. What makes food intolerance likely is if you have two, three or more of these symptoms, especially if your doctor has been unable to find any cause for them.

No-one with food intolerance will have *all* these symptoms – most patients have two or three major symptoms and several minor ones, but some people have just one symptom. No two patients with food intolerance are the same, and each one has a different collection of symptoms, acquired in a different order, and at a different time of life. Food intolerance can begin at any age, and it may disappear in a child as it grows up, only to reappear later, often in a different form.

The digestive system

This is the 'front line' as far as food is concerned, and it is hardly surprising that many of the symptoms of food intolerance occur here. Most patients show some disturbances of the digestive system, although they may be quite minor – but not all patients are affected in this way.

Mouth ulcers

An ulcer is an area where the top surface of the mouth lining is lost, producing a small 'crater'. Mouth ulcers are painful, especially when acidic fruits or spicy foods are eaten. There are two main types of ulcer – those caused by injury, and those caused in other ways. The first type is larger and can be caused by a rough edge to a tooth, badly fitting dentures, or careless brushing of the teeth. Those of the second type is smaller, about 2–3 mm across. Most people suffer from mouth ulcers of this type from time to time. They are only unusual if you have large crops of ulcers that recur frequently – roughly one person in ten is affected in this way.

Viral infections are probably the most common cause of mouth ulcers generally, but they are *not* found in cases of recurrent mouth ulcers. No-one knows exactly what causes this problem, but it is thought to be some sort of infectious agent that induces the body to make antibodies against its own mouth cells. The infectious agent itself has not been tracked down yet, because it is not present in large numbers. According to this theory, the ulcers are produced by the body's immune system attacking the lining of the mouth. Heredity seems to play a part – recurrent mouth ulcers often 'run in the family'.

JOHN

For the past 15 years, John had suffered from regular bouts of mouth ulcers. Sometimes these were so painful that he could not eat for several days. Eventually the ulcers would clear up, only to come back again a few weeks later. During a long holiday in Southeast Asia, John's mouth ulcers were much less of a problem, and this made him wonder if food might be the culprit, because he was eating a very different diet on holiday. Soon after his return, the mouth ulcers began to trouble him again. His doctor suggested that being on holiday, and free from stress, could have effected the cure, but John pointed out that they had never got better on holiday before. The foods he had eaten very little of in Southeast Asia were bread, milk, butter and cheese, so he decided to try cutting these foods out for a while. There was no improvement, so the doctor suggested that John should also cut out other foods containing wheat, such as biscuits, pastry and pasta. When he did so John's mouth ulcers improved considerably but did not disappear. The doctor then advised a gluten-free diet, cutting out oats, barley and rye, as well as wheat. On this diet, John has not suffered from mouth ulcers for over two years.

MAGGIE

Like many mothers with young children, Maggie found it difficult to make time for a proper breakfast or lunch. She made up for this by eating a large evening meal with her husband, after which she usually suffered indigestion. By sucking indigestion tablets she could settle her stomach in time for bed, but then the pattern would be repeated the next day. Eventually the pain in her stomach became quite severe and she began to feel generally unwell. Once the children went to school this improved, but she still suffered indigestion most days. She now had a job as receptionist at a doctor's surgery, and the doctor noticed Maggie constantly sucking indigestion tablets.

He discovered that Maggie had never consulted a doctor about her problem, which had now been going on for almost eight years, and suggested that she should do so. After examining her carefully, her own doctor decided that there was nothing seriously wrong, and suggested that she try to relax and eat more slowly. She also recommended a bland diet, so Maggie began to eat more cottage cheese and drink warm milk instead of tea. Within two weeks her indigestion was a great deal worse, which provided a clue to the cause of the poblem. As an experiment, Maggie switched to a diet containing no milk at all, and her indigestion cleared up completely a few days later.

Some vitamin and mineral deficiencies can also produce this symptom (see p271), and those with Crohn's disease (p118), ulcerative colitis (pp137–8) and coeliac disease (see p142) also tend to suffer from persistent mouth ulcers.

In general, food intolerance is a relatively unlikely cause of recurrent mouth ulcers – but there are certainly some cases where such ulcers clear up during an elimination diet. Those with classical allergic symptoms, such as hay-fever or asthma (atopics), are more likely to fall into this group than others. In most of those whose recurrent ulcers are due to food, there are other food-related symptoms as well, but sometimes recurrent mouth ulcers are the sole symptom of food sensitivity.

How foods might produce mouth ulcers is not known, although in atopic patients, mast cells probably play an important part. Any food can be responsible, as in all forms of food intolerance, but there is some evidence that **gluten** – the mixture of proteins found in wheat, rye, barley and oats – is a common offender here. So anyone who has mouth ulcers as their main symptom, or sole symptom, could try a gluten-free diet before embarking on the main elimination diet.

Nausea and indigestion

Everyone gets indigestion at some time or another. By far the most common cause is unwise eating habits – eating too much, eating too quickly, trying to eat when you are anxious, excited, angry, upset or tense, eating standing up, rushing about after a meal, eating late at night, or having too much rich food. Smoking makes matters worse, as does too much alcohol, very acid food, spicy food, or too much oil and fat. The fashion for drinking large quantities of fruit juice is likely to produce indigestion in some people: when fruit is eaten, the stomach has time to adjust to the influx of acid – drinking a large glass of orange juice all at once is a different matter. For some people, there are specific foods that cause indigestion, and these should simply be avoided. In some cases, nausea and indigestion are purely psychosomatic (see p150).

More seriously, a peptic ulcer (stomach ulcer or duodenal ulcer) can be at the root of nausea and indigestion. Other possibilities include gallstones, a hiatus hernia, and, very rarely, cancer of the stomach. If your indigestion becomes more severe, or very frequent, if you lose your appetite, lose weight, or begin vomiting regularly, then there may be something seriously amiss, and these possibilities should be investigated by your doctor.

Food intolerance can cause nausea and indigestion, although this is rarely the sole symptom. It seems that if the food affects the stomach in this way, then it affects the digestive system as a whole. So there is usually diarrhoea or other bowel symptoms as well. In babies, the equivalent of indigestion appears to be **colic** (see p203).

Stomach (gastric) ulcers

A stomach ulcer, like a mouth ulcer, is a crater-like area where the upper layer of the stomach lining is missing. But it is much larger than a mouth ulcer, and a far more serious problem. The main symptom is a burning pain that extends across the chest and upper abdomen. The pain lasts for between half an hour and three hours, and episodes of pain tend to come and go.

No-one is sure what causes stomach ulcers, but the acid that the stomach produces to help in digestion may be a factor – if there is an eroded or inflamed area in the stomach lining, then the acid could begin to break it down. A tendency to suffer from stomach ulcers runs in some families. Smoking, drinking too much alcohol and taking aspirin and similar painkillers (see p327) can all contribute to the development of a stomach ulcer. So can stress, particularly if this means hurried, irregular or unrelaxed meal-times.

Whether food intolerance can ever produce stomach ulcers is a controversial issue. Certainly, there are case-histories of patients with persistent or recurring stomach ulcers who have recovered remarkably well on an elimination diet. However, these people are probably a minority of all patients with this problem. What might arouse suspicion is if the symptoms *get substantially worse* during the conventional treatment. Such treatment relies heavily on milk, as a safe, bland food. For anyone who is sensitive to milk, this sort of diet will make matters worse.

The presence of allergic symptoms, such as asthma, hay-fever or urticaria, makes it more likely that a stomach ulcer is due to food sensitivity. Some patients of this type (atopics), who also have stomach or duodenal ulcers, turn out to have high IgE levels for certain foods. Objective evidence that foods are causing their ulcers comes from direct observation of the stomach lining in contact with a few drops of food extract. This can be achieved by lowering an observation tube into the stomach, a method that has been developed by a Polish allergist, Dr Bogdan Romanski. Dr Romanski reports that inflammation occurs rapidly in the stomach lining where the food extract touches it – the action of stomach acid on such inflamed areas is the likely cause of ulceration. A drug that prevents mast cells from reacting, sodium cromoglycate (see p320), is an effective treatment for these people. All this points to the ulcers being produced by IgE antibodies and mast cells – in other words, being truly allergic. At present, however, stomach and duodenal ulcers are not generally accepted as a possible symptom of food allergy, which is why they are dealt with here, rather than in Chapter Three.

There is little doubt that psychosomatic factors (see p150) play a part in stomach ulcers, even where there is some other underlying cause. Research has shown that by learning to relax, patients can reduce the likelihood of their ulcer recurring after treatment.

Duodenal ulcers
These are very similar to stomach ulcers, but occur in the first part of the small intestine – the duodenum. The main symptom is pain, several hours after eating. This pain is usually felt in the upper abdomen, although sometimes it appears to be in the back.

Most duodenal ulcers result from excessive acid production in the stomach. All the causative factors described above for stomach ulcers are also operative in duodenal ulcers, particularly anxiety, tension, smoking and drinking too much alcohol. Wine and spirits are the main offenders. Duodenal ulcers also seem to be linked with eating a lot of pickled food, and eating refined carbohydrates; that is, sugar and white flour. Duodenal ulcers tend to heal themselves, provided the original causes are removed.

Again, a small minority of patients with duodenal ulcers may be suffering from food allergy or food intolerance – but there is little hard evidence to support this belief, only individual case-histories.

Diarrhoea

Bowel function varies a great deal from one person to another, making it difficult to say exactly what diarrhoea is. For most people, one bowel movement a day seems to be the norm, but some people only go once every three or four days, while others go twice a day or more. An important question here is whether 'average' is the same thing as 'normal and healthy'. One survey of 301 apparently healthy adults found that almost a third of them reported bowel symptoms of some sort (diarrhoea, constipation etc), although most had not consulted a doctor for their problem. This study can be interpreted in two ways. It either shows that everyone's bowel function is different and there is no such thing as a normal pattern – or it shows that a large percentage of the population are suffering from minor bowel complaints. We would lean towards the latter view, and suggest that some of those people, at least, are sensitive to the food they eat.

In general, a healthy bowel pattern *feels* healthy, whether you go three times a day or twice a week. There is a regularity to the pattern – it is not erratic. The stools are fairly firm and well-formed and there is no particular urgency, nor any great difficulty in going. There is no sense of malaise or pain, either before or afterwards, and the movement feels complete – not as if you still have some faeces left to pass. In diarrhoea, soft, loose or semi-liquid stools are passed several times a day; there is usually a sense of urgency and, usually, some feeling of malaise. Diarrhoea is basically a means of ridding the body of toxins, harmful bacteria or other unwanted substances – it is a healthy reaction to infection, and should only be considered a problem when it serves no useful purpose. However, acute diarrhoea can lead to dehydration because so much water is lost, and this can be dangerous (see p211).

Diarrhoea can be caused in many different ways. Infections are the most common cause – they tend to bring on an acute attack of diarrhoea that clears up of its own accord within a few days, as long as no further food is taken. Sometimes a temporary deficiency in the enzyme lactase (see p207) follows on from the infection, and this can perpetuate the diarrhoea if milk is consumed. One form of infection that often goes unrecognized is infestation with the parasite *Giardia* (see pp197–9). Disturbance of the gut flora can also produce diarrhoea, usually with other symptoms as well (see p193).

Coeliac disease numbers diarrhoea among its symptoms, and in mild cases there may be few other signs (see p142). Crohn's disease (p118) and ulcerative colitis (pp137–8) also result in diarrhoea, but they are serious conditions that

JENNY

Jenny had been in excellent health until she went on holiday to Morocco and picked up a very unpleasant stomach infection. This resulted in severe diarrhoea that lasted for over a week. Although she recovered from this illness, her bowels never really got back to mormal, and she continued to have mild diarrhoea most of the time. When this had gone on for a couple of years, Jenny consulted her doctor, who suggested she try a wholefood diet, with plenty of brown bread and vegetables. She did so for two months, but had to report that she was no better – in fact she was worse than before. This prompted her doctor to try Jenny on an elimination diet, cutting out wheat, milk and eggs. Avoiding these foods proved very effective, and, when she reintroduced each of them in turn, it was clear that wheat was the source of her problems. After avoiding wheat for a year, Jenny is now able to eat the occasional slice of bread without ill-effects.

produce other symptoms as well. Psychosomatic illness can result in diarrhoea (see p151) and intense stress can produce diarrhoea directly, by stimulating the sympathetic nervous system (see p150). Finally, cancer of the colon can cause diarrhoea, although this is the least likely of all the causes listed here.

One potential cause of recurrent diarrhoea that is often overlooked is poor food hygiene. People vary greatly in their ability to resist food-borne infections: some have a 'cast-iron constitution' and remain well however filthy the kitchen, while others need far more stringent hygiene. Judging hygiene standards by the way other people live is not necessarily a good policy.

Many people are unaware that food which has been kept for a long time is not always rendered safe by thorough cooking – some bacteria produce toxins that are not destroyed by heat, even though the bacteria themselves are killed. These toxins can produce a short-lived bout of diarrhoea. So anyone in the habit of keeping food or leftovers for long periods of time may be regularly exposed to this sort of 'food poisoning'. Food should be eaten as fresh as possible, and other basic hygiene measures adopted. These include washing the hands *with soap* after visiting the lavatory and before preparing food – water alone does not remove bacteria. Kitchen worktops should also be kept clean, knives and chopping boards should be washed in hot soapy water after cutting up meat, and raw meat should never be stored alongside or above cooked meat. Pets should be kept off surfaces used for food preparation. Any leftovers should be heated for 20 minutes or more to kill bacteria.

Another potential cause of diarrhoea is the natural laxative effect of some fruits (see p15). Prunes, rhubarb and figs are well known for such properties, but other fruits can have similar, if milder, effects, and so can avocado pears. Eating too much of foods such as these may produce diarrhoea in the susceptible person. Eating beans, lentils, chickpeas or other legumes can also cause problems, especially if they have not been properly cooked (see p80). Shellfish are another common cause of diarrhoea – they quite often contain toxins that are not destroyed by cooking.

These are common reactions to food, or to food contaminants, which anyone might have. In food intolerance, there is a more specific reaction to one or more foods, which do not produce diarrhoea in most people. The sort of diarrhoea caused by food intolerance is likely to be fairly mild, although with occasional more acute attacks, perhaps in reponse to a change in diet, or to stress. There might also be periods when the bowel reverts to normal function for a while, or brief episodes of constipation. Opinions vary, but some doctors would classify this sort of chronic diarrhoea, *without* any pain, as a form of irritable bowel syndrome. It is therefore dealt with below, under that heading. For diarrhoea in children, see pp210–11.

Constipation

The difficulty of deciding what is 'normal' or 'healthy' in terms of bowel function is just as much a problem here as for diarrhoea (see above). In general it is not a question of how infrequently the bowels are opened, as the accompanying symptoms – if there is a feeling of bloating and discomfort, of wanting to go and not being able to, of straining or incomplete evacuation, then this really is constipation.

Over-use of laxatives makes the bowel dependent on them, and this is one possible cause of chronic constipation. Other medicines may have a similar effect, notably cough mixtures. Lack of fibre in the diet is another common cause – but the answer is *not* to eat mountains of bran (see p269). Haemorrhoids can cause constipation, and so can various psychological problems. In rare cases, constipation is the main symptom of coeliac disease.

Whether food intolerance can ever be a cause of constipation, as some doctors believe, is an open question. There may be some individuals that do respond in this way, and occasionally constipation might be the sole symptom. Quite often, patients taking large quantities of bran for constipation improve markedly when this, and all other forms of wheat, are eliminated.

Irritable bowel syndrome

Irritable bowel syndrome or IBS (also called 'irritable colon' or 'spastic colon') is a diagnosis that means different things to different doctors. However, it usually denotes abnormal bowel function – either constipation or diarrhoea – without any sign of infection, or other physical cause (*eg* bowel cancer), and without any structural damage to the wall of the bowel. Within this group there is plenty of scope for variation – some patients suffer diarrhoea most of the time, others are usually constipated, while in others these symptoms alternate. Most patients suffer pain that is relieved by defecation, but not all do. In effect, IBS is little more than an umbrella term for various minor bowel disturbances of unknown origin. In some cases, there may be a more serious underlying problem, or a very simple problem that is easily cured (see above, under *Diarrhoea* and *Constipation*).

Since there is no damage to the gut in IBS, there is usually no blood in the stools. Neither is there any weight loss or night-time diarrhoea – either of these symptoms indicate more serious conditions such as Crohn's disease or ulcerative colitis. IBS is a fairly minor problem in the sense that it does not affect general health, does not usually get any worse as the years go by, and does not predispose the sufferer to any other illnesses.

There appear to be two distinct subgroups within IBS patients. The first group suffer from mild diarrhoea most of the time, often with pain, and sometimes with brief episodes of constipation. The second group suffer from constipation for some or most of the time, with bloating, and occasional bouts of mild diarrhoea. They may also suffer pain. For people in this second group, food sensitivity is unlikely to be at the root of their symptoms. For those with chronic diarrhoea – the first group – food sensitivity *is* worth investigating, especially if they have bloating and wind as well. Some studies have shown that as many as 70 per cent of IBS sufferers may be food-intolerant (see p94).

Alternative explanations for IBS are very thin on the ground. The most widely accepted theory is that the complaint is usually psychosomatic, an idea which is discussed further on p158. Another theory suggests that lack of fibre in the diet is responsible. Although this idea is now largely discredited, extra bran and other bulk-forming agents are still prescribed for IBS, regardless of whether diarrhoea or constipation is the main symptom. The latter might be helped by this strategy, but not the former. Indeed, there is evidence that *some* people with IBS are made worse by eating bran, suggesting a sensitivity to wheat or other grains.

Exactly what goes wrong in IBS is far from clear. In many cases it may be that the muscles of the gut are contracting too much, or too little, or are simply unsynchronized. The muscles that control the bowel are **smooth muscles**, like those in the bladder and the bronchi (the tubes leading to the lungs).

Some patients with IBS have to urinate frequently, and this can be a sign that smooth-muscle spasms are at the root of the symptoms, although frequent urination can also be a straightforward psychological problem.

What causes these spasms? It could be an effect of the sympathetic nerves, if IBS really is psychosomatic. Or it could be mediators released by mast cells (see p26), if there is a true allergic reaction. The term 'asthma of the gut' is sometimes used to describe this sort of reaction – in just the same way as there are spasms of the bronchial muscles, producing asthma, there could be spasmodic contractions of the smooth muscles of the gut, producing diarrhoea.

Another important causative factor in IBS may be the **gut flora** – the menagerie of bacteria and yeasts that live in our intestines and are harmless, or beneficial, in most people. Research done by Dr John Hunter at Addenbrooke's Hospital in Cambridge suggests that many IBS sufferers have a disturbed gut flora: some bacteria or yeasts are over-represented while others are lacking (see Chapter Ten). How a disturbed gut flora might be treated is discussed on p199.

There are various other ways in which adverse reactions to foods might bring on diarrhoea and pain, but at present there is too little evidence to choose between them. In the end, it may turn out that several different factors are at work.

Crohn's disease
This is a serious bowel disorder that produces patches of inflammation in the intestines, mostly in the second part of the small intestine (the ileum) or the large intestine (the colon). These patches have a characteristic appearance under the microscope. They may heal themselves in time, and some patients recover after just one or two attacks of Crohn's disease. Others suffer recurring attacks throughout their lives. As they heal, the inflamed areas may develop scar tissue that narrows the intestine, making passage of food difficult. In terms of actual symptoms, Crohn's disease produces diarrhoea, and cramps or more generalized pain in the abdomen, especially after eating. There is usually a general feeling of malaise and, sometimes, a slight fever. If left untreated, there is weight-loss and the health deteriorates because nutrients are not absorbed properly. Other symptoms, such as joint pains and mouth ulcers, often go with Crohn's disease.

Despite intensive study, doctors still have no clear idea of what produces Crohn's disease. The damaged areas of intestine, when studied under the microscope, contain a great many immune cells – it is these that produce the inflammation. The obvious explanation is that some infectious agent attracts them there – but there is no evidence that Crohn's disease is infectious, and the fact that the disease mostly affects people in their twenties makes an infection unlikely. However, some researchers believe that they may now have found an infectious agent – a slow-growing bacterium related to the one that causes tuberculosis. Attempts to show that this bacterium really does produce Crohn's disease are now in progress.

Another line of research has pinned the blame for Crohn's disease on substances produced by bacteria that are a normal part of the gut flora. These substances are peptide molecules (see p240) that happen to act as attractants for certain cells of the immune system. It is believed that most people have bacteria that generate these peptides, but that they can neutralize them, by means of a special enzymes (see p18) which breaks them down. What goes wrong in Crohn's disease, according to this theory, is that the patient lacks the enzymes to break down these peptides. It has been shown that the peptides attract the immune cells known as **phagocytes** ('eating cells') and that these come pouring through the gut wall into the intestine. Once there, they can set up an inflammation reaction.

Although interesting, all this research has not resulted in any new form of treatment for Crohn's disease as yet. The conventional treatment is to use drugs such as **corticosteroids** (see pp323–5) to suppress the inflammation. Surgery may also be used if parts of the bowel are so badly scarred that they are causing congestion.

In the first edition of this book we wrote that the proposed link between food intolerance and Crohn's disease was 'highly controversial'. We are pleased to report that, in the three years since then, the idea has become respectable, thanks to the excellent scientific work of Dr John Hunter at Addenbrooke's Hospital in Cambridge. With his own Crohn's disease patients, Dr Hunter finds that over 80 per cent recover on an elimination diet, and then react to specific foods when these are reintroduced. By cutting out the incriminated foods, these patients can remain well. Some relapse later – as is common with Crohn's disease – but after two years, 80 per cent of those still on their diet remain well.

The latest trial, instigated by Dr Hunter, but carried out at nine different hospitals under the supervision of several different doctors, has vindicated the original results. The long-term recovery rate, at 50 per cent, was not as good, but still much better than a comparable treatment using steroid drugs. The doctors assessing the patients were totally impartial, in that they did not know whether their patients were receiving the dietary treatment or the drug treatment.

Because patients with Crohn's disease are often very ill, carrying out an elimination diet is not all that easy, and other doctors have been reluctant to try this new approach. The technique that Dr Hunter uses is to feed his patients on an elemental diet (see p263) during the first part of the elimination diet, or to feed them in some other way – using an intravenous drip, which puts nutrients straight into the bloodstream, for example. Other doctors, who are sceptical about food intolerance, suggest that the Crohn's disease symptoms clear up simply because the patient's gut is being given a rest from digesting real food, or because the patient's nutritional status is improved. But if this were the case, one would not expect the patients to remain well afterwards, on a normal diet that just excluded certain food items. And in the latest trial, this possibility was investigated, by giving the elemental diet to *all* the patients involved. Of those who recovered on the elemental diet, half were then told to return to their normal diet, but given corticosteroid drugs. The other half tested out foods on a one-by-one basis, noted which ones they reacted to, and then avoided those. They were not given any drugs, yet twice as many in this group were still well two years later.

How specific foods might cause Crohn's disease is not clear. Dr Hunter believes that an abnormal population of bacteria in the gut might be the problem, as in IBS (see p117). The discovery that bacterial peptides attract immune cells into the gut (described above) could fit in quite well with this explanation, and Dr Hunter suspects that enzyme deficiencies might play a part. It certainly looks as if several different factors could be at work in producing this puzzling disease.

Given that corticosteroids have some side-effects, including making the patient more susceptible to infections, an alternative non-drug treatment with a good success rate should seem very attractive. At present, however, elimination diets are not widely used for Crohn's disease, and the serious nature of this illness makes it unsuitable for self-help treatment. *If you have Crohn's disease, you should not consider trying an elimination diet without full medical supervision.* If your doctor is willing to help, he or she can prescribe an elemental diet for you.

Bloating and flatulence (wind)

Bloating of the abdomen after meals is usually caused by overgrowth of certain bacteria or yeasts in the gut. These feed on food residues, and produce gas in the process. Certain foods are notorious for producing this effect, notably kidney beans (haricot beans, baked beans etc) and Jerusalem artichokes. In the case of Jerusalem artichokes, they contain an unusual type of sugar which human beings cannot digest and which therefore passes through to nourish bacteria in the hind part of the gut.

Where belching is the main problem, it may be due to swallowing air when eating. Wind can also indicate more serious problems, such as gallstones, hiatus hernia or malabsorption of food, but there will usually be other symptoms as well. A possible cause of flatulence and bloating, that is not widely recognized, is an imbalance in the gut flora (see p185). Infection with *Giardia* can also have this effect (see p197). Alternatively, food intolerance may be the cause of the problem, although there will usually be other symptoms as well, such as diarrhoea, abdominal pain, nausea or indigestion.

The skin
Itchiness
Itchy skin is usually accompanied by a rash of some sort, as in eczema (p45) and urticaria (p44). Itchiness, *without* any spots or rash, can be caused by all sorts of things. The most likely sources of trouble are clothing, toiletries and cosmetics. Woollens and synthetics are the most common offenders, while cotton or silk clothes are the least irritating. Changing to unscented brands of soap and using the minimum of cosmetics may relieve the itching. Adding baby oil to the bathwater can also help. Some people are sensitive to traces of detergent or fabric conditioner left on clothes, and simply rinsing clothing more thoroughly may be the answer. If the itching is mainly on the hands, then cleaning agents may be the culprit, and you should wear rubber gloves for housework, preferably with cotton gloves inside them, or cotton-lined PVC gloves (see p338).

Various parasites cause itching, including scabies, threadworms, lice and ringworms. Generalized itchiness is also one of the symptoms that may clear up on a no-sugar, no-yeast diet (see Chapter Ten). Itchiness of the vulva or vagina is likely to indicate a *Candida* overgrowth, and an itchy anus may also be due to *Candida*. However, anal itching could be due to some other problem with the gut flora, food intolerance, or even piles. In general, itchiness in other parts of the body does not seem to be a common symptom of food intolerance, but it is reported in a few cases.

The joints and muscles
Muscular aches (myalgia)
It is unusual to experience aches in the muscles that are not the result of over-using the muscles, or of a viral infection such as influenza. However, they are a feature of post-viral syndrome (see p237) or, if severe, they may indicate a disease known as polymyalgia rheumatica. Tension can produce muscle aches, especially in the neck, shoulders and face. Misaligned vertebra can also produce aches and pains in the back, shoulders and neck, and these may respond to treatment by an osteopath.

More generalized, but mild, muscle aches may also be a symptom of food intolerance, although this is unusual. One group of food-intolerant patients who regularly include muscle aches among their symptoms are hyperactive children (see p212).

Aching joints (arthralgia)

The joints are a very vulnerable part of the body, and misuse or overuse can easily produce pains in the joints. Too much kneeling can produce bursitis, for example, commonly known as housemaid's knee or parson's knee. Sports enthusiasts may also suffer joint pains in certain susceptible joints.

Generalized joint pain can accompany some illnesses, such as rheumatic fever, or it may follow on from influenza, *Salmonella* poisoning and other infections. *Giardia* (p197) and a gut flora imbalance (p186) may also produce joint pain among their symptoms. Diseases that make the gut wall more permeable to food molecules may also produce aching joints – these include Crohn's disease, coeliac disease and ulcerative colitis. If the underlying disease is sorted out, the joints tend to get better. In children, vaccination sometimes results in an attack of joint pain. Rarely, generalized joint pain may be an indication of a serious **autoimmune disease**, called systemic lupus erythematosus or SLE (see p73).

In many of these disorders, the pain is produced by immune complexes (see p73) forming in the blood, and then becoming deposited in the joint. These immune complexes consist of masses of antigens and antibodies. In the examples mentioned above, the antigens are either bacteria (in an infection), the vaccine (in vaccination), food molecules (in Crohn's disease and coeliac disease) or the body's own proteins (in autoimmune diseases such as SLE). Because so many immune complexes are formed at once, the system that normally mops them up cannot cope.

Food intolerance can apparently cause aching joints in some people. It is likely to be the most heavily used joints, such as the knees, that are afflicted first, but it may later spread to other joints. Assuming that all the disorders mentioned above have been ruled out, then food intolerance is a very likely cause for joint pain, especially in patients with a variety of other minor symptoms as well. Studies have found that between 50 per cent and 85 per cent of patients respond to an elimination diet.

Since immune complexes are known to produce joint pain in several other diseases, they are a logical suspect in food intolerance as well. In this case, the immune complexes might well consist of food molecules (absorbed intact into the blood from the gut) and antibodies to the food. At present there is no evidence to show whether this idea is right or not, and it is possible that food produces joint pain by some completely different mechanism.

An acute, immediate *allergic* reaction to a food, with characteristic symptoms such as swelling of the lips, can also include transitory pain and swelling in the joints, especially those of the hand and wrist. Other atopic

GEORGE

George was in his mid-forties when his joints began to feel painful and stiff. The affected joints were red and swollen and he also felt feverish at times. After running some blood tests, his doctor diagnosed rheumatoid arthritis. George was a landscape gardener, who had always done a lot of the hard physical work himself, and the gradual loss of mobility affected his business badly. Although the drugs he was given helped a little, the disease gradually got worse and by the time he was 50 simply getting out of bed in the morning was difficult. His shoulders were so stiff that he could not comb his hair or put on a tie, and gripping a tea mug was difficult because of the stiffness in his hands. At this stage, his doctor suggested that George might like to try an elimination diet, which was said to help some people with rheumatoid arthritis. She told him to cut out grains, dairy produce, eggs, citrus fruit and other common foods, but this produced little improvement. In fact, his symptoms got slightly worse in the first few days, but he stayed on the diet anyway. By the end of the second week he began to feel better in himself, and some of his joints were less swollen and painful. Over the next week, things improved noticeably every day, and after three weeks he was almost back to his former good health. When he tried reintroducing foods, George found that milk, potatoes and yeast triggered off his joint symptoms again. By avoiding these he is fairly well, although he still has a few aches in his joints and his shoulders are a little stiff. He suspects that some of the foods he is still eating may be at the root of this, but rather than restrict his diet further he relies on low doses of an anti-rheumatoid drug to reduce the inflammation. His gardening business is expanding again and he feels better than he has done for years.

('allergic') patients experience more long-lasting joint pain, which may be due to food – whether this is food allergy or intolerance is a debatable point, but mast cells do seem to be involved in some of these patients.

Rheumatoid arthritis

Rheumatoid arthritis is characterized by painful, swollen joints that feel warm to the touch and are often stiff. The stiffness and pain are usually worse in the morning. Various blood tests are used to confirm the diagnosis – they look for certain factors in the blood that are characteristic of rheumatoid arthritis.

Inflammation is the cause of the problem, and the part to be affected first is the **synovial membrane**, although the inflammation later spreads to other parts of the joint. The synovial membrane has an important role to play in the joint, because it produces the fluid that lubricates the joint. The **synovium**, which surround the joint, is filled with this fluid. In rheumatoid arthritis the synovial membrane is invaded by large numbers of immune cells which cause the inflammation.

The presence of all these immune cells suggests that there is an infection in the membrane, and early theories about rheumatoid arthritis invoked some bacteria or virus. But despite many years of searching, no infectious agent has been found. An alternative theory suggests that the body is mounting an immune reaction against its own proteins – in other words, that rheumatoid arthritis is an **autoimmune disease**. Some recent discoveries tend to support this idea. A third theory suggests that there is an overgrowth of cells in the synovial membrane which attracts the attention of the immune system – this idea is currently being tested.

The standard treatment for rheumatoid arthritis at present is to use drugs that suppress inflammation, such as aspirin, ibuprofen, gold salts and penicillamine (see pp327–8). Unfortunately, these can all have various side-effects, and they do little more than suppress – or partially suppress – the symptoms. Corticosteroids, the most effective anti-inflammatory drugs, are only used in severe attacks.

The idea that food intolerance can play a part in causing rheumatoid arthritis is not widely accepted among rheumatologists. However, some specialists in this field report excellent results when they try their patients out on an elimination diet. One of these is Dr Gail Darlington, whose work is described on p91. According to Dr Darlington, about three-quarters of patients show some improvement when they identify culprit foods and eliminate them from their diet. Some of these patients lose their symptoms entirely – a dramatic improvement which drug treatment rarely achieves.

How food intolerance might trigger the inflammation in the joint is still an open question. The idea that immune complexes (consisting of food molecules and their antigens) are deposited in the joint is tempting, but there is no evidence for this at present.

Backache

Most backache is a result of injury or misuse of the back. Very occasionally, however, long-term back pain has abated as a result of an elimination diet. In all these cases, there are other symptoms as well, such as joint pain, aching muscles or irritable bowel syndrome.

The heart and blood vessels

Irregular heartbeat

There may be many causes for an irregular heartbeat, (sometimes called **palpitations**) and since any condition affecting the heart can be serious, it is wise to seek medical advice without delay. If there is no serious underlying problem, then over-consumption of caffeine (p165) or hyperventilation (p162) should be considered. Some doctors have reported that sensitivity to foods or to chemicals (see Chapter Nine) may cause irregularities in the heartbeat, and these factors may be worth investigating if other possible causes have been ruled out.

Chest pain

Chest pain is reported as a symptom of food intolerance by some doctors, but this is certainly not common. There are a great many other possible causes, some of which may be serious and require immediate attention. If the doctor can find no underlying cause for the chest pain, then the possibility of hyperventilation (p162) is worth considering.

The head

Headaches

The brain itself has no pain receptors. But the blood vessels supplying the brain, and the membranes that surround it (the meninges) do feel pain. It is these that produce a 'headache'.

Most people experience headaches from time to time, and they are usually nothing to worry about. The possible causes are too numerous to list, but tension, anxiety, overwork, irregular meals, eyestrain and alcohol are the most common ones. Regular headaches are a sign that something is amiss, and simply suppressing this warning sign with a painkiller, and ignoring the underlying cause, is a mistake. Mild or moderate headache that is continuous is generally regarded as psychosomatic (see p150). A sudden attack of severe recurrent headaches, or daily headaches, may be a sign of some serious underlying illness, such as meningitis or brain tumour – medical help should be sought without any delay.

Recurrent headaches are often reported as a feature of food intolerance, and in some people they may be the sole symptom, although there will usually be some other problems as well. Hyperventilation (p162) and abnormalities of the gut flora may also cause headache, among other symptoms.

Migraine

Defining migraine is no easy task. It is generally described as a severe, throbbing headache that is usually restricted to one side of the head and is often accompanied by nausea and a dislike of loud noises and bright lights – or any light (photophobia). Some people also experience split vision, half vision, flashing lights or other visual disturbances – this sort of migraine is called **classical migraine**. Where there are no visual phenomena, the term **common migraine** is used. In both types of migraine, there may be indications that an attack is imminent – visual effects or just mood changes.

Doctors differ in their interpretation of these criteria. Some will tell you that it is not migraine unless you feel nauseous and your head throbs. Others

TOM

Tom was in his late thirties when he first started to get migraines. With a demanding job as a social worker in a hostel for alcoholics, and three young children to bring up, he put his symptoms down to stress. Over the next ten years the problem gradually got worse, until he rarely had a day without some sort of head pain. He was also very tired and lacked the energy to join in with family activities or help look after the children at weekends. This inevitably led to friction, and his marriage was in danger of breaking up.

In the hope of improving his health and keeping the family together, Tom and his wife decided to move to the country and he gave up social work for a job in a garden centre which did not pay as well, but was much less taxing. Moving house involved registering with a different doctor, who asked all his new patients to come in for an initial check-up. The doctor spent some time with Tom, and asked him what he thought the cause of his headaches and tiredness might be. 'Stress,' Tom replied, without hesitation, 'That's why we've moved out here.' The doctor suggested that he come back and see him after a year, when he had had time to settle in and judge the effects of a slower pace of life.

Tom did so, and had to

maintain that the pain has to be incapacitating for it to qualify – if you are walking about, it's not a migraine. In reality, migraine refuses to fit into these rigid definitions. Many patients with migraine experience varying symptoms. Sometimes their attacks are incapacitating, or make them vomit violently, at others they are fairly mild but have that same essential 'migrainey' quality. Whereas a headache is just a pain in the head, migraine seems to disrupt the mental functioning and perception of the world – even if the visual disturbances of classical migraine are lacking. There is a spaced-out, cut-off-from-things, groggy, disorientated quality to a migraine that sets it apart from a headache, even when the pain is mild, and there is no throbbing or nausea.

One characteristic feature of migraine is that patients recognize certain things that tend to trigger off attacks. For some people it is alcohol, or certain foods. For others it is bright lights, flashing lights, television, very hot baths, strong winds or changes in climate, loud noises, strong smells, excitement,

---

report that, while there was some improvement, it was not nearly as much as he had hoped, and he was still very tired, with migraines several times a week. The doctor then suggested that he try changing his diet, for an experimental period, and told him to eat nothing but meat and vegetables, and drink only spring water for ten days. Tom felt very ill on this diet at first, with stomach pains and a severe migraine. But after a week he noticed a remarkable improvement, his energy restored and his head without any pain. The doctor then explained to Tom that he should test foods individually, which he did. To test wheat, he ate some spaghetti. Within an hour of eating the pasta he was his 'old self' again, and with a vengeance – exhausted, depressed, nauseated, and with a throbbing pain on one side of his head. Cow's milk, oranges and rye had similar effects. After avoiding these foods for a year, he finds he can now eat them occasionally without ill-effects. His children are amazed and delighted with the transformation in their father, who now plays football with them, takes them swimming and is a lot more fun to be with. The family have decided they like country life, but Tom is planning to go back into social work as soon as he can get a job locally.

anxiety, shock or sleeping too long. Although this might seem like a very miscellaneous list, it is striking how often migraine patients report the same sort of triggers – especially bright lights and oversleeping. Where stress is a factor, the migraine attack often develops *after* the pressure is off – weekend migraines, or ones that spoil the first few days of any holiday, are commonly reported.

Migraine attacks usually begin between the ages of 20 and 30, but there are a few unfortunate people who develop migraine in childhood. Sometimes children suffer more in their stomachs than in their heads, with vomiting as the main feature of an attack. They may have these bouts of vomiting without any head pain at first, only developing a one-sided headache as they grow older.

As a result of extensive research into migraine, doctors have a fairly clear idea of what happens during an attack. They know that there are two distinct phases. During the first one, the blood vessels throughout the body – including those in the brain – become constricted. In the second phase, there is a 'backlash' reaction, and the blood vessels open out (or **dilate**) more than is normal. It is the expansion of blood vessels in the brain, during the second phase, that causes the pain. The premonitions of migraine, which some sufferers feel, occur during the first phase, and may be caused by a reduced blood flow to certain parts of the brain as the blood vessels narrow.

Playing a central part in this reaction are tiny 'cells' in the blood known as platelets. These are very numerous – there are 15 million of them in a single drop of blood – and their main function is to help the blood clot around a wound. During clotting the platelets clump together and release a substance called **serotonin** or **5HT** that makes the blood vessels constrict. This reduces blood flow so that less blood is lost from the wound.

What happens in a migraine attack is that the platelets clump together and release serotonin when it is not needed. During the first phase of a migraine attack something makes the platelets in the blood clump together – they do not actually form clots of course, but they do release large amounts of serotonin. The serotonin makes the blood vessels constrict and so reduces the blood-flow to the brain. The body has control mechanisms that counteract the effect of the serotonin, but when these come into play they cause a violent swing in the opposite direction. The blood vessels in the brain open out too much and this brings on the throbbing pain that is a feature of the second phase of the attack. Pressure on certain parts of the brain might produce the feelings of nausea.

But what makes the platelets clump together in the first place? The answer to this question may be two **vasoactive amines**, known as **tyramine** and **phenylethylamine**, that are found in certain foods. These substances are usually broken down by the platelets, which produce various enzymes for the purpose. Doctors suspect that some people with migraine do not produce enough of these enzymes – or produce defective versions of them. So if they eat foods that are rich in these substances they cannot break them down fast enough – and platelet clumping follows. The foods that are rich in these amines are well known as migraine triggers – principally chocolate, cheese and red wine.

However, studies of the enzymes involved in breaking down tyramine and phenylethylamine have produced rather puzzling results. Many migraine patients *are* defective for one of the enzymes involved, called a monoamine oxidase. But those who are sensitive to triggers such as chocolate or cheese are no more defective than other migraine patients. If tyramine and phenylethylamine *are* involved in migraine (and it is by no means certain that they are) then the underlying enzyme deficiencies are obviously not simple ones. For more on enzyme deficiencies in migraine, see p244.

There must be other factors that can make the platelets clump together, because it is only a minority of patients whose migraines are triggered by these foods. The hormone adrenaline is known to have similar effects on platelets, and other substances produced by the body may act in this way. Presumably the migraine-sufferer produces too much of these substances, or lacks the control mechanisms that normally keep them in check.

Although the blood vessels play an important part in migraines, many doctors believe that they are not the whole story. Some things are difficult to explain on the basis of blood vessels alone – why the pain is usually on one side of the head, for example, or why bright lights should trigger migraine off. These facts suggest that the nervous system is involved as well, but exactly how is not known.

The conventional view of migraine is that it cannot be cured, except in rare instances where a misaligned vertebra, usually in the neck, is at the root of the problem – and this may not be true migraine anyway. For such patients, treatment by an osteopath may be effective. (How a misaligned vertebra might *cause* migraine in the first place is something of a puzzle, but one that we will return to at the end of this section.) Given that there is no 'cure', the main form of conventional treatment is drug therapy, using drugs that can stop an attack, or at least alleviate it (see pp328–9). Patients are also advised to identify their particular 'triggers' and avoid them.

The relevance of food intolerance to migraine is hotly debated. The conventional wisdom is that certain foods (chocolate, cheese etc) can act as *triggers* but that commonly eaten foods, such as wheat and milk, are unlikely to play a part in migraine. However, several carefully conducted scientific trials have produced good results, using elimination diets to treat migraine sufferers. One of these studies, involving children with severe migraine, is described on p96. Studies with adults have shown that about 70 per cent of patients recover very well when treated in this way. Doctors working in this field in fact achieve a better success rate than this, because patients who do not respond to a simple elimination diet often turn out to have chemical sensitivities, or they respond to a no-sugar, no-yeast diet (see Chapter Ten). When this much broader approach is taken, then the success rate rises to 80 or 90 per cent.

The foods identified by an elimination diet seem to be acting in a different way from the accepted food 'triggers'. When they are eliminated from the diet, the migraines usually clear up completely – whereas excluding trigger foods only makes the migraines less frequent. Following an elimination diet, and the avoidance of culprit foods, patients often find that they can once more tolerate their triggers – both food and non-food. It looks as if the milk, wheat or whatever was creating some serious underlying problem which made the body vulnerable to any external change. Thus bright lights, stress, the flickering of a television screen, or the drug-like substances in chocolate could upset the delicate balance and tip the whole system into a migraine attack. Once the underlying food intolerance has been sorted out, the system is far more stable and can better cope with external circumstances.

How food intolerance might create this underlying instability is not known. One study suggests that migraine patients, although not apparently atopic, have a mild IgE/mast-cell reaction to the food when it comes into contact with the lining of the gut. This may set up inflammation locally, make the gut wall more leaky, and thus allow more food molecules through. These might then provoke an immune response in the blood, although it is not clear how this could make the person susceptible to migraines.

Another possibility is that certain naturally-occurring chemicals in the foods, which require detoxification by enzymes, are to blame. If the patient has a deficit in certain detoxification enzymes, this could be made much worse by overloading them with particular foodstuffs. There might then be less spare enzyme capacity to deal with 'triggers' such as tyramine. At present this is just speculation, and much more research is needed in this area.

Although elimination diets do seem to be useful for many people with migraine, they are probably not worth trying for those who only get migraines occasionally – once a month or less. In such circumstances, it would be difficult to tell if excluding foods had had any effect, unless there were other symptoms as well. Testing might also be rather inconclusive. But for anyone who has migraines at particular times – during the monthly period for example – then it might be worth carrying out an elimination diet, timed to coincide with the moment when migraines usually occur.

There is one final puzzle in relation to migraine. Within the past few years, several dentists have apparently discovered a 'miracle cure' for migraine. Being dentists, they did not set out to treat migraines, of course. What they were doing was treating people who habitually ground their teeth together in their sleep. This habit, which is usually due to stress and tension, tends to leave tell-tale marks on the teeth – a polished area where they rub together. Anyone whose teeth has these marks is usually offered a dental plate to wear in bed – this is designed to stop the grinding action. Surprisingly, some patients reported that they previously suffered migraines, but that these had cleared up since they began wearing the dental plate.

Further research was carried out, involving patients with classical migraine, all of whom experienced migraines on waking up – the theory was that such migraines are far more likely to be due to nocturnal tooth-grinding. Some of these patients showed signs of grinding on their teeth, but not all did – it seems that only the most enthusiastic grinders actually manage to wear the teeth down. The effect on the patients of using dental plates at night was remarkable – almost all of them suffered far fewer attacks.

How can this discovery be reconciled with the finding that food intolerance is at the root of most migraine? One possibility is that the subgroup of patients being studied by the dentists are uncharacteristic of migraine patients as a whole – they are part of the 10 or 20 per cent of patients who cannot be helped by an elimination diet, chemical avoidance or by a no-sugar, no-yeast diet. Another possibility, and a more likely one, is that tooth-grinding is a trigger, just like bright lights or chocolate. The underlying tendency to get migraines is already there, and probably remains there after the dental treatment.

Dr Phillip Lamey, of Glasgow University, who carried out this research on dental plates, suggests a way in which tooth-grinding could produce a migraine. The continuous tensing of the jaw muscles during sleep might well produce toxins – overworked muscles do this. These toxins might then affect the blood vessels in the vicinity, precipitating a migraine attack. A misaligned vertebra can also cause migraines, as mentioned earlier – again, excess muscle tension, due to the skeleton being awry, could spark the migraine off.

Generalized muscle tension, due to psychological stresses, also contributes to migraine, probably because the tension tends to focus on the muscles of the shoulders and neck. Learning to relax can be very beneficial for migraine sufferers, even if food intolerance *is* the root-cause of the problem. Mental factors can also play a part in migraine by means of adrenaline production, which affects the blood vessels as described above. Feeling angry or afraid, or being under constant stress, boosts adrenaline production and can trigger migraines. An elimination diet may work wonders, but for many migraine sufferers it is only part of the solution. They also need to adopt a calmer approach to life to attain real physical health, and to protect them from other stress-induced illnesses.

Mental symptoms

The question of whether food intolerance can cause mental symptoms is discussed fully in Chapter Eight. In general, mental disorders are much more likely to be caused by emotional or social problems than by foods. Where they are a result of food intolerance, there will usually be physical symptoms as well, although a few patients have mental symptoms only.

The mental symptoms most often mentioned in connection with food intolerance are anxiety and depression – often accompanied by excessive fatigue (see pp134–5). Other minor symptoms that are reported include dizziness, confusion, tension, 'nervousness', insomnia, emotional instability, mental exhaustion, sleepiness, lack of concentration and memory lapses. In children there may be various mental and behavioural problems that are described as the 'hyperkinetic syndrome' (p212).

The possibility of hyperventilation should always be kept in mind, where there are minor mental symptoms – see p162 for further details. Finally, abnormalities of the gut flora (see Chapter Ten) can cause lethargy and depression.

The eyes, nose, throat and lungs
Red, itchy or watery eyes

Assuming there is no infection causing these symptoms, then the most likely explanation is sensitivity to airborne allergens – see p37 and pp62–3. Occasionally, however, food sensitivity can produce symptoms in the eye, or along the margins of the eyelids.

Other symptoms
Bed-wetting and other forms of incontinence

Most children wet the bed until they are three or four. Thereafter about 25 per cent of children continue to wet the bed, and some may also wet themselves during the day. In some children, this may continue until they are ten or more. Sometimes a urinary infection causes bed-wetting, and so can diabetes. However, in the vast majority of cases, the cause is probably psychological, with anxiety or insecurity at the root of the problem.

In many children with food sensitivity, bed-wetting has unexpectedly stopped when they were treated for other symptoms, and recurred, along with those other symptoms, when certain foods were reintroduced.

At first this was put down to coincidence, but most doctors now accept that food sensitivity (either allergy or intolerance) can cause bed-wetting.

It probably does so by making smooth muscles throughout the body contract. As well as being found in the bronchi (where their spasms can cause asthma) and the bowels (where they can cause diarrhoea), smooth muscles

ANNA

Anna had suffered from an allergy to house-dust mite since she was a child. If she breathed in too much dust she suffered with a streaming nose and watery eyes. By keeping her house scrupulously clean and dust-free she had remained well for many years. In her thirties, however, she began to be troubled by a new problem. When she ate certain foods her face flushed scarlet and remained hot and itchy for an hour or two. This caused her a great deal of embarrassment if she had to eat out. She kept a record of the foods responsible, and these included onions, wine, vinegar and cheese. But even when she avoided these foods, she still had episodes of flushing that she could not explain. The doctor suggested that she try a very simple diet, avoiding all commonly eaten foods for a while. This seemed to help considerably, and Anna reported feeling much more energetic and cheerful as well. When she reintroduced foods, she found that wheat, milk and sweetcorn caused her to flush and brought on a headache. By avoiding these foods, she is able to eat other things, including wine, vinegar and onions, which no longer make her face flush.

make up the wall of the bladder. If they contract excessively, the bladder empties much more frequently, and with less control.

Some adults with food sensitivity have to empty their bladder very frequently, and the mechanism is probably the same.

Water retention (oedema)
The symptoms of oedema are a sudden gain in weight, and a general puffiness all over the body, most noticeably around the eyes, on the face generally, and around the ankles. The most common cause of oedema is kidney disease, and it is important that anyone with these symptoms should see their doctor without delay.

Oedema sometimes occurs in food allergy (see pp44 and 75–6). It is also reported in some patients with food intolerance.

Epileptic fits
There are two types of epileptic fit. In *grand mal* epilepsy, the sufferer falls to

the ground unconscious, goes very stiff, and then jerks and twitches uncontrollably. In *petit mal* epilepsy, the sufferer does not usually fall, but simply stares blankly for a few seconds, and is unaware of external events. It is mostly children who suffer from *petit mal* epilepsy, and they usually grow out of it by their teens. Epilepsy is a disorder of the brain, in which one group of brain cells becomes over-active and sends out strong electrical signals that overwhelm other parts of the brain.

Children with severe migraine sometimes suffer from seizures, probably epileptic in nature. Studies at Great Ormond Street Hospital in London have shown that eliminating certain foods can help these children (see p96), and the seizures often clear up along with the migraine. So it is probably worth investigating the role of food in epileptic children, but only if they also have migraines, or some well-recognized allergic condition, such as asthma, allergic rhinitis or eczema. How foods might provoke a seizure is a mystery, but they may affect the blood vessels supplying the brain, as they are thought to do in migraine.

Flushing, sweating and chilling

Flushing and sweating are natural reactions to being too hot – both help to cool the body off. They also occur as a nervous reaction to various emotions – fear, embarrassment, anger or excitement – and they are a symptom of the menopause, which usually begins during the forties or fifties, but can start earlier in some women. Flushing and sweating are only a cause for concern if they occur regularly for no obvious reason.

People with food intolerance sometimes report flushing or sweating, or both, among their symptoms. They often say that they also get chilled easily or 'feel the cold'. A few patients seem to have a slight fever, either intermittently or for much of the time. The general impression given by these symptoms is that they have difficulty in controlling their body temperature – or in adapting to normal changes in air temperature. It is unlikely that this would be the sole symptom of food intolerance, and it is not obvious how food might produce such an effect.

Fatigue

Excessive tiredness, that is not relieved by rest, is usually a sign of some mental disorder, such as depression. It can also be caused by many infectious diseases, by anaemia, or by an underactive thyroid gland. Sometimes fatigue persists following a viral infection, and this is now known as **post-viral syndrome** or **chronic fatigue syndrome** (see p237).

Fatigue is very often reported as a symptom of food intolerance, especially in connection with migraine and irritable bowel syndrome. Early-morning tiredness is the most frequent problem. Looking back over case-histories, it seems that fatigue may be an early warning sign as food intolerance develops. How food might produce fatigue is not known, but exorphins (see p240) may play a part, or it may be a side-effect of some generalized immune reaction, as is suspected in post-viral syndrome.

No-one should embark on an elimination diet without first consulting their doctor, but this point should be emphasized for anyone with severe fatigue. There can be several other causes for this problem, and some of these are serious diseases.

Hypoglycaemia

What petrol is to a car, **glucose** is to the body – an energy-rich fuel that keeps every part of the body alive and powers our muscles. Glucose is carried around the body in the blood, and cells that need glucose can absorb it from the blood. It is very important that the level of glucose in the blood is always kept at about the same level. The brain is the organ most sensitive to a change in glucose level – too little produces tiredness, confusion, irritability, aggression and other symptoms, while too much may result in loss of consciousness.

The body keeps glucose at the right level with the help of several hormones, the main ones being glucagon and insulin. Glucagon releases glucose from the liver, where it is stored, when the blood sugar is low. Insulin comes into play when the blood sugar is too high – it takes glucose out of circulation and puts it into store. The level of glucagon is kept fairly steady, whereas the level of insulin changes rapidly in reponse to changes in blood glucose. After a meal, especially one containing a lot of sugar or starch, large quantities of glucose pass into the blood. Insulin is therefore produced to keep the blood glucose down. In diabetics, too little insulin is produced. They must compensate with injected insulin, and avoid foods that release a lot of glucose at once – mainly sugar and other sweet foods.

Hypoglycaemia is the medical term for 'low blood sugar', and it is usually a result of too much insulin being produced (or too much injected, in the case of diabetics). Everyone suffers from this condition to some extent – especially when they eat meals containing a lot of sugar and starch. Drinking alcohol with the meal makes matters worse. Extra insulin is produced to cope with this onslaught of high-glucose food, and in an excess of zeal it reduces the blood sugar to a very low level, producing symptoms of tiredness, confusion and hunger about two to five hours after the meal. If the blood sugar drops to a very low level, then adrenaline (see p151) is produced, to help the body cope with what is a major crisis. The effect of the adrenaline is to make the subject irritable and aggressive. He or she will also sweat more, tremble and look pale

– and there may be a change in the heart rhythm. Since this type of hypoglycaemia is a response to too much sugar, it is known as **reactive hypoglycaemia**.

In the past, doctors often advised people with reactive hypoglycaemia to drink a cup of sweet tea, or suck sweets or glucose tablets, whenever they felt the symptoms coming on. This may relieve the symptoms temporarily, but in the long term it just perpetuates the problem. The influx of sugar will simply stimulate the body to produce more insulin, and so make matters worse.

People who are overweight and eat a lot of starchy or sugary food may suffer from reactive hypoglycaemia on a daily basis. Their body cells become more responsive to insulin, because they have to cope with such a high glucose load, so they easily become hypoglycaemic, especially if they miss out on one of their usual sugary snacks. Simply changing their diet will help such people, although they may find it quite difficult to wean themselves off the high-sugar diet that their body has become accustomed to. They should eat more meat, fish, eggs, cheese and vegetables, and cut out sugar and honey entirely. White flour and bread should be replaced by wholemeal, since this is digested more slowly and does not release a lot of glucose at once. Even so, the amount of bread, pastry and potatoes should be restricted, and no cakes, biscuits, sweets, puddings or jam must be eaten. If there is an improvement, then some sweet foods can be reintroduced to the diet later, once the body has regained its natural equilibrium.

Various things can make hypoglycaemia more likely. Alcohol, tea and coffee can all do so, especially if drunk in excess. Smoking increases the amount of both glucagon and insulin, producing a rise in blood sugar followed by a fall, about an hour later. The thyroid hormone plays an important part in controlling glucose levels, and either too much or too little thyroid hormone can cause hypoglycaemia. Some vitamin and mineral deficiencies make people more prone to hypoglycaemia. Drugs can cause hypoglycaemia, and stress makes it a great deal worse. Gut flora overgrowth or imbalance can also be at the root of hypoglycaemia (see p189). Finally, there are some people who simply produce too much insulin, regardless of their diet or other circumstances – it seems, however, that these cases are quite rare.

The relationship between hypoglycaemia and food intolerance is a very tangled one. For one thing, the standard laboratory test for hypoglycaemia uses glucose that is derived from maize (known as dextrose). This is fed to the patient, and the level of glucose in the blood is measured some time later. In North America, where maize (corn) is a common food, many people are intolerant of it – and although maize sensitivity is less widespread in Britain, it does occur quite often. Someone who is very sensitive to maize may well react badly to the traces of maize protein in the dextrose, and that could mean that their blood glucose falls, regardless of whether they are hypoglycaemic or not. So there is a suspicion that the tests for hypoglycaemia may sometimes be measuring food intolerance, without anyone being aware of this. Patients may be told that they are hypoglycaemic when in fact they are intolerant of maize.

More importantly, some doctors claim that hypoglycaemia can sometimes be a *symptom* of food intolerance. The basis for this is that many patients, previously diagnosed as hypoglycaemic, have found that such problems disappear following an elimination diet – although in most cases they were undertaking the diet for other symptoms, and did not expect any improvement in their hypoglycaemia. In children, there seems to be a link between hyperkinetic syndrome and hypoglycaemia – a great many hyperactive children handle glucose abnormally. If the proposed link between food and hyperkinesis is a reality (see p213), then it may be that food sensitivity is causing the hypoglycaemia in such children. Some of the children's symptoms, such as poor concentration and irritability, could be due to low blood sugar. The craving for sugary 'junk food' that is common in these children may also be a result of hypoglycaemia. Some doctors believe that a high proportion of hypoglycaemia cases might be caused by food intolerance, but at present there is no hard evidence to support this. How foods might cause hypoglycaemia is an open question, but a small group of doctors in the United States are investigating the idea that food sensitivity can make the insulin-producing cells in the pancreas over-active.

Pre-menstrual syndrome
Some doctors report that a proportion of patients with severe premenstrual problems improve considerably following an elimination diet. These patients usually embark on the diet because they have some other symptoms, such as migraine or irritable bowel syndrome. On avoiding the foods that bring on these symptoms, they find that their premenstrual problems also disappear, or become much less troublesome.

Symptoms that have been reported in food intolerance
Many other symptoms have been attributed to food intolerance over the years. Those discussed below are ones that are mentioned fairly regularly in connection with food.

Ulcerative colitis
Ulcerative colitis is an inflammatory disease that affects the large intestine (also called the **colon** – hence **colitis**, inflammation of the colon). It causes bouts of abdominal pain and diarrhoea, often with blood and mucus in the stools. There were reports in the 1960s and 1970s that ulcerative colitis patients

'recovered' on a milk-free diet, and this was attributed to food intolerance. But subsequent experience has not borne this out.

Dr John Hunter, who pioneered the study of food intolerance in Crohn's disease, has had little success in treating ulcerative colitis by the same methods. When all food is withdrawn, and elemental diets (see p263) or intravenous feeding used instead, the ulcerative colitis patients do not make a sustained recovery. Perhaps the milk-free diets in the original studies *seemed* to be effective because the patients were short of lactase, the enzyme that breaks down milk sugar (see p207). Diarrhoea often makes the gut deficient in lactase temporarily, and by drinking milk the patients may have been perpetuating their attacks of colitis.

One form of ulcerative colitis, known as **proctitis**, produces inflammation mainly in the lower part of the large intestine, near where it opens at the anus. It is possible that food allergy plays a part in this disorder, as a great many IgE antibodies have been found in the vicinity. So far, however, there has been little investigation of this possibility.

There is one type of colitis which *is* commonly due to food, and that is **infant colitis**, especially when it affects children under a year old. This rare condition is regarded as a form of ulcerative colitis by some doctors, but not by others. The main symptom is diarrhoea containing blood and mucus. A sample is taken and examined under the microscope (a **biopsy**) to assess the degree of inflammation in the gut. Dr Peter Milla, of the Institute of Child Health in London, has made a special study of infant colitis, and finds that the symptoms are caused by food in about 75 per cent of cases. There are clear signs of immune-system involvement, so this is in fact food *allergy*. In some babies, IgE and mast cells are involved, in others it is a different type of immune reaction.

This condition is known as **food-allergic colitis** or **FAC** and most of the babies suffering from it are are bottle-fed. However, some are breast-fed infants responding to foods that the mother is eating (see p252). For bottle-fed infants, switching to a hydrolysate feed (see p221) is the usual treatment. For those being breast-fed, it is usually enough for the mother to eliminate certain foods from her diet – the most common culprits being milk, egg, soya and wheat. Where this alone does not work, the mother can also be treated with the drug, sodium cromoglycate (see p320) to reduce absorption of intact food molecules by suppressing her own allergic reactions to them. Some babies are best treated by taking them off the breast and giving a hydrolysate feed instead.

A few babies with colitis have a type of autoimmune disease – they are making antibodies to their own cells. These antibodies start to attack various body cells, including those in the large intestine, and this sets off the

KATE

'I had lots of headaches, particularly migraines and sinus pains, and I just felt tired all the time. I always woke up feeling sick, had stomach aches after eating, asthma, diarrhoea and lots of menstrual problems. My doctor was quite sympathetic at first, but every time I went it was a different diagnosis, and eventually he began to get fairly irritable with me.

At one point he thought I might have ME, then hyperventilation, and then he said perhaps it was the early stages of multiple sclerosis, because I kept going numb in one leg, and had trouble moving about and kept falling over. I used to have quite bad bouts of this, then it would go away. I had joint pains too, but I didn't even tell the doctor about those – there were too many other things.

I tried various alternative treatments, such as acupuncture, but they didn't really make any difference. In the end I came across something about diet, and thought I would try cutting out certain things. I stopped eating wheat, dairy products, chocolate and sugar, and cut out all alcoholic drinks. The effect was pretty astonishing. Almost all the symptoms went, even my asthma, which I'd had for years. I've never had another bout of numbness or falling over since then either. I think I was just lucky in guessing what foods might be a problem.

It's only since coming off these foods that I've really recognised how ill I felt before. When I felt better I dashed round and cleaned the whole house and just ran about outside in the garden for joy – it was really amazing to feel so well.'

inflammation that causes the bleeding and diarrhoea. By looking for auto-antibodies in the blood, doctors can tell if colitis is being caused in this way. Interestingly enough, Dr Milla has found that changing to a hydrolysate feed or chicken-based feed helps these babies considerably. Some still need immuno-suppressant drugs to control the inflammation, but others do not. It would seem that immune reactions to foods are aggravating the autoimmune reaction in such cases. Some babies with food-allergic colitis grow out of it, but others are still sensitive to the same foods five or more years later. For other causes of diarrhoea in babies and children, see p210.

Multiple sclerosis

Multiple sclerosis is a degenerative disease affecting the nerves and brain. The cause is not known. Several doctors have tried investigating MS patients for food intolerance. They claim that, by treating them for supposed 'candidiasis' (see Chapter Ten), and eliminating suspect foods, the patient's symptoms can sometimes be greatly alleviated.

Some patients treated in this way have recovered sufficiently to be able to walk again, when previously they had been confined to a wheelchair. However, it is very difficult to know if these improvements have anything to do with the treatment, because MS is characterized by natural periods of remission anyway. As yet, there is no hard evidence that these measures make any difference in MS.

One new theory is that chocolate plays a part in developing MS. Clearly it does not produce MS in everyone, but there may be a small number of people who are unusually susceptible to something in chocolate. The limited evidence available suggests that the reaction is a slow one, perhaps taking as long as a week, so it may not be obvious that eating chocolate (or an especially large amount of chocolate) has triggered a deterioration in the condition of an MS patient.

Some MS patients have halted the progress of their disease by cutting out chocolate. While the existing damage to the nerves does not disappear, no further decline occurs. Since chocolate is not an essential part of anyone's diet, nutritionally speaking, there can be no harm in trying this out. Some doctors also advise cutting out coffee, cola and strong tea at the same time, as they contain some of the same drug-like chemicals that are found in chocolate.

Because of the natural cycle of remissions, described above, it may be necessary to live without chocolate for some time to assess the effects realistically.

Diabetes

Diabetes is a shortage of the hormone **insulin** that controls the level of glucose in the blood (see p135). There are two types of diabetes. One form comes on in childhood, and is due to the body forming antibodies against its own cells. In this case, the cells under attack are the islet cells in the pancreas, which produce the insulin. The second type of diabetes comes on in adults, usually those who are overweight, and is probably due to exhaustion of the islet cells, through over-consumption of sugar and starch.

It has been suggested that diabetes might be due to food intolerance, but this seems very unlikely. It is possible, however, that immune reactions to food may aggravate any **autoimmune disease** – a disease in which the immune system attacks the body's own cells. One such autoimmune disease is systemic lupus erythmatosus (see p73). Some patients with this disease fare much better if they are investigated with an elimination diet and treated for reactions to food and other environmental factors – which suggests that these sensitivities may make the underlying disease worse. In the same way, food sensitivity *might* make the autoimmune type of diabetes worse.

Alcoholism

This is a very controversial area. The putative link between food intolerance and alcoholism is based on case-histories of dried-out alcoholics, many of whom were seeking treatment for other symptoms. Regardless of what these other symptoms were, most also complained of extreme tension, great fatigue, continuous headaches, or other such symptoms.

These symptoms had begun when they gave up drinking, but had not cleared up despite many years 'on the wagon'. Some sought treatment because these symptoms had become so unbearable that they felt they were about to hit the bottle again.

According to the doctors treating these cases, the case-histories show a common pattern. For many of these patients, the elimination diet was apparently very successful – it brought relief from the tension, fatigue and other symptoms. More surprisingly, the craving for a drink, which is the bane of reformed alcoholics, also disappeared for the first time. When they began to reintroduce foods, they experienced unusual reactions to some of them: in some patients, certain food items supposedly produced symptoms akin to drunkenness. It invariably turned out that the food concerned was a major ingredient of the drink the patient had formerly favoured – potatoes for the vodka alcoholic, wheat, barley or maize for the whisky alcoholic, grapes for the confirmed brandy drinker.

These discoveries were first made by Dr Theron G. Randolph, one of the founders of the clinical ecology movement in the United States. Dr Randolph interpreted the findings as follows:

The patients concerned were primarily intolerant of/addicted to a *food*. (Addictive eating is often a feature of food intolerance, as explained on p108.) Small amounts of food protein remain in an alcoholic drink, and can pass through the gut wall and into the blood much more readily than food proteins that are eaten in the ordinary way – simply because of the alcohol. The alcoholic is addicted both to the food *and* to the alcohol. When the potent combination of the two is withdrawn, the reformed alcoholic is still eating the culprit food. So his 'addiction' is kept alive, and he continues to crave his favourite drink – the 'jet-propelled' version of his addictive food, in Dr Randolph's words. If he can identify the culprit food, and avoid it for some time, this lingering addiction is broken.

The revolutionary implication of Dr Randolph's theory is that reformed alcoholics *can* drink again, as long as they avoid the drinks that contain their culprit foods. Because this goes against the conventional wisdom on alcoholism – which forbids the reformed alcoholic to ever drink again – Dr Randolph's work has been rejected out of hand by organizations such as Alcoholics Anonymous. There have been no scientific studies of his claims, although his basic findings have been confirmed by several other doctors working in this field.

Other reported symptoms

Some of the other symptoms attributed to food intolerance are excessive hunger or thirst, twitching muscles, muscle cramps, numbness, insomnia, sleeping too much and sexual impotence. Experience suggests that none of these are very likely indicators of food intolerance, although excessive hunger and thirst are often reported in hyperkinetic syndrome (see p212). Numbness is a common symptom of hyperventilation (see p162).

COELIAC DISEASE

Coeliac disease is not usually thought of as 'food intolerance', although it *is* an adverse reaction to food. In this disease, there is just one type of food at fault – wheat and related grains (rye, barley and oats). Moreover, the symptoms are very specific. In babies they consist of pale, foul-smelling stools, wind, bloating and poor growth. These symptoms usually develop a few weeks after cereals are introduced into the diet. In those infrequent cases where coeliac disease begins in an adult, the symptoms are diarrhoea, pain, bloating, weight loss, malaise and weakness. In rare cases, however, constipation may be the main symptom. When the lining of the small intestine is examined under a microscope, it shows clear signs of damage.

The offending element in wheat is the main protein, commonly known as **gluten**. In fact, gluten is a mixture of dozens of different proteins, which fall into two main types, the glutenins and the gliadins. It is the gliadin that is responsible for producing coeliac disease, but exactly how it does so is still not clear. There is definitely an inherited component because coeliac disease runs in families. And the immune system is involved in some way, as shown by the large numbers of immune cells found in the coeliac's gut lining.

At present, the only treatment for coeliac disease is to eliminate the foods that contain gluten, namely any food containing wheat, rye, barley or oats. Most sufferers have to avoid all traces of gluten, but some can get away with eating a small amount occasionally, and some do not have to avoid oats, which contain far less gluten than the others. However, it is very risky for coeliacs to experiment with eating gluten, even if they have avoided it for some years and are fully recovered. Some have an acute reaction to even the smallest amount, known as **coeliac shock**. There is also evidence that coeliac patients who stick religiously to their gluten-free diet are less likely to develop certain cancers, compared to coeliacs who eat gluten.

A few patients do not get better, even though they are very careful to avoid gluten. This may be because their gut lining is badly damaged and needs time to repair itself. Zinc deficiency can contribute to this problem, and a zinc supplement (see p333) may be useful. Continuing symptoms can also be due to lactase deficiency (see p207), a consequence of structural damage to the gut lining. Avoiding milk may help in such cases. Soya milk can be used instead, and yoghurt or cheese made from cow's, sheep or goat's milk can be eaten, but not cottage cheese.

Alternatively, persistent symptoms may be due to some other problem, such as a tumour, or a defective pancreas. More commonly, however, the patient turns out to have sensitivities to other foods, besides wheat. The damage done to the gut lining by coeliac disease makes it much more leaky, so other food molecules get through into the bloodstream, paving the way for food sensitivity. Soya is a common culprit, perhaps because it is so widely used in gluten-free products. Milk, fish, rice and chicken have also been known to cause this problem. They can perpetuate the damaging reactions in the gut lining long after gluten has been eliminated from the diet. In theory, any food might have this effect. An elimination diet should help to track down the offender, but this should only be tried under medical supervision.

Chapter Eight

MIND AND BODY

Can food allergy or intolerance cause mental symptoms? This is, without doubt, the most controversial aspect of food sensitivity. Reports of mental disorders that were apparently caused by foods began with the work of the early clinical ecologists in America. Since then, many other doctors who treat food intolerance and chemical sensitivity have claimed that such sensitivity can produce a wide range of mental problems. The most common are anxiety and depression, but many more serious illnesses, including psychosis and schizophrenia, have also been attributed to food.

For the most part, objective evidence to support these claims, in the form of scientific trials, is still lacking. But this may simply reflect the tremendous difficulties involved in such trials. For doctors specializing in the treatment of food sensitivity, the many positive responses they have seen in their patients are sufficient evidence that food can cause mental symptoms. But the case has been greatly overstated in some popular publications, and genuine psychological problems have been wrongly attributed to food sensitivity, both by patients and fringe practitioners.

This is just one of the mind-body controversies that beset the question of food sensitivity. Equally acrimonious are the disputes over the purely physical symptoms of food intolerance, which some regard as psychosomatic – conditions where the mind produces genuine physical symptoms in the body. On the one hand, there are those who see most 'food intolerance' as misdiagnosed psychosomatic illness, and on the other hand, those who see most 'psychosomatic illness' as unrecognized food intolerance.

The effect of the mind on the body, and the problem of disentangling physical and emotional causes in chronic health problems, are also considered in this chapter. The mind has the power to produce health, as well as illness, and ways in which its healing powers can be harnessed are described here.

Psychological problems in food allergy

Some doctors believe that true, IgE-mediated allergy can produce mental symptoms as well as physical ones, but others would dispute this. Certainly, some studies have shown that those with serious allergic disorders, such as asthma, tend to have more emotional and social problems. The difficulty lies in separating cause and effect. The disabling symptoms of the allergy, and the restrictions incurred by having to avoid certain allergens, is bound to cause mental suffering. Indeed, studies that have compared asthmatic children with children suffering from other physical handicaps find little difference in the level of psychological problems.

However, there are innumerable reports of children with allergic disorders, such as asthma or perennial rhinitis (runny or congested nose), who also show a cluster of symptoms that includes an inability to keep still, excitability, clumsiness, poor memory and short attention span. These symptoms, often known collectively as **hyperactivity** or the **hyperkinetic syndrome** are dealt with more fully in Chapter Eleven. Some of these children show an interesting reaction when the allergenic foods are removed from the diet and other allergens avoided: their mental and behavioural symptoms clear up at the same time as their physical ones. Reintroducing those foods brings the bad behaviour back along with the wheezing or runny nose. Although the mental symptoms could be a result of the physical ones, this seems unlikely.

One study showed that some such children had high IgE levels for foods that caused behavioural problems, so it seems that this could sometimes be a true allergic symptom. However this is a controversial area, and conventional allergists do not seem eager to welcome behavioural disorders such as hyperactivity into their domain.

Less controversial is the notion that some allergic *symptoms* may affect the brain and cause mental problems, these being 'secondary' to the allergic response itself. In those with severe asthma, for example, the reduction in oxygen reaching the brain can cause changes in mood and abnormal behaviour. Lack of concentration, poor memory, 'slowness', drowsiness, depression, anxiety and irritability can all result from lack of oxygen.

Hay-fever and non-seasonal rhinitis (constant runny nose) can also have secondary effects on the brain. The congestion in the nose may result in the normal breathing pattern stopping entirely during sleep (**sleep apnoea**). This wakes the patient up and breathing starts again, but if there are repeated attacks during the night this can produce severe fatigue and drowsiness during the following day.

Overall, the evidence suggests that IgE-mediated allergy probably *can* affect the brain, either directly or indirectly. But the mechanism of direct action is unknown and the subject remains highly contentious. Nevertheless, there is considerable evidence that the immune system interacts with both the nervous system and the hormones. This evidence, which will be looked at in the next section, is an indication that a direct link between allergy and mental problems is not impossible.

Interlocking systems

One of the newest and most exciting fields of biological research at present concerns the relationships between the immune system, the nervous system and the hormones. The realization that these three systems can interact, and the identification of the mechanisms involved, has only come within the past few years. This new science has been given the rather daunting name of **psychoneuroimmunology**.

Among the discoveries made in psychoneuroimmunology is that stressful events can make the immune cells far less responsive to infection. Bereavement can have devastating effects on our defensive cells, but even something as minor as taking an exam can make us more vulnerable to infection. With long-term stress, it appears that a sense of being in control makes all the difference – feelings of helplessness and inability to improve matters are the most damaging. Controllable stress, on the other hand, can actually improve immune status. (However, expecting to have absolute control over external events is obviously unrealistic, and can eventually increase stress levels.) Another important factor in reducing stress is having the support of family, friends and colleagues. Having little social contact, or not turning to others for comfort, sympathy or advice when in difficult circumstances, tends to magnify stress.

The mechanisms behind the interactions of mind and immune system are still waiting to be unravelled, but there are indications that small messenger molecules may be important. These small messengers include the major chemical signals produced by the body (**hormones**), messenger substances released by the nerves for communication with adjacent nerves (**neurotransmitters**) and mediators released by immune cells which stimulate or suppress other immune cells (**lymphokines**). Some of the hormones known to affect the nervous system, such as the **endorphins** (p240), now appear to bind to immune cells as well, and probably influence their behaviour. Conversely, mediators produced by immune cells can influence nerve cells – histamine and prostaglandins both have this effect. One lymphokine with marked effects on both body and mind is **interferon** (see p237). The hormone, **noradrenaline**, also acts as a neurotransmitter for some nerves. In other words, these are three closely interconnected systems.

There are also direct links between the nerves and the immune system that do not rely on messenger substances. Detailed anatomical studies have revealed nervous connections that were not previously suspected. It turns out that several parts of the immune system – including the lymph nodes, the spleen, the thymus gland and the bone marrow – are connected by nerve fibres to the central nervous system. Exactly what effect the nerves have on these organs is as yet unknown.

So far, research into psychoneuroimmunology has done no more than scratch the surface of this potentially important topic. But it indicates that the idea of allergies affecting the mind – and vice versa – is not implausible.

Food intolerance and mental symptoms

Most of the British doctors now working on food intolerance trace their interest back to a book, published in 1976, with the intriguing title *Not All in the Mind.* Written by Dr Richard Mackarness, a psychiatrist at Basingstoke District Hospital, it described the good results of dietary change on a patient called 'Joanna' whose severe mental disturbance had been variously diagnosed as 'schizophrenia, schizo-affective psychosis, presenile dementia, temporal lobe epilepsy, neurotic depression and anxiety hysteria.' During seven years of illness she had been admitted to hospital 13 times, often compulsorily during episodes of violent behaviour when she was a danger both to her children and herself. She had made determined attempts at suicide by slashing her wrists several times.

The outlook for this patient was very poor. Although his fellow psychiatrists were thoroughly sceptical about the usefulness of an elimination diet – which Dr Mackarness had learned about from clinical ecologists in America – they were desperate enough to try anything. During a five-day fast, Joanna showed a 'very marked improvement in her condition' and when subsequently challenged with individual foods, she responded sharply to some but not others. In follow-up tests, the same foods were given by a tube leading straight into the stomach (thus avoiding the taste-buds) to check whether she would still respond in the same way. By using the stomach tube, and portions of liquefied food identified only by a code number, the test could be carried out without either the patient or the nurse giving the test food knowing its identity. (This sort of test – known as a **double-blind test** – is a must if the observations are to be verified objectively. Even if the patient does not know the identity of the food – as in a **single-blind test** – the expectations of the experimenter can still influence the outcome.) In Joanna's case, the double-blind test confirmed the severe mental reactions to culprit foods already identified in open testing.

This is how one of the more sceptical psychiatrists involved later described the patient's case: 'I must admit that such a remarkable response has been a surprise to me. However, it has been so dramatic that I think it would be difficult for us to say that it was due to anything but the dietary changes, especially in view of the double-blind trial.'

These and other well-documented case-histories lend support to the idea that food sensitivity can *sometimes* be at the root of serious mental illness. But it seems unlikely that it is often so, and it would be a mistake to extrapolate to other cases of mental illness which have been given the same diagnostic labels. There is little doubt that a variety of different diseases are concealed under umbrella terms such as 'psychosis' and 'schizophrenia'. No-one is suggesting that the mental hospitals are full of food-sensitive individuals who simply need

ROSEMARY

Rosemary was 67 and lived alone. From time to time she suffered from bouts of depression, as she had done for many years. At one stage, in her early fifties, the depression had been so bad that she had been admitted to hospital. But this was not her reason for seeking medical help now. She suffered from diarrhoea with pain and bloating, which had been diagnosed as irritable bowel syndrome. Her doctor had told her that there was nothing he could do for this problem, so she decided on private treatment from a doctor that a friend recommended. He put her on an elimination diet, and within two weeks her bowels were functioning normally, for the first time in many years. She also reported feeling much more cheerful, alert and confident than before, and the doctor assumed that this was an effect of losing her unpleasant bowel symptoms. What surprised them both was Rosemary's reaction on retesting food. Milk taken at breakfast time produced itchy skin by lunchtime, and severe bloating and diarrhoea in the afternoon. A profound depression set in at the same time, despite the fact that she knew her bowel symptoms could now be controlled quite easily. The depression took two days to clear, but afterwards Rosemary felt as well as before, both mentally and physically. Two years later she is still very healthy on a milk-free diet, and no longer suffers from depression.

an elimination diet to set them free from their illness. Nor is it possible to say what percentage of cases might be attributable to food, because nobody has even attempted to find out. For obvious reasons, it is extremely difficult to set up a large-scale trial of dietary treatment among patients who are seriously disturbed.

Less serious forms of mental illness, such as depression and anxiety, are commonly reported among those with food intolerance, usually accompanied by some physical symptoms. Doctors who treat food intolerance have observed the mental symptoms to clear up at the same time as the physical ones during an elimination diet, and to reappear when the patient tests particular foods. In many cases, it was the physical symptoms alone that were the target of the treatment, and both doctor and patient were pleasantly surprised at the change in mood that occurred simultaneously. It is possible, of course, that the depression or anxiety is felt in response to the physical symptoms – rather than being directly caused by the food itself – or that the person experiences certain mental responses to certain foods simply because they expect to do so. But the pattern of response that is observed is not easily explained in this way: with most patients there is a strong impression that the food itself is directly responsible for the symptoms.

Proving this is not easy, however. It involves administering food in such a way that the patient cannot taste it, and somehow assessing their mental symptoms objectively. The food must not only be disguised, but also given in sufficient quantity, a task that has taxed the ingenuity of many a researcher (see p95 and p96). For the present, mental responses to food must be regarded as 'unproven', but with considerable circumstantial evidence in their favour.

Apart from depression and anxiety, the following mental symptoms are reported in cases of food intolerance: fatigue, mental exhaustion and confusion, inability to concentrate, poor memory, insomnia, tension, dizziness, disorientation, over-excitement, 'nervousness', irritability, violent mood-swings and aggressive behaviour. In children, hyperactivity is frequently reported (see p213), while in adults the most common symptom is excessive fatigue that is not relieved by rest. Children may also show great lethargy and drowsiness. Some doctors interpret both fatigue and hyperactivity as part of a common set of reactions which they describe as the 'tension-fatigue' syndrome, in which the patient may be profoundly tired or tense and irritable, or both. For many, the fatigue is worst in the morning, so that the patient has difficulty in waking up and feels ghastly on getting out of bed. As the day progresses the fatigue begins to clear.

Schizophrenia

One mental disorder, schizophrenia, deserves special mention here because it has been strongly linked with food sensitivity by some doctors. The idea originated with the observation that it was more common among those with coeliac disease than among the population at large. Coeliac disease is an extreme sensitivity to wheat that causes damage to the structure of the small intestine (see p142). Because of the damage to the gut wall, there is often a greater absorption of intact food molecules, which creates the potential for further food sensitivities.

The earliest studies designed to test this idea gave promising results. A gluten-free, milk-free diet produced fewer symptoms in some schizophrenics, while feeding extra gluten made the symptoms worse. Later studies failed to find any response, for the most part, although one found that two out of 16 schizophrenics responded. It may be that gluten *is* important, but only in a fairly small proportion of schizophrenia cases.

Psychosomatic illness and hypochondria

A large proportion of those with food intolerance are diagnosed as having psychosomatic illness by their family doctors, or by consultants to whom they are referred. Although this is distressing and frustrating for the patient, the confusion is understandable because the two disorders do present a very similar picture in terms of symptoms. **Psychosomatic illness**, like **hypochondria**, is a term that is frequently misused, by the public and the medical profession alike. The term 'psychosomatic' is derived from the Greek words *psyche* meaning soul, and *soma* meaning body. It denotes an illness in which the action of the mind creates a damaging reaction in the body, with physical symptoms that can be observed or measured. There is no sense in which the symptoms are imaginary or 'all in the mind', as is often implied in both medical and casual use. Nor is it possible for the sufferer to 'snap out of it' as is often suggested with varying degrees of tactfulness.

There are several ways in which psychosomatic symptoms can be generated. One major route is via the **autonomic nervous system** which regulates the bodily functions that are not under conscious control, such as digestion, circulation of the blood, breathing and sweating. The autonomic system consists of two parts, the **parasympathetic** and the **sympathetic**, which have largely opposing effects. The parasympathetic is responsible for the day-to-day running of the body, for keeping things ticking over nicely. The sympathetic system comes into force when there is an emergency to deal with. It increases the heart rate and blood pressure, and mobilizes glucose, the body's energy source. It diverts blood from the gut and increases the flow to the muscles, preparing the body for action. The sympathetic system can also cause bowel movement so that the contents of the gut are voided promptly, making the body lighter and therefore faster-moving. The benefit of these reactions have to be understood in terms of life in the wild, where fighting off predators, or fleeing from them, may literally be a matter of life or death. The reactions produced are often summed up as the **flight or fight** response.

The sympathetic nerves achieve their effects by releasing the hormone **noradrenaline** from the nerve-tips, which are located close to the organs that they influence. A very similar hormone, **adrenaline**, can also be generated by a pair of glands known as the adrenals that sit above the kidneys. The sympathetic nerves control the adrenals' activity, so they are really part of the same system. The inner part of the gland, the adrenal medulla, produces adrenaline, while the outer part of the gland, known as the adrenal cortex, is responsible for producing **corticosteroids** ('steroids derived from the cortex'). As the bloodstream carries these hormones around the body, the adrenaline produces the 'flight or fight' reaction already described, while the corticosteroids have a great variety of effects. They too are capable of mobilizing glucose, but they also suppress inflammation (see p323) and inhibit some immune functions. Their main function in emergencies is to release glucose and thus perpetuate the 'flight or fight' reaction initiated by adrenaline and noradrenaline – they have a longer-lasting effect on the body.

Over-stimulation of the sympathetic nervous system can produce psychosomatic symptoms such as diarrhoea, nervousness, tremors, high blood pressure and abnormal heart rhythms. To make matters worse, adrenaline production is encouraged by smoking and by too much sugar, alcohol or coffee.

TABLE 1 SOME COMMON SYMPTOMS OF PSYCHOSOMATIC ILLNESS

Body system affected

Digestive system	Dry mouth or excessive saliva production. Spasm of the oesophagus (the tube leading from the throat to the stomach). Nausea and vomiting, stomach ulcers, frequent indigestion, loss of appetite. Diarrhoea or constipation.
Nervous system	Headache, fatigue, insomnia, tremors, 'nervousness', dizziness and loss of balance.
Circulatory system	Abnormal heart rhythms, pain in chest.
Respiratory system	Runny or congested nose, constant sore throat, catarrh or post-nasal drip, difficulty in breathing, hyperventilation.
Skin	Excessive sweating, skin irritation.

Overactivity by the parasympathetic can also result in bowel disturbances, or contraction of the bronchi producing asthma, or over-secretion of acid by the stomach eventually leading to stomach ulcers.

A third way in which symptoms can be produced is through mental tension being translated into muscle tension, especially in the muscles of the neck, jaw and head. Prolonged tightening of these muscles can produce headache, and possibly migraine (for more on this see p131).

The full range of symptoms attributed to psychosomatic mechanisms are shown in Table 1. In addition there are conditions where the psychological component is only a small part of the story – it can make the symptoms worse but not initiate the illness. This is true of eczema, psoriasis and most cases of asthma. Exactly how the mind affects such symptoms is not known, except in the case of asthma where the autonomic nervous system can make the bronchi contract in reponse to anxiety or emotion.

Diagnosing psychosomatic illness

A diagnosis of psychosomatic illness should not be made lightly. Firstly, the possibility of any organic illness must be ruled out. (**Organic** in this sense means 'of the body', and organic illness includes infections, autoimmune disorders, allergies and other problems with an identifiable cause.) Even if all organic diseases have been ruled out, there are still other criteria to satisfy. The patient should have the right sort of symptoms and should have been subject to some stressful emotional experience before the onset of the illness. A typical pattern in psychosomatic illness is for the disease to fluctuate with periods when the symptoms disappear only to return again at a later date. If this pattern is present, and if other members of the family have had psychosomatic complaints, then the diagnosis is strengthened.

Unfortunately, a diagnosis of psychosomatic illness is often arrived at by a much shorter and less strenuous route than this, particularly with female patients, who tend to be perceived as more 'nervy'. All too often, doctors use 'psychosomatic' as a diagnosis of convenience, to cover any illness with no obvious cause. What is more, little is offered in the way of treatment. This is paradoxical because physical illness is taken seriously and given adequate treatment, and mental illness with mainly mental symptoms is taken seriously and treated (if not always very effectively or humanely). For some reason, mental illness that produces physical symptoms is relegated to the status of an 'imaginary' disease.

Hypochondria

The same is also true of hypochondria, an anxious preoccupation with the body, or a part of the body. The patient characteristically believes that the part is diseased or not fully functional. He or she generally reports pain, and other bizarre sensations of bodily disturbance and internal movement. There are few physical symptoms that can be observed, apart from vomiting, fainting and sweating in some cases. Hypochondria is thought to be a result of repressed emotions and secret fears, and it is far more likely to develop in families where there is a preoccupation with illness, or in people who have a great deal of contact with invalids as children.

In earlier centuries, hypochondria was recognized as a 'real' illness, with a distinctive set of characteristics. And it was considered to be worthy of treatment. The dismissal of hypochondria by most doctors is a relatively new attitude, and one which is lamented by those that have studied this disorder. Robert Meister in his book *Hypochondria* writes: 'Those physicians who shrug off a suffering patient because they regard his condition as psychosomatic or hypochondriacal are not acting as professional healers . . . The cultural and social norms that affect considerations of health and illness have established what might be called an unspoken "Acceptability Index" of various forms of illness. On such an index, bacterial pneumonia, which is regarded as a "real" illness, would indubitably outrank peptic ulcers, which are viewed suspiciously as being of "psychosomatic" origin, and all illnesses known to man would outrank hypochondria . . . The prevailing negative attitudes towards hypochondria are largely unexplained, unjustified and certainly unjust to victims of the condition.'

The best type of treatment for both psychosomatic complaints and hypochondria is some form of psychotherapy, cognitive therapy or hypnotherapy (see p161) which should make it possible for the sufferer to identify the underlying emotions that are responsible for the symptoms. Once aware of the source of the problem, the patient can come to terms with these emotions and the physical symptoms should then diminish.

In some cases, however, the symptoms are a vital element in the way the patient deals with the world and with his or her own conflicts about life and relationships. For such people, the symptoms are indispensable and the best hope is to keep the condition within limits so that it causes the least possible disruption to the patient and his family.

The placebo effect

One intriguing aspect of illness is that it can often be 'cured' – at least temporarily – by *any* form of medical attention. A medical investigation or injection can work wonders, and a course of tablets is almost as good. This phenomenon is known as the placebo effect, *placebo* being a Latin word that means 'I shall be pleasing'.

Research shows that over a third of people in pain get relief from inert

LYNNE

Lynne suffered constant diarrhoea and nausea, and became convinced that foods were causing these symptoms. She tried cutting out wheat and milk, and felt a little better for a while, but then the symptoms came back. So she tried cutting out a few more foods, and again felt better – but only for a short while. This led to more and more foods being cut out, until she was on a very restricted diet of lamb, pears, plums, celery, rice and some fish. Although she still felt ill on this diet, she refused to consider eating other foods, saying that they would make her worse. At the same time, she began to suffer panic attacks and feelings of utter exhaustion, which she blamed on sensitivity to perfume and exhaust fumes. There was a danger of her losing her job, so she reluctantly took her doctor's advice and went to see a psychotherapist.

Over the following weeks Lynne began talking to the therapist about things that had happened to her as a child – the violence at home, the constant arguments, and, later, the sexual abuse by her father. For years she had felt very blank and unemotional about these events and had therefore concluded that they had not had any lasting effect on her. In talking to the therapist she gradually began to recognise that she had erased the feelings of terror and anger from her mind, leaving just a sense of numb despair. Bringing these feelings to the surface and acknowledging them was painful and difficult, but when she had done this the relief was tremendous. Her panic attacks stopped, the feeling of exhaustion lifted, and her diarrhoea and nausea disappeared. In retrospect, Lynne saw that blaming her physical illness on food had been a way of not confronting the real source of her problems.

tablets that they believe to be painkillers. Headaches, migraine, insomnia, epilepsy and rheumatoid arthritis are among the conditions that are susceptible to placebos.

In some cases, the symptoms may have been psychosomatic in origin, which would account for the good effect of the placebo. It may be that the patient feels gratified by someone taking his or her illness seriously, or it may simply be the power of suggestion – because they feel they are being offered a cure, they actually begin to get better. In other cases, there may be a mixture of organic illness and psychosomatic illness behind the symptoms – the two can coexist, one feeding on the other. Again, the placebo could be powerful because it meets some psychological need for attention and treatment.

With diseases such as rheumatoid arthritis, it is less obvious how the placebo effect works. However, the immune system plays an important role in rheumatoid arthritis (see p124), and this may provide a clue. A new form of treatment, or a new and more enthusiastic doctor, may act as a morale-booster which has a beneficial effect on the immune system – the sort of effect that the psychoneuroimmunologists are currently studying. Placebo effects are also seen in allergy, perhaps for the same reason.

A characteristic feature of the placebo effect is that it does not last all that long: it is usually only a matter of weeks, and two to six months is about the most that can be expected. If a patient responds to a new treatment and is still well after a year, it is unlikely to be a placebo effect.

Psychogenic reactions to food

The other side of the placebo coin is that people can be made ill by something they _believe_ will make them ill. Some patients are more suggestible than others in this respect, but a fair proportion of food-sensitive people will react with symptoms if they _think_ they have eaten one of their culprit foods. This reaction in no way invalidates their food sensitivity – it is real, even if the symptoms of the moment are mentally generated or **psychogenic**.

Such reactions are not really surprising, if you remember Pavlov's famous experiment with the dog and the dinner bell. The dog was 'conditioned' by a bell being sounded every time it was fed. Even before it was given the food, the dog began to produce saliva in response to the appetizing smell. After a time, the dog would salivate whenever it heard the bell, whether food was present or not.

An experiment with guinea pigs has shown that immune reactions can be conditioned in exactly the same way. The guinea pigs were sensitized to an antigen by having it injected into them, and they were simultaneously exposed to a strong odour. Later, the odour alone was enough to make them release large amounts of histamine. If guinea pigs can do this, then why not humans? Certainly anyone who has ever had a severe, immediate reaction to a food is likely to react in the same way if they are told that they have consumed some of the same food. And people whose intolerance of a food has long since cleared up may continue to react to that food for purely psychological reasons.

Occasionally people develop psychogenic reactions to food when there is no physical response. This can happen if someone becomes convinced that they are food-allergic or food-intolerant without undergoing proper diagnosis. They may decide that they react to particular foods, on the basis of a bogus diagnostic test or an elimination diet that is not properly carried out. Thereafter the reaction occurs obligingly every time they eat the food – but the response is a psychogenic one. This response is one of the pitfalls of self-treatment, but it can occur just as readily – if not more so – with treatment by fringe practitioners who use ineffective methods of diagnosis.

Psychogenic reactions of this type are most likely to occur in those whose symptoms are purely psychosomatic, but who prefer to think they are 'allergic' to food, because they see this as being a more respectable sort of illness. The medical neglect of psychosomatic illness and hypochondria must shoulder some of the blame in such situations, because the stigma attached to these disorders owes much to doctors' negative attitudes.

Patients who mistakenly believe that they are sensitive to food often put themselves on increasingly strict diets as their symptoms persist, and they may become seriously malnourished. They are in need of sympathetic professional help to identify the true causes of their malaise, and should be persuaded to undertake psychotherapy or some other form of psychological treatment. Such treatment can be valuable even where foods are a major cause of symptoms (see p160), so undertaking this type of therapy is worthwhile for a whole range of patients, not just for those whose problems are purely psychosomatic.

Psychogenic reactions to food are important in the diagnosis of food allergy and intolerance, because a challenge with *any* food may produce symptoms if the patient is expecting symptoms. In order to separate real responses from psychogenic ones, dummy challenges, with foods that are known not to cause any reaction, are included in the double-blind trials. Most patients are expected to respond to some of these dummy challenges, but they should respond to significantly more of the real ones. These dummy challenges are also known as placebos.

Food intolerance or psychosomatic illness?

It will be clear from Table 1, that many of the symptoms seen in psychosomatic illness are also features of food intolerance. Indeed, 'opponents' of food intolerance would maintain that most supposed food intolerance *is* psychosomatic illness. But doctors specializing in the treatment of food allergy and intolerance would disagree. They see innumerable patients who have been told that their symptoms are psychosomatic or 'all in the mind' by one doctor or another. Yet a high proportion of these patients respond to an elimination diet. They get better when foods are eliminated from the diet – and they stay better, which is the important thing.

A diagnosis of psychosomatic illness or hypochondria is very largely a diagnosis of exclusion – it requires all other possibilities to be excluded first. With many patients suffering vague, multiple symptoms, food intolerance must be regarded as one of those possibilities. Unless steps are taken to 'eliminate it from the enquiry' – and that must mean a diagnostic diet – then there is no sound basis for saying that a patient's symptoms are psychosomatic.

Things are not necessarily done in this order, however, and for good reason. Many of those attending the doctor's surgery with physical symptoms, such as headache or diarrhoea, actually have serious emotional, sexual or family problems that they want to discuss with the doctor, but find it difficult to start on such sensitive topics. Family doctors are trained in the art of discovering what the patient has *really* come to see them about. If you have symptoms that you think may be caused by food intolerance you should not feel affronted if the doctor's initial questions seem rather personal and irrelevant to the aches and pains being suffered. Answering the questions calmly and reasonably will do much to convince the doctor that your problems are not psychosomatic.

The question of how many psychosomatic cases the average family doctor sees is an interesting one. One survey concluded that a full third of patients have some psychological element in their illness, with 18 per cent showing purely psychiatric or psychosomatic symptoms. Other studies put the figure even higher, some as high as 50 per cent. Such studies have received a lot of publicity, so it is small wonder that the average family doctor suspects a psychological cause rather than a physical one, especially where patients complain of multiple symptoms.

Doctors who are aware of food intolerance and experienced in diagnosing it have a different statistical outlook. They vary in their estimates of how many patients might trace some or all of their symptoms to food, but most come up with a figure of 20-30 per cent. The surveys described above, that showed large numbers of patients suffering from psychosomatic symptoms, *took little account of the possibility of food intolerance*. Many of those classified as 'psychosomatic' may in fact have been sensitive to food.

On the other hand, more objective methods of assessing psychological disorders have also pinned the 'psychosomatic' label on problems such as irritable bowel syndrome and migraine – diseases that are claimed as prime indicators of food intolerance. And forms of treatment that address the mind rather than the body – including psychotherapy and hypnotherapy – have been successfully used to treat them. In the next section we will look more closely at these apparently conflicting claims in relation to one particular disorder, irritable bowel syndrome or IBS.

Mental factors in IBS

One study that is often quoted by 'opponents' of food intolerance was carried out by Dr David Pearson of Manchester University and Dr Keith Rix of Leeds University. They studied 27 patients suffering from irritable bowel syndrome who believed themselves to have food allergy or intolerance. The study only found evidence of food reactions in 15 per cent of the patients, compared with 70 per cent in another major study. The main reason for this discrepancy was probably their method of testing which only used very small amounts of the test foods (see pp94-5).

Dr Rix, who is a psychiatrist, examined half the patients. He identified a variety of mild psychiatric problems, principally neurotic depression and anxiety neurosis, in 86 per cent of them. The conclusion the doctors reached, given the apparently poor response to food testing, was that the psychological problems were affecting the bowel, rather than the other way round, in the majority of patients.

Doctors with an interest in food intolerance take a different view – that the psychological problems, where they exist, are largely a *result* of the illness, or of its rejection by the medical profession, or a mixture of the two. But they would agree that anxiety, tension or depression can make the physical symptoms worse.

It is not difficult to imagine how a disorder such as irritable bowel syndrome could affect a patient psychologically. For those with diarrhoea – one form of IBS – the symptoms are highly disruptive to normal life. Any outing revolves around the need to find a lavatory at short notice, and many outdoor activities, such as hiking or climbing, are virtually impossible. Apart from the pain which many patients suffer, the continual diarrhoea does great damage to the self-image and feelings of self-disgust are common. If the diarrhoea comes and goes, there is an understandable tendency to blame 'germs' and a neurotic concern about food hygiene may result. Where constipation is the predominant symptom, there may be considerable discomfort which again is damaging to morale.

Given these difficulties, it is hardly surprising that many patients with IBS show signs of neurotic depression and anxiety neurosis. Lack of understanding by family members and doctors is likely to compound the problem. Dr Joseph Miller, a clinical ecologist working in Alabama, writes: 'These patients are not basically neurotic, but they are less able to cope with daily problems because their symptoms distract and bewilder them. They shop for relief from physician to physician, their self-esteem diminishes, and their anxieties increase when they are told repeatedly that their symptoms are "only due to nerves". They receive symptomatic and supportive care rather than specific treatment. Many . . . become secondarily depressed from the feeling of being hopelessly trapped.'

Dr Pearson and Dr Rix point out that the level of psychiatric disorder in patients with a variety of other bowel complaints is much lower – only 34 per cent compared to 86 per cent. One factor in this difference is probably the attitude of the medical profession, since the other bowel·complaints studied were all recognized conditions which are not dismissed as psychosomatic. Unpleasant symptoms are a lot easier to cope with if you know you have Whatsisname's Syndrome than if you've been told that it's 'all in your mind'.

The idea that the psychological symptoms could be largely a *result* of the physical symptoms, rather than the *cause* of them, is substantiated by one of the patients that Dr Pearson and Dr Rix studied. This patient was sensitive to yeast and reacted to it in very small amounts, so that she produced a positive reaction even with the minute quantities that they used for testing. This patient was put on a yeast-free diet, and given a second psychiatric assessment when her bowel symptoms had resolved. Before the diet her score on the psychiatric assessment was 20 – well over the critical score of 12 that indicates significant psychiatric disturbance. With IBS a thing of the past, her score was one – a marked improvement.

The usefulness of treatments such as psychotherapy and hypnotherapy in treating IBS is entirely compatible with this view. If such treatments could eradicate the symptoms in a large proportion of patients it would be a different matter, but they do not: in most patients, they simply reduce the symptoms to a more manageable level. For the patients who respond to such treatment, there is probably a subtle interplay of mental and physical factors – the distressing symptoms lead to anxiety or depression, and the disturbed state of mind makes the symptoms worse. In some patients, psychological disorders may be even more important. Mental and emotional problems, which began long before the food intolerance, could make a significant contribution to the symptoms, once the gut has become sensitized and over-reactive. Even quite ordinary forms of stress can have an exaggerated effect on an irritable bowel. A stressful situation, such as having to catch a train or make a speech, might make a normal person's stomach churn a little, but in the IBS sufferer it can provoke a violent attack of diarrhoea.

During psychotherapy or hypnotherapy, the patient should acquire new insights into his or her own problems, which can help to modify unhealthy ways of thinking and behaving. If the treatment is successful, imbalances between the different arms of the autonomic nervous system – the sympathetic and the parasympathetic – should be corrected. This helps to tone down the bodily reactions to mental stress, and can therefore moderate a symptom such as diarrhoea, even though the primary cause of that diarrhoea is a reaction to food.

No doubt there are *some* patients with IBS for whom mental and emotional factors are the major cause of their illness, but the research done at Addenbrooke's Hospital in Cambridge (see p94), and recently confirmed by a team of doctors at the Radcliffe Infirmary in Oxford, show that food intolerance can account for between 50 per cent and 70 per cent of cases. Where food turns out to be the cause of the symptoms, lasting and complete relief is often possible, which compares favourably with the damping down of symptoms that hypnotherapy and similar treatments offer.

To sum up, IBS is probably a general term for a variety of conditions. These look similar, in terms of symptoms, but can be caused in a number of different ways. Some are largely caused by stress or emotional problems, others are due largely to food intolerance or some other physical cause, some are a 50–50 mixture of the two. To regard all cases of IBS as psychosomatic, as some doctors still do, is unhelpful to the patient. But it is equally unhelpful for anyone with IBS to decide firmly that *their* IBS must be due to food and food alone. To consider the possibility of a psychological cause is a sign of strength, not weakness, and to acknowledge such a cause could be the route back to good health.

Mind over matter

Thanks to the action of the autonomic nervous system, any disorder of the digestive system can be exacerbated by the emotions – IBS is not unique in this respect. The bronchi and the blood vessels are also controlled by the autonomic system, so they too can be affected, aggravating conditions such as asthma and migraine (due to expansion and contraction of blood vessels in the brain). Although the mechanism is not understood, mental stress also seems to make eczema and urticaria worse. Indeed, most of the physical symptoms of food sensitivity can probably be influenced by the mind.

If an illness has multiple causes it makes sense to attack it on several fronts at once. By coming to terms with basic personal problems and achieving a calmer approach to life, the symptoms of food sensitivity can sometimes be much reduced. It may still be necessary to avoid certain food items or undergo other forms of treatment, but it should speed the body's recovery, and make it possible to return to a more normal diet sooner. And in the long run it will help to ensure continuing good health.

The approach used can vary considerably. For those who can afford it, a course of treatment with a professional psychotherapist may be the best answer, although it is important to select the person and the approach carefully. At its simplest, psychotherapy consists mainly of talking through past events and present problems, with assistance from the therapist or counsellor. Hypnotherapy is also useful, except with those susceptible to depression, since this can be brought on or made much worse by hypnosis. A professional hypnotherapist should assess each potential patient carefully and advise against treatment where necessary. Some useful addresses are given on p339.

For those who cannot afford this sort of treatment, but have plenty of time to spare, co-counselling may represent a viable alternative. After a period of training, co-counsellors are paired off, and thereafter act as both counsellor and client to each other. The idea may sound strange at first, but it often works very well, and the co-counselling movement has many enthusiastic adherents. Contact addresses can be found on pp339–40.

For some people it can be enormously helpful just to write things down on paper. The process of recording how you feel sets up an internal dialogue that can offer new insights into old difficulties. Yoga or meditation may also be helpful in learning to relax. For the less spiritually inclined, biofeedback offers a 'scientific' route to relaxation.

There is one ailment where learning to relax is of special importance, and that is asthma. The fear of suffocation that accompanies an asthmatic attack is understandable, but the anxiety itself can make the attack worse – or even bring one on unaided. Asthmatics should learn a relaxation technique and practise it every day so that it can be 'turned on' at will, whenever an attack seems imminent. Hypnotherapy is often used to teach this sort of instant relaxation, and is particularly effective with children. They learn to feel that they are able to control the asthma, which reduces their feeling of helplessness and panic. In the case of children, it is very important for the parents and other adults to stay calm as well – anxiety is infectious. For children who are too young to learn a relaxation technique, a reassuring presence and a warm drink can often stave off an attack.

Physical health – mental health
Maintaining good mental health is a vital part of the fight against physical disease, and is especially important in long-term or 'chronic' illnesses such as food intolerance. While some sufferers will quickly be restored to perfect health, for others it may be a long haul. This is particularly true for those with multiple symptoms who have been ill for many years. Patience and perseverance are needed, and a positive frame of mind is essential. The following suggestions should help to improve your general health and maintain a well-balanced mental outlook.

If you are undertaking an elimination diet, you should be cutting out tea, coffee, alcohol and sugar anyway. Assuming you are not sensitive to these items, you may later reintroduce them, but avoid taking any of them in large quantities, and in particular avoid strong coffee or tea. Caffeine can be very damaging – see pp165–6. If you smoke, make every effort to give up.

Eat regular, adequate meals and make sure you get enough sleep. Try to keep to a regular timetable of waking and sleeping. Keep your surroundings tidy and well organized.

Get out of doors as much as possible and take some exercise – preferably fairly strenuous – every day. Feeling fit does wonders for the morale. If you suffer from morning fatigue, taking some exercise before breakfast is often very helpful. It need not take very long, but it should be fairly strenuous – running up and down stairs a few times will do. You will probably find that you perform very badly and feel dreadful for the first few minutes. Take a rest and try again – it is amazing how much better you do the second time around. Exercising before breakfast seems to 'clean the slate' for the body, before it has to deal with a new dose of food.

Try to spend plenty of time with other people, especially people outside your immediate family. If you find yourself endlessly talking about your illness or your diet, as you may begin to do, make a big effort to occupy your mind with other things.

Restrict yourself to one news bulletin a day, or avoid the news and newspapers altogether. The constant exposure to doom and gloom that most of us take for granted can be a source of hidden stress – if you have real problems to contend with you do not need this extra mental burden. Television programmes or books that make you laugh will do you far more good.

Hyperventilation

Some of the typical symptoms of food intolerance can also be caused by simply breathing too deeply. When we breathe we take oxygen into the body and expel the waste gas, carbon dioxide, or CO_2. Our normal breathing pattern keeps oxygen and carbon dioxide at a level to which our bodies are well adjusted. But we have to have some spare capacity in case we want to run for the bus or climb Everest (where the air is less oxygen-rich). So we have the ability to breathe faster or take deeper breaths, as required.

The problem, in those who hyperventilate, is that they have got into the habit of breathing faster all the time. Yet they are unaware of doing this. The level of CO_2 in their blood falls below the normal level, and this alters the pH (acidity-alkalinity) of the blood, producing a wide range of mental and physical symptoms. The type of symptoms produced by hyperventilation are shown in Table 2.

The importance of hyperventilation depends very much on your point of

TABLE 2   MAIN SYMPTOMS OF HYPERVENTILATION

Brain	Migraine and headache. Poor memory. Spaced-out feeling, confusion, anxiety or depression, tension, dizziness, panic attacks, hallucinations, delusions, mood swings, phobias, stupor, convulsions. Waking up with symptoms, having vivid or frightening dreams. Fear of sudden death.
Ears	Ringing sounds in ears, vertigo, sensitivity to loud noise, sounds seeming very distant.
Eyes	Blurred vision, double vision, sensitivity to bright lights.
Breathing	Shortness of breath, tightness and aching in chest, frequent sighing or yawning, dry throat, cough, asthma-like attacks, 'lump in the throat'.
Heart	Abnormal heart rhythm, chest pains.
Digestive system	Stomach pain, bloating, belching, intermittent diarrhoea.
Muscles	Sudden loss of strength, tremors or twitches, exaggerated twitching when falling asleep, cramps, aching muscles.
General	Tingling or numbness in the tongue, lips, fingers or toes. Coldness or sweating, flushing, poor circulation, fatigue, fainting. Feeling of pressure in the throat, difficulty in swallowing, husky voice, swelling below the jaw ('swollen glands').

(Reproduced by kind permission of Dr L. M. McEwen.)

view. Some of those who are dismissive of food intolerance, see hyperventilation as a widespread cause of vague, multiple symptoms. They claim that large numbers of those who are diagnosed as food-intolerant are actually hyperventilators. The belief that they are 'allergic' to a particular food or environmental chemical makes these patients hyperventilate when they encounter it – breathing more deeply is a natural reaction to fear or anxiety. The hyperventilation brings on the symptoms, but the patient perceives them as a consequence of the food or chemical – so the pattern of behaviour is reinforced.

Those who specialize in treating food intolerance regard hyperventilation as a somewhat less common problem, but one which can masquerade as food sensitivity. More importantly, they recognize a minority of patients who are both food sensitive *and* hyperventilators. They suspect that the anxiety caused by the food reactions was originally responsible for the change in breathing pattern, and that the two disorders aggravate one another. A number of these patients are very seriously ill and appear to react to almost every imaginable

EDITH

Edith's medical problems dated back to her teens, but her symptoms had always been rather vague – excessive tiredness, headaches and indigestion. At the age of 38 she suffered premature menopause, and her health then deteriorated very rapidly. She suffered from migraine, diarrhoea with wind and bloating, and stiff, painful joints. Hormone replacement therapy, the standard treatment for symptoms associated with the menopause, was tried. She seemed to have more energy as a result, but she developed nettle-rash and a vaginal discharge, which turned out to be due to thrush (Candida infection). Apart from this she had a great many 'mental' symptoms – floating feelings, panic attacks, irrational bouts of crying, dizziness, numbness and tingling in her hands and arms.

Her doctor was convinced that most of Edith's problems were psychosomatic, but he referred her to a specialist who was interested in such cases. She immediately recognized the signs of hyperventilation and retrained Edith's breathing pattern, which cleared most of the mental symptoms very promptly. Suspecting that her diarrhoea and wind might be due to a yeast overgrowth, she put her on a no-sugar, no-yeast diet and a course of anti-fungal drugs. Her bowels were much improved by this, but Edith still had migraine attacks and trouble with her joints. So she was asked to undertake an elimination diet, which cleared these symptoms within a week.

On testing foods, she found that wheat brought her stiff joints back, while milk and cheese produced a migraine within a few hours. By avoiding these foods, she has remained very well, and has far more energy in her fifties than she had as a teenager.

food and chemical. Some doctors call them 'universal reactors', and they will be discussed more fully in Chapter Nine.

Another school of thought maintains that a mild form of hyperventilation can be a feature, perhaps a symptom, of food intolerance. According to these doctors, when the incriminated foods are avoided, or neutralization therapy provided (see p297), the hyperventilation automatically disappears, without the patient even being aware of it. They suggest that the adverse reaction to the food has some direct effect on centres in the brain which control breathing.

Anyone who shows a large number of the symptoms listed in Table 2 should consider the possibility that they are hyperventilating. The most characteristic symptoms are numbness, tingling and a 'spaced-out' feeling. Hyperventilation can be tested for, but not necessarily treated, at home. To test yourself, choose a time when your symptoms are severe, take a fairly large, clean paper bag, and hold it over your mouth and nose. Breathe as you normally would for a few minutes. If you begin to feel better, then it is likely that hyperventilation is the cause of the trouble. By rebreathing expelled air from the bag, you are increasing your intake of CO_2, which raises its level in the blood.

If you are hyperventilating, but also have food intolerance, you may find that the hyperventilation clears up spontaneously when you undertake an elimination diet. If it does not, then you need to be retrained into a normal breathing pattern, and your family doctor should be able to refer you to someone (*eg* a physiotherapist) who can do this.

Caffeine

One important dietary component, that can have a powerful effect on both mind and body, is caffeine. This drug is found in coffee and tea, and, in lesser amounts, in chocolate, Coca-cola, Pepsi-cola and other cola drinks. Some experts advise a maximum dose of 350–500 mg per day, but according to others, a dose of 250 mg a day is potentially toxic. Two to six cups of coffee (depending on its strength), three to seven cups of tea, or seven cans of cola supply this amount. Children are more susceptible to caffeine than adults and should probably not drink more than one or two colas a day. Some individuals are far more sensitive than others and should not consume caffeine at all.

Taking excess caffeine can produce anxiety, mood swings, tremors, insomnia, abnormal heart rhythms (palpitations), sweating and weight loss. Hyperventilation sometimes accompanies these symptoms, producing breathlessness, chest pains, tingling in the toes and fingers, dizziness and fainting. Some patients who drink too much caffeine show none of these symptoms, but vomit violently instead – this is particularly common with tea

KEN

Ken was in his forties when he was first found to have high blood-pressure. He was given drugs which controlled this well and had no more health problems for the next four years. Then he experienced pains in the chest, faintness, sickness and sweating. Suspecting a mild heart attack, his doctor had him admitted to hospital but tests were negative and he was discharged after a few days. This seemed to be a turning point for Ken. After leaving hospital he was tired, anxious and depressed, apparently losing all interest in life. He also experienced panic attacks from time to time. Hypnosis and electroconvulsive therapy were tried but had no effect, and he became heavily dependent on tranquillizers.

Eventually Ken was referred to a doctor who had an interest in dietary factors in disease, and asked him about his diet. It emerged that Ken drank 20 cups of tea or coffee, both very strong, in the course of the average day. He was told to gradually cut these out, along with all other drinks containing caffeine. Within a few weeks he began to feel better, and his depression, anxiety, tiredness, panic attacks, fainting and sweating are now a thing of the past. Problems due to too much caffeine are fairly common, but not everyone has the sort of symptoms that Ken experienced. Some suffer severe headaches, others abdominal pain or vomiting, or a variety of other symptoms (see p165).

drinkers. Abdominal pain and diarrhoea can also be produced by too much caffeine, and in children it can produce hyperactive behaviour.

Those who drink large amounts of coffee during work hours may suffer from caffeine withdrawal at weekends, or if they miss their morning cup of coffee. They may be irritable, lethargic, depressed, drowsy or nervous. Nausea, sneezing and a runny or congested nose are other possible symptoms, and a headache may follow. Some cases of 'weekend migraine' may be due to caffeine withdrawal.

Another symptom that has been attributed to excess caffeine is the **restless legs syndrome**. Extreme discomfort in the legs, and sometimes the arms, leads sufferers to constantly move their legs around in bed, resulting in insomnia for themselves and anyone unfortunate enough to have to share a bed with them. Although not all doctors would agree that restless legs are attributable to caffeine, anyone suffering this condition should try avoiding caffeine for a while to see if it makes any difference. The amount of caffeine should be reduced gradually, over a period of two to three weeks, to minimize withdrawal reactions. Remember that some painkillers contain caffeine (eg Anadin) and cut these out as well.

Psychological effects of allergy drugs

Some of the drugs used to treat allergy may have side-effects that involve the mind and behaviour. It is easy to mistake these for direct effects of the allergy itself, so it is important to be aware of the possible effects of particular drugs.

Antihistamines tend to cause drowsiness, but some are better in this respect than others (see p321). If you or your child are affected it is worth asking the doctor to change you to another type of antihistamine.

Corticosteroids, if used for a prolonged period, can cause a type of dependency. When they are withdrawn the patient may suffer fatigue, headache, depression, weakness, and aches and pains. These drugs are only likely to cause such problems if they have been taken continuously, at high doses, for some months.

Ephedrine (see p322) can cause anxiety, insomnia and restlessness. Although it is less widely used than it once was, it is found in some bronchodilators and cough mixtures. Some of these can be bought without a prescription.

Pseudoephedrine (see p322) can produce euphoria and delusions, if taken in very large doses, and even in normal doses it may cause nightmares and behavioural problems in children. It is widely found in cough mixtures (eg Actifed) and hay-fever medication, some of which can be bought without a prescription.

Consult the list of drugs on pp329–33. If the medicine you are taking is not listed there, ask to speak to the pharmacist at the shop where you buy it – he or she will be able to tell you if it contains any of these drugs. Consult your doctor before discontinuing any prescribed medicines.

Chapter Nine

CHEMICAL SENSITIVITY

Hazel had been ill, in one way or another, for most of her life. As a child she had pains in her stomach a lot of the time, and shooting pains in her arms and legs. She was sick when she ate certain foods, notably fish. Despite this, she was a bright child and did well at school. At 17, she suddenly became very lethargic, put on weight and suffered 'swollen glands' (enlargement of the lymph nodes, which are part of the immune system). These symptoms looked just like those of glandular fever, and that was what her doctor diagnosed. But the illness lingered for over a year, and in the end the doctor decided that she must be suffering from depression. Her tiredness was such that Hazel could no longer study and she failed all her school exams. She remained unwell, with recurrent headaches, sleepiness, fatigue and inexplicable bouts of fainting. Alcohol made these symptoms worse, she noticed, so she gave up drinking at the age of 20. Her family doctor remained convinced that all her problems were in her mind.

When she was 22, Hazel consulted a doctor who felt that her illness might be brought on by something in her diet or her environment, rather than a psychosomatic problem. He tried out an elimination diet, and got a reasonably good response. Six common foods were identified as causing symptoms, but even when she avoided all these Hazel was still not particularly well. So she was admitted to a special hospital with controlled environmental conditions (described later, on p178). Here she blossomed, recovering a great deal of her former vitality and alertness. She was then exposed to various synthetic chemicals in turn, and reacted badly to diesel fumes, cigarette smoke, natural gas, chlorine and alcohol. Some made her drowsy or faint, others produced a severe headache or nausea. Tap water and filtered tap water also affected her, whereas mineral waters caused no problems.

By avoiding her culprit foods, and removing a number of synthetic chemicals (see page 172) from her home, Hazel managed to maintain a reasonable state of health once she left the environmental unit.

Problems with chemicals

Hazel is one of those unfortunate patients who not only have food intolerance, but also seem to be sensitive to various everyday chemicals as well. A few of these people react to a great variety of chemicals and foods, and are quite severely ill. They are sometimes called 'universal reactors' by doctors working in this field. A few cases have attracted public attention – such as that of Sheila Rossall, a pop singer, who was flown to America for treatment in the 1970s, before such problems could be treated in Britain. The newspapers invented the misleading name 'total allergy syndrome' for her problem, as well as the melodramatic headline 'Allergic to the Twentieth Century'.

Patients of this sort were first discovered in the late 1940s by Dr Theron G. Randolph, one of the founders of clinical ecology in America, and they have been reported by many other doctors since. People with a milder form of chemical sensitivity have also been found – they may become dizzy and nauseated if they breathe too many car exhaust fumes, have headaches when there is a strong smell of paint, or develop a sore throat and catarrh when they use particular cleaning fluids. In children, hyperactivity (see page 213) is among the symptoms, and food colourings appear to be common culprits.

The range of chemicals that have been identified as causing problems is enormous – Table 3 shows a representative selection. The range of symptoms is also vast, and includes many of those linked with food intolerance: headache, migraine, fatigue, nausea, vomiting, diarrhoea, abdominal pain, rhinitis (runny or congested nose), wheezing, coughing, epileptic seizures, eczema, urticaria (nettle-rash or hives) and hyperactivity. Despite these many similarities, patients with chemical sensitivity *are* noticeably different – for one thing, mental and behavioural symptoms are very common with chemicals. Depression, excessive sleepiness, severe mental confusion, uncontrollable anger and 'drunken', clumsy behaviour have all been reported. Another characteristic of reactions to chemicals is that they come on very promptly after the exposure – which helps in the diagnosis.

Recently, the problem of hyperventilation (see page 162) has been diagnosed in some people with alleged chemical sensitivity – particularly the 'universal reactors'. This has led some doctors to dismiss the whole idea of chemical sensitivity and claim that *all* such patients are hyperventilating. The truth is probably more complex than that. Careful investigation often shows that these people have a dual problem: they are sensitive to foods and chemicals on the one hand, and they are hyperventilating on the other. Which came first is anybody's guess, but the two are now working together to make the patient even more ill.

Chemical controversies

The question of chemical sensitivity is no less controversial than that of food intolerance – if anything is more hotly debated. But whereas there is good evidence to support the idea of food intolerance (see pp89–100), there is almost no scientific data about chemical sensitivity. Belief that the phenomenon exists is simply based on seeing individual patients who get well when they avoid certain chemical exposures.

A great many doctors feel that chemical sensitivity is improbable – a dubious diagnosis that probably covers up for psychosomatic illness, hyperventilation, or purely psychological symptoms. Convincing them otherwise would take double-blind trials and a plausible explanation of how the sensitivity might arise. Double-blind trials (see p147) are difficult to perform with chemical-sensitive patients for a variety of reasons. Firstly, it would be impossible to try out many of the gases and solvents 'blind' because they have a powerful smell – the patient would know what was being tested. Secondly, many of the symptoms produced are highly subjective – headache, confusion or nausea, for example. These are very difficult to measure objectively.

Looking for a plausible mechanism is slightly easier, but the search has only just begun, and there are few clues to go on at present. Later in the chapter, we will consider the various possibilities in this area. First we need to look more closely at 'chemicals' and discover exactly what they are.

WHAT ARE 'CHEMICALS'?

All living things are made up of chemicals – chemicals and water and nothing else. So are rocks and the air and other inanimate objects. But when people use the word 'chemicals' that is not what they usually mean. Colloquially, it means man-made chemicals or **synthetic chemicals** – ones that do not occur in nature, or which only occur naturally in very small quantities, compared to the amounts that we manufacture.

Synthetic chemicals are not intrinsically different from naturally-occurring ones – their basic chemistry is much the same, although there are some novelties (eg chlorinated hydrocarbons – hydrocarbons are fundamental to life, but adding chlorine to them was a human innovation). What is more, many naturally-occurring chemicals are highly toxic: the natural foods we eat are stiff with potentially damaging chemicals – plants, in particular, spike their products with an armoury of defensive substances (see p15), fungi on the plants contribute their own toxins, and the bacteria in our gut add to the number we absorb. Human beings are well equipped to detoxify these natural chemicals, with a powerful array of **enzymes** (see p18).

For the most part, the enzymes that our ancestors evolved to tackle natural chemicals work pretty well on synthetic ones – as long as they are not overwhelmed by the amount they have to detoxify. However, the initial products of the enzyme reactions are sometimes more toxic than the original chemical. In other words, the body's detoxification enzymes have evolved to deal with a certain range of naturally occurring chemicals – they can go to work on synthetic ones, but on the way to breaking them down they may produce intermediates that are harmful. For this reason, such changes are known as **biotransformation** rather than detoxification.

Chemicals from oil and coal

Most of the synthetic chemicals, that we come into contact with – including pesticides, petrol, plastics and most solvents – are made from oil or coal. These are known as **organic chemicals** – which probably sounds like a contradiction in terms to anyone who buys 'organic' vegetables! The word organic is being used in two different ways – but with the same etymological root. It means 'of living things'.

The chemicals that make up living things are all based on chains of carbon atoms, with hydrogen atoms attached to them all along the chain – such molecules are known as **hydrocarbons**. Until 1828 it was thought that *only* living things could make such molecules – hence the name 'organic'. Chemists now know how to make most organic molecules in the laboratory, but the name has stuck.

In the case of 'organic' farming, the name was originally used to show that crops were grown using fertilizers derived from living things – manure or compost – rather than *inorganic* fertilizers such as nitrates, which are made by chemical processes. As pesticides became more widely used by most farmers, 'organic' farming took on a broader meaning – the crops were not sprayed with synthetic pesticides either. So an 'organically' grown carrot is one that has *not* been sprayed with synthetic pesticides – despite the fact that these are 'organic' chemicals.

Geologists believe that oil and coal are composed of organic molecules because they themselves are derived from living things. In the case of coal, this is undoubtedly true: it is the partially decomposed remains of forests, which were made up of giant clubmosses and other extinct trees. These forests covered the earth about 300 million years ago. Oil is derived from the remains of microscopic sea creatures, and is even older, according to most geologists. A novel theory about the origin of oil suggests that it is actually a product of the earth's core, and not of living organisms at all, but this is not widely accepted.

TABLE 3   SUBSTANCES THAT MAY CAUSE PROBLEMS IN CHEMICAL SENSITIVITY

GASES AND AIRBORNE DROPLETS	Fumes from chlorinated water and bleach Natural gas Industrial air pollution Aerosols Pesticide sprays
SMOKE AND OTHER COMBUSTION PRODUCTS	Tobacco smoke Coal smoke Fumes from gas- or paraffin-burning stoves/heaters Petrol and diesel exhaust fumes

SOLVENTS* AND OTHER VOLATILE* COMPOUNDS	Petrol and oil vapours, also lighter fuel and paraffin
	Perfumes and after-shave
	Scented soaps and toiletries, scented cleaning materials
	Paint
	Varnish
	White spirit, meths, paint-remover
	Disinfectant
	Mothballs
	Air-fresheners
	Polish (furniture, brass etc)
	Formaldehyde (from cavity wall insulation, chipboard, foam rubber)
	Smells given off by:
	    plastics (*eg* when warm)
	    rubber and foam rubber
	    coated (shiny) paper
	    newsprint
	    new fabric

NON-VOLATILE* COMPOUNDS	Food additives Pesticide residues in food Pollutants in water Plasticizers (escaping from cling-film and some flexible plastics) Waxes (on some vegetables and fruit) Medicinal drugs

The origin of these substances is worth considering here, because there is so much misinformation on the subject. It is part of the folklore of clinical ecology that coal and oil are both derived from 'ancient pine forests'. In fact, both were deposited many millions of years before the first pine tree grew on earth. The clubmosses, which created most of the coal seams, are more closely related to ferns than they are to pine trees, and oil – from which most synthetics are obtained – is not derived from plants at all. These distinctions are important, because the 'ancient pine forest' myth has led to the idea that chemical-sensitive patients are also likely to react to pine wood and pine products. Perhaps chemical-sensitive patients *are* affected by pine resins – which contain a lot of natural toxins to protect the tree – but it has nothing to do with the origins of coal and oil.

The 'ancient pine forests' concept is linked to another myth about chemical sensitivity – that patients who are 'universal reactors' are reacting to all synthetic organic chemicals *because they come from a common source*. In other words, they are reacting to the 'coalness' or 'oilness' of the chemical, rather than the chemical itself. This theory stretches credibility considerably, because synthetic compounds go through so many chemical reactions, distillations and purification procedures that they bear little relationship to their raw materials, let alone to each other. And in any case, those raw materials – coal and oil – are not at all similar in their own origins.

Again, these misconceptions are important, because the 'common origin' idea is the basis for some forms of therapy used with chemical sensitive patients. Doctors employing the 'neutralization technique' (see p297), often give ethyl alcohol in **sublingual drops** (under-the-tongue drops) as neutralization therapy for mild forms of chemical sensitivity. **Ethyl alcohol**, also known as **ethanol**, is the alcohol we use as a social lubricant in wines,

---

* A *volatile* chemical compound is one that readily gives off vapour at room temperature – so although it may be a liquid or a solid, some of its molecules escape into the air as a gas.

A *solvent* is a substance in which other things dissolve – water is a solvent, as is alcohol, white spirit, turps and acetone (nail-varnish remover). Solvents are used very widely in the chemical industry and they are present in a huge variety of substances. Such solvents are mostly very volatile. It is solvents that give paint and varnish their smell as they evaporate, *ie* as the paint dries. Solvents and other volatile chemicals will mostly enter the body *via* the nose and lungs, but liquid solvents can also get through the skin.

Non-volatile compounds mostly enter our bodies in food or drink.

beers and spirits. But what is used in sub-lingual therapy is industrial alcohol. This is made by adding water to ethylene gas, which itself is obtained from oil. The theory is that industrial alcohol can desensitize someone to *all* synthetic organic chemicals, because it is derived from oil. It will be clear from the facts given above that this is highly unlikely. Which is not to say that ethyl alcohol drops do not work – they could help a chemical-sensitive patient by stimulating the liver to produce more detoxification enzymes.

The chemical environment

Exposure to synthetic chemicals comes in three main forms – by mouth, through the nose and lungs, and through the skin. The sort of synthetic chemicals we eat and drink are described in Appendix VI, p313. Those that we commonly breathe include solvents (see Table 3), exhaust fumes, cigarette smoke and aerosol droplets. In addition to these, many people are exposed to fumes at work – from industrial processes, photocopier machines or dry cleaning solvents, for example. Those living in industrial areas, or near rubbish incinerators, are exposed to other airborne chemicals from these sources. The third source listed above – the skin – is far less important. The number of synthetic chemicals that get into our bodies through the skin is relatively small, but solvents such as white spirit can enter in this way, as can oils and solvents used in cosmetics.

Someone eating an average diet and drinking unfiltered tap water is likely to ingest at least a hundred different synthetic chemicals every day – see pp313–17. Exposure to airborne chemicals will vary more widely, depending on where people live, what work they do, how well-ventilated their homes are, and what sort of household products they use. A smoker in the house will increase the variety of quantity of air pollutants considerably. In all, we are probably exposed to at least two hundred different synthetic chemicals every day – and some people will encounter many more.

WHAT CAUSES CHEMICAL SENSITIVITY?

Why are some people apparently made ill by everyday synthetic chemicals? There are two types of explanation on offer, which can be summed up as 'allergic explanations' and 'deficiency explanations'. The first type of theory proposes that these people make an inappropriate immune response (allergic response) to certain synthetic chemicals, in the same way that a hay-fever sufferer reacts adversely to pollen (see Chapter Two). The second type of explanation suggests that these people have some sort of defect that makes them less able to cope with environmental chemicals. It is usually assumed that this is a deficiency in the **enzymes** (see p18) that detoxify foreign chemicals. We will look at the evidence – such as it is – for each of these explanations.

The allergic explanation

This assumes that the affected person makes IgE antibodies to the synthetic chemical concerned (see page 25), or responds with some other inappropriate and damaging immune reaction. Since the chemicals concerned are too small to act as antigens in their own right, they would have to combine with body proteins and act as haptens (see p31).

It has been suggested that this can happen with some food additives, particularly preservatives and synthetic colours. These cause chronic urticaria (nettle-rash) in some people, and urticaria is sometimes due to an allergic reaction. There are also isolated cases of tartrazine (a synthetic colouring) causing acute asthma attacks, or a severe reaction that resembles anaphylactic shock (see page 29) in some very susceptible people. Other food colourings, particularly the synthetic ones, have been known to cause allergic dermatitis, mainly in food workers exposed to large amounts. The preservative, sorbic acid, has occasionally caused allergic dermatitis when used in medicinal creams.

In most of these cases, the tests to show that the reaction really is an allergic one have not been carried out. And when a group of patients who were apparently allergic to tartrazine were tested for IgE antibodies, none were found. So it looks as if these are not allergic reactions at all, even though they produce allergy-like symptoms. Doctors suspect that tartrazine produces symptoms in these people by directly affecting the immune response in some way – perhaps by stopping the synthesis of immune regulators called prostaglandins (see p28), or by triggering mast cells directly. In the case of synthetic chemicals apparently causing asthma, the effect may be due to irritation rather than an allergic reaction. This is well known for metabisulphites and sulphur dioxide (see p301).

These are cases where the symptoms provoked by chemicals at least *looked* allergic symptoms. In the majority of chemical-sensitive people, the symptoms are not those commonly associated with allergy. So it seems unlikely that chemical sensitivity is allergic in origin. It is possible, however, that synthetic chemicals might affect the immune response in some way. This has indeed been shown for some chemicals, but the usual effect is to lower resistance to disease, rather than to make allergies more likely.

The deficiency explanation

Some synthetic chemicals are excreted from our bodies unchanged – in urine, for example, or on our breath when we exhale. Some, such as DDT, are stored unchanged in the body's fatty tissues. But the vast majority are acted on by enzymes, which change them chemically in **biotransformation** reactions (see p171). Ultimately, these reactions lead to the detoxification of the chemical.

In recent years, minor enzyme deficiencies have been found in some people, which do not normally make them ill unless they take a particular medicinal drug. Studies of such drugs in food-intolerant patients have shown that a large proportion of them suffer from these minor enzyme deficiencies (see p243). In one study, some of the patients also had chemical sensitivities, and when the results for these patients alone were considered, 99 per cent were found to be deficient in a particular enzyme system. Such a high percentage is unusual in medical research, and suggests strongly that there is a link between chemical sensitivity and enzyme deficiency. This result was for just one set of enzymes – and hundreds are involved in detoxification.

In another study, described on pp243–4, certain artificial food colourings have been found to inhibit crucial detoxification enzymes. It is possible that enzyme inhibition by these artificial colours contributes to the problem in people whose enzymes are partially defective. This could account for the frequency with which food colourings have been identified as the source of adverse reactions.

If enzyme deficiencies are at the root of the problem in chemical-sensitive patients then one might expect them to show the same sort of reaction to *small* amounts of a chemical as normal people show to *large* amounts of that chemical. Occupational medicine – the study of how exposures in the workplace affect workers' health – is the main source of information here. This branch of medicine studies the effects of brief high-dose exposures (as during an industrial accident) and long-term exposures at a lower level (but still much higher than most people would encounter). It is the latter which are relevant to the chemical-sensitive patient, and they do provide some interesting and revealing parallels.

In the case of organic solvents, for example, the prime symptoms seen in workers exposed to regular 'low' doses are mental ones. For example, toluene (found in paints and glues) produces fatigue and vague feelings of malaise, while styrene (used in the manufacture of polystyrene) produces fatigue, a sense of ill-health and irritability. Trichloroethylene (an industrial solvent that is a common contaminant of drinking water) may produce tiredness, dizziness, headache, irritability and digestive problems. White spirit, which is a mixture of solvents, produces fatigue and general feelings of ill-health. These are very much the sort of symptoms seen in many chemical-sensitive patients when they are exposed to organic solvents. (See Table 3.)

It is known from occupational medicine, that exposure to two chemicals at once can be far more damaging than being exposed to each chemical individually. This **cocktail effect** commonly occurs when the same enzymes are involved in detoxifying both chemicals – the two then 'compete' for the same enzyme, which is only present in limited amounts. Even chemicals that are broken down by different enzymes may 'compete': some enzymes need substances known **cofactors** to help them do their work, so the two chemicals are 'competing' for cofactors, rather than for the enzymes themselves. Many organic solvents interact with each other in this way, and it may be the *combination* of chemicals surrounding them that causes illness in chemical-sensitive patients. Most of the vitamins are enzyme cofactors, and some doctors believe that a lack of vitamins can make people more sensitive to environmental chemicals (see pp269–70). The alcohol in alcoholic drinks is itself an organic solvent, and it 'competes' with several other solvents for detoxification enzymes, slowing their breakdown. Not surprisingly, perhaps, most chemical-sensitive patients cannot tolerate alcohol – this is often one of the earliest symptoms. Many food-intolerant patients, with little or no sign of chemical sensitivity, are also unable to drink, which supports the idea that enzyme defects are important to food intolerance as well (see pp242–3).

The multiple role of many detoxification enzymes would explain one of the curious features of chemical-sensitive patients – the fact that they are usually affected by a whole range of chemicals, not just one. This has nothing to do with the chemicals all being derived from oil and coal (see p173) as is often suggested. But it could be due to defects in an enzyme that is responsible for detoxifying a variety of environmental chemicals.

In general, enzyme defects are inherited – passed on from parents to children in the form of an abnormal gene. So one might expect chemical sensitivity to run in families, if enzyme defects are a common cause of the problem. But what about patients who are apparently fit and healthy until they suffer a massive exposure to toxic man-made chemicals? Many patients with severe chemical sensitivity trace their problems back to such an incident.

It is possible that such people had minor enzyme deficiences before their damaging exposure, but that these were not causing any symptoms at that stage. Some parts of the liver could have sustained *mild* damage during their exposure – not enough to cause characteristic symptoms such as jaundice, but enough to leave a legacy of inadequate detoxification systems. Liver damage is known to occur when the breakdown product of a chemical is highly toxic. Because the chemical is being dealt with in the liver, the toxic intermediates (the initial products of the biotransformation reaction) accumulate there. So damage is concentrated in the cells of the liver.

Canaries of the chemical age?

One enzyme system, involved in detoxification, was found to be defective in 90 per cent of patients with chemical sensitivity (see p175). But that same enzyme system is defective in 20 per cent of normal, healthy people. This suggests that there is some other deficiency as well in those with chemical sensitivity – perhaps a defect in another enzyme. But it also suggests that many 'normal, healthy' people are not as immune from everyday chemicals as they might appear to be. One in five apparently has a potential problem, considering this one enzyme system alone.

Many of the symptoms shown by food-intolerant and chemical-sensitive patients are symptoms that we all suffer from at times – headaches, tiredness and indigestion for example. Which is why some doctors feel that such patients are 'not really ill', simply over-reacting to everyday symptoms. But to look at the problem from another angle, none of us lives in an environment free from synthetic chemicals – if we did, would we still suffer from those 'everyday symptoms' such as headaches?

Sceptics will argue that the chemicals we are exposed to have all been tested for safety, and should have no ill-effects at the concentrations we encounter. But the fact is that such tests are done on single chemicals, never on mixtures. So any 'cocktail effects' will have gone unnoticed in such tests. Given the mixture of 200 or more chemicals that we may encounter everyday, cocktail effects could be very important. It is also the case that the tests use animals such as rats, not human beings. How does a rat tell the experimenter that it has a headache or feels a bit off-colour? Quite apart from these objections, there are many other doubts about the effectiveness of safety testing – some of these are discussed in Appendix VI, in relation to food additives and pesticides.

Perhaps the chemical-sensitive patient is like the miner's canary, carried along in a cage to detect dangerous accumulations of gas in the pit. This may sound alarmist to some people, especially those in the chemical industry who have a large financial stake in the continuing use of their products, but there is worrying evidence that we *are* being made ill by the chemicals around us. One study of Parkinson's disease, an incurable nervous condition, showed that the use of garden pesticides was associated with a higher incidence of the disease. Another study, carried out in America, showed that the children of parents who used pesticide sprays were more likely to suffer from leukemia. Yet these products are supposedly 'safe' for domestic use. The recent *volte-face* by the British government on the dangers of pesticide residues (see p316) raises doubts about official assurances on other safety matters.

TREATING CHEMICAL SENSITIVITY

For those who think they may be sensitive to synthetic chemicals, the only sound method of diagnosis is to avoid chemical exposure as much as possible and see if the symptoms improve. Individual chemicals can then be tested to discover which ones are to blame for the symptoms.

Those who are seriously ill may be 'universal reactors' (see p169) and they will only recover fully if they can be protected from the majority of synthetic chemicals. This is achieved with 'environmentally controlled units', which were first developed in America. Ideally, these should be built and furnished using wood, metals, cotton and other natural products – no plastics or other synthetic materials, which might release solvent fumes, are allowed. Air going into the unit is filtered, as is the supply of water used for washing. Spring water only is used for drinking and cooking food. All foods are organically grown, except when foods with pesticide residues are used for testing. Two environmental units are now in use in Britain, one a purpose-built unit of this type.

Needless to say, treatment in such units is costly. Fortunately, there is much that can be done at home to reduce the level of chemical exposure – for the majority of patients, these simple measures will be enough to alleviate the symptoms considerably.

Reducing chemical exposure

The following measures will reduce the level of chemical exposure experienced. The list begins with the simplest measures, and works through to more difficult ones. Try the first three measures for a couple of weeks, and see what effect this has. If there is some improvement, add the next two measures and wait another two weeks, and so on. If there is none, it may be that workplace chemicals, or generalized exposures (eg air pollution) are the problem. Consider whether this is likely, and if it is, try out the appropriate avoidance measures.

Cigarette smoke

If you smoke, even only occasionally, you should stop. If other people in your household smoke, try to persuade them to give up, or to smoke in the garden shed for a while. Wash curtains and other furnishings that harbour smoke residues, and air all rooms thoroughly. If cigarette smoke is unavoidable, you could consider hiring an air filter for a while (see p337). Cigarette smoke at work is more of a problem, but if your colleagues smoke you might try asking your employer to provide you with a smoke-free environment.

Household chemicals

Clear out all cleaning materials, white spirit, turps, meths, dry cleaning fluids, polish, bleach, aerosols, air-fresheners, moth balls and disinfectant. Rags and dusters with polish, window-cleaning liquid or white spirit on them should also be removed. Banish all these items to a garage, shed, garden or balcony for a while. If you live in a flat, and this is impossible, throw away all those that you do not really need, and store the remainder in large biscuit tins or other airtight containers. Stick to an unscented washing-up liquid (see p338) for all cleaning purposes.

Painting, gluing, varnishing, soldering and similar activities are banned for a while. If magazines or books smell strongly (usually the 'glossy' magazines and books with shiny paper), read something else. Do not use felt-tip pens, especially the strong-smelling ones. The rule here is – if it smells, avoid it.

Some furnishings, pot-holders and ornaments have a very strong-smelling varnish coating, particularly cheap bamboo products with a glossy surface. If you have any items of this sort, banish them or put them in an airtight container. Also evict any smelly plastic items – certain plastic bags, for example.

Open all windows whenever you can, to blow away residual smells. If you have gas or coal fires, and can avoid using them for a while, it would be a useful addition to this list. Make sure electric heaters are clean and free from dust before turning them on.

Avoid places such as dry cleaners and petrol stations while you are testing out these measures. Do not use any insecticide sprays in the house, or pesticide sprays in the garden.

Perfumes and cosmetics

Do not use perfume, after-shave or any strongly scented toiletries for a while. If you have to use deodorant, use the unscented, roll-on variety and try not to breathe the fumes. Do not use aerosols or talcum powder.

Water pollutants

For details of these, see pp316–17. You can either buy bottled mineral water, or use a filter to improve the quality of tap-water. Filters do not remove all contaminants however – see pp317–18. Rather than investing in a filter, it may be better to use bottled water if you are just avoiding tap-water for a few weeks.

Food additives

Avoid all packaged foods and drinks with additives listed on the label. Remember that 'flavourings' count as additives, even though they have no E-numbers, and that 'No Artificial Additives' can be very misleading – some 'natural' additives are potentially harmful (see pp314–15). Bear in mind that bread from a bakery can contain additives, although it does not have to be labelled – buy bread from a healthfood shop or make your own. Unwrapped cakes, sweets and delicatessan foods are exempt from detailed labelling, as are alcoholic drinks. Do not drink alcohol, unless you have home-made wine brewed from pure fruit and sugar (no Campden tablets), or can buy organic wine (see p336 for suppliers). Restaurant, cafeteria, or take-away food, including fish-and-chips, is often very rich in additives. Also avoid tinned foods, because the phenolic resin that is used to line the tin can contaminate the food. If you are taking any vitamin tablets with coloured coatings, give these up – an uncoloured supplement is suggested on p339. If you are taking medicines that appear to contain colourings, ask your doctor if he can prescribe an uncoloured version.

Pesticide residues

If you are able to get organic foods, and can afford them, then try to use these as much as possible. Addresses of suppliers are given on pp335–6. Growing your own vegetables is much the cheapest way of avoiding pesticides in the long run, but in the short term is may be possible to get unsprayed produce from someone with a large garden or allotment. If none of these options are open to you, then shopping at a large supermarket is probably the best solution. Two supermarket chains – Sainsbury's and Tesco – have their own systems for checking that fresh foods do not contain significant pesticide residues.

One major source of pesticides in our diet is potatoes, because these are sprayed *after harvesting* with a pesticide called thiabendazole, to prevent them from going mouldy. Significant amounts of this pesticide remain on the potatoes we eat. There are no legal limits on the amount of residue, although some large retailers (*eg* Marks and Spencer) set their own limits. If you can only afford to buy a certain amount of organic produce, potatoes would be a good choice. Fortunately potatoes are among the easiest vegetables to grow, and a small garden can provide a surprisingly large harvest. As long as you buy good quality seed potatoes you should not need to use any pesticides – planting ordinary potatoes is not recommended as they can succumb to viruses. For information on organic gardening methods, see p336.

Thiabendazole and other fungicides are also used to prolong the storage life of oranges and lemons. It is a good idea to wash such fruit in hot soapy water, and rine them thoroughly, before grating the peel, or adding slices of lemon to drinks. Oranges that are to be peeled and eaten should also be washed, because the fungicide is contained in a wax layer which comes off on the hands during peeling and then contaminates the fruit. Some supermarkets now sell unwaxed oranges and lemons, and these do not have extra fungicides applied to the peel after harvesting. (There may, of course, still be residues of sprays used when the fruit was grown, but these should be less concentrated and more easily rinsed off.)

Washing other fruit and vegetables thoroughly will help to reduce the amount of pesticide eaten, and peeling fruit will reduce the quantity further. When fruit is cooked in an open pan, some of the pesticides are boiled off, so this can help to lessen the amount that you eat.

Formaldehyde

The main sources of formaldehyde in the home are cavity-wall insulation and chipboard. There is little one can do about the former. The latter can be replaced or 'sealed in' with gloss paint – get someone else to do this for you if you can, and stay out of the way until the smell of paint has dispersed. If you have cavity wall insulation as well, the only way you can test for its effects is to go away for a while, to a house without sources of formaldehyde. Simple stone cottages with solid walls are a good bet. Plush modern hotels are likely to be oozing formaldehyde vapour.

Other sources of formaldehyde include foam rubber, new textiles, paper (including newsprint), photographs, leather luggage, antiperspirants, some cosmetics and shampoos, plywood and blockboard. It is only worth eliminating these if you have strong reasons to suspect formaldehyde.

Plastics and other synthetics

Plastics and other synthetic materials release small amounts of volatile chemicals – a process known as 'de-gassing'. By evicting smelly plastic items (see p179) you have already got rid of the worst de-gassers. Removing those that remain is a fairly drastic step, which you should only embark on if you have good reason to suspect chemical sensitivity. Bear in mind that soft plastic items de-gas more than hard items. With synthetic fabrics, it may be sufficient to just stop wearing them and using them as bedding for a while, to see if this is beneficial. One common source of fumes is the foam-backing on carpets – this tends to break down due to constant wear, and formaldehyde (see above) may interact with its to produce toxic airborne chemicals that can irritate the airways causing symptoms similar to bronchitis.

If you *are* sensitive to certain plastics, you should avoid keeping food or drinks in plastic containers. This applies to mineral water as well – substances in the plastic bottle can leach out into the water. Choose a mineral water that is available in glass bottles, but do not consume too much Perrier, as it seems to cause problems for some people.

Natural gas, oil fumes etc

The idea that people can be sensitive to natural gas is a contentious one, but it is claimed that some people have made dramatic recoveries after removing the gas supply from their house. Just turning gas appliances off is not sufficient apparently – small amounts of gas still escape from the joints of pipes.

The sort of symptoms reported in gas-sensitive patients are faintness, mental confusion, irritability, aggression, lack of coordination and facial flushing. A holiday in a gas-free house is the best way to test if gas is a problem. Sensitivity to oil fumes, coal smoke, paraffin fumes and other odours from heating systems can be tested for in the same way.

Exhaust fumes

For most people, a couple of weeks 'away from it all' is the only way to test for sensitivity to exhaust fumes. But for anyone who does a lot of travelling by car or lorry, simply reducing the amount of travelling can significantly lessen exposure to exhaust fumes. This may be enough to alleviate the symptoms.

Exposure to chemicals in the workplace

For anyone working in the chemical, pharmaceutical, engineering or food-processing industries, exposures at work should be a prime suspect. The fact that symptoms come on after work does not rule out occupational illness – the effects can be delayed. Not everyone gets better at weekends either – sometimes it can take a week or more to recover from the effects of chemicals at work. Taking a long holiday in an unpolluted environment, while avoiding other chemical exposures, is the best way of testing for this possibility.

Hairdressing salons, dry cleaners, photographic developers and petrol stations are other places of work that may cause ill health. Those working in offices may also be suffering from workplace exposure – to photocopier fumes, for example, or to solvents released by erasing liquids (Tippex etc), glue, carbon paper, chipboard and plywood. Such airborne chemicals are likely to accumulate if the ventilation is poor. Sometimes it is simply dry air that causes symptoms in modern air-conditioned offices. Or it may be fungi and other microorganisms growing in humidifiers and being circulated with the air – typical symptoms in such cases are cough, tightness in the chest, fever, aches and pains, and general feelings of malaise. Whatever the cause, a holiday in a clear environment should be sufficient to show if the workplace is the source of trouble. The difficulty here is that simple lack of stress may also alleviate the symptoms – so an improvement while on holiday may be a slightly ambiguous result.

Outside air pollution

This is only likely to be a problem in heavily polluted areas. Symptoms that regularly appear in close humid weather, or when the wind is in a particular direction, are an indication of air pollution problems. Again, a holiday in an unpolluted environment is the only test.

Living with chemical sensitivity

If you find that you are sensitive to various chemicals, then avoiding them is the best treatment. Complete avoidance is often very difficult, but fortunately it is rarely necessary. For most people, reducing their overall chemical 'load' makes them far more robust and able to cope with everyday exposures. So simply avoiding cigarette smoke, household chemicals, food additives and tap water may be enough to eliminate symptoms, or reduce them to a bearable level. You should also avoid exposure to large doses of synthetic chemicals, such as from household timber treatment or crop-spraying (see pp258–9).

There are also other measures that can improve overall health and make the body more resilient. These include correcting nutritional deficiencies (see p271), taking regular exercise, eating a good, healthy diet and reducing stress. Tackling underlying problems such as hyperventilation (see p162) will also help considerably. Try to get outdoors, to somewhere with clean air, as often as you can, and take some strenuous exercise to improve your general health and fitness.

For those with severe chemical sensitivity, creating a chemical-free 'oasis' in the house can be very valuable. For preference, this should be the bedroom, but there should be comfortable chairs, a table, and whatever else is needed for everyday living. A space in which you can do some simple exercises may also be useful if you have difficulty getting exercise out-of-doors. The idea is to retreat to the oasis whenever you can, thus reducing your overall exposure. The oasis is also useful when you are feeling ill and need to recover.

All synthetic fabrics, plastics, chipboard, plywood, foam rubber and other man-made materials are excluded from the oasis. This means old-fashioned armchairs, cotton blankets or a feather duvet, and a traditional type of mattress or a futon. (If you are also allergic to feathers, see p337.) Nothing that has been painted or varnished recently should be allowed in, nor should cosmetics, cleaning materials or any of the other items mentioned in Table 3. If you must, have a television in the room, but it is best not to watch it for too long, as the warmth of the set makes its plastic components give off fumes. Books and a radio-set are a better choice. If the air is polluted, an air filter may be a useful addition to the oasis (see p337).

It is very important for chemical-sensitive patients to keep their problem in perspective, and not get unduly paranoid about the world around them. The twentieth century may seem threatening at times for someone with these problems, but at least you are not likely to be struck down in your prime by cholera, smallpox or bubonic plague, and there is little risk of being eaten by lions. Life has always had some risks attached to it. Rather than focusing on the hazards of the world around you, try to think what you can do to make your body stronger and more resistant to environmental chemicals.

Above all, make an effort not to develop psychological reactions to chemicals – never assume that you are going to react to a chemical just because you have in the past. If you allow yourself to become fearful of certain chemicals and imagine that they are harming you, you will just be perpetuating the problems rather than solving them.

Chapter Ten

BUGS IN THE SYSTEM: 'CANDIDA' AND GIARDIA

THE CANDIDA QUESTION

For several years a strong link has been reported between food sensitivity and overpopulation with a yeast, *Candida albicans*. Again, this is a highly controversial topic, and there is considerable disagreement, even among those doctors who treat food intolerance. Some deny that *Candida* is a common problem, while a few claim that it underlies the majority of cases of food intolerance. A third group suggests that there is a genuine problem with unsuitable yeast or bacteria in the gut, but that *Candida* itself is not the guilty party, and the real culprits have still to be identified. It is difficult, at present, to decide which of these ideas is correct, but scientific opinion is tending towards the third option.

The gut flora

All of us have millions of bacteria and yeasts living harmlessly inside us, natural inhabitants of the large intestine. They are known as **gut flora**. (A curious name, perhaps, but naturalists used to think that bacteria and yeasts belonged to the plant kingdom; 'flora' can mean not just flowers, but plants in general, as in 'flora and fauna'.)

The gut flora feed on the remains of our meals, but they do us no harm. In fact, we have got so used to them being there, during the course of our evolution, that we would suffer without them. They have become essential to the well-being of the gut.

In the normal, healthy person, the gut flora is a balanced community of different organisms. There are hundreds of different species to be found, and the proportions of each vary from person to person, and from time to time. But in general, a particular balance of different species is established, which results in a healthy bowel.

These bacteria provide us with some vitamins and may aid digestion in some way. More importantly, however, because they occupy all the available surfaces in the bowel, they prevent unfriendly, disease-causing bacteria from gaining a 'foothold'. Of course, they cannot withstand a massive onslaught, such as produces a bout of food-poisoning. But in the ordinary way, low levels of harmful bacteria find themselves unable to secure a cosy niche in the face of the regular inhabitants. Not being attached to the gut wall, they are ejected far more quickly.

The members of the gut flora also produce toxins, but our bodies are used to these, and they are broken down in the liver. (This safety mechanism may be ineffective in people with cirrhosis of the liver, who are then 'poisoned' by the toxins their gut flora produce.) As for our immune system, it has learned to regard these microbes as harmless fellow-travellers. But it keeps them firmly in their place – within the digestive system. The gut flora are prevented from penetrating the gut wall and making themselves at home elsewhere in the body. Only when the immune system is severely impaired, as in AIDS, do some members of the gut flora threaten to invade the body as a whole.

Bugs in the system

Until relatively recently, the gut flora was largely taken for granted by the medical profession. It is still a neglected area, in many ways, and most family doctors probably know little about it. But a few research workers are studying the gut flora in healthy people, and comparing it with that in patients suffering from irritable bowel syndrome (IBS) or similar diseases. It would seem that there *are* differences in the relative proportions of different bacteria. Abnormalities have been identified in IBS, Crohn's disease, rheumatoid arthritis, ankylosing spondylitis and atopic eczema. Some early evidence suggests that, by re-establishing the right mix of bacteria, IBS (or at least those cases where diarrhoea is the main symptom) can be successfully treated. The same success has been claimed with atopic eczema. At present, these forms of treatment are still at an experimental stage, and are not widely available. (The only 'home therapy' that might be tried is eating live yoghurt, see pp199–200.)

If there are imbalances, what might have caused them? One answer is a severe bout of diarrhoea, which flushes a lot of the resident microbes out of the bowel. Many people date the onset of irritable bowel syndrome to such an infection. A second likely cause of trouble is antibiotics, taken by mouth. These could, potentially, kill off useful members of the gut flora and allow others to proliferate. But it seems unlikely that an ordinary one-off course of antibiotics would produce a lasting imbalance – the gut flora should re-establish itself normally afterwards. Where there might be problems is with repeated courses of antibiotics (as were once prescribed for acne) or a single course at a very high dose. The main evidence on this point has been gathered by Dr John Hunter of Addenbrooke's Hospital in Cambridge. Dr Hunter noticed that a number of his women patients had first suffered from IBS after having a hysterectomy operation. This seemed puzzling, until Dr Hunter discovered that antibiotics were always given before such operations, to help prevent infections. An experiment followed in which some hysterectomy patients had the antibiotic treatment while others did not – 11 per cent of the first group developed IBS, but none of the second group did.

The Candida controversy

Candida albicans is a yeast that we all have living in the gut, and in women it is also found in the vagina. Normally, its numbers are controlled by other microbes, and by the body itself, and it causes no trouble. Where it can become a nuisance is in the vagina, if Candida escapes the usual control mechanisms and multiplies excessively. The main symptom is a maddening itch, but there can also be a creamy discharge. This type of Candida infection, known as **thrush**, is easily treated by creams or pessaries containing anti-fungal drugs (yeasts are a type of fungus). There is now also a type of drug that can be taken by mouth, which is useful for anyone who becomes sensitive to the creams or pessaries. Occasionally women become over-sensitive to Candida itself, and may experience the itching even when the yeast is not present in excessive numbers (as defined by laboratory tests). Such cases are more difficult to diagnose, because the laboratory test is negative (which may lead the doctor to a diagnosis of 'psychosomatic'), but they respond to the normal treatments used for vaginal thrush. If Candida gets into a woman's urinary tract or bladder it can produce a form of cystitis – characterized by a burning sensation when passing urine.

Candida can also infect the throat, producing soreness, and either tiny red spots inside the mouth, or creamy yellow patches that leave a sore area when they are rubbed off. Babies are very susceptible to such infections, especially in the mouth, where Candida produces a creamy or grey-coloured 'skin' over the tongue. In newborn babies, the infection is usually picked up from the mother's vagina during birth. The baby's immune system cannot keep Candida in its place as well as an adult's, so the yeast flourishes. Some cases of nappy rash are also due to Candida.

Diabetic women run a higher risk of developing Candida overgrowth in the vagina, because of the sugar in their urine – sugar feeds the yeast. Thrush in the mouth is also more common in diabetics, although the reason for this is unclear.

When the immune system is weakened, then Candida may become a more serious problem. People with AIDS suffer greatly with *Candida* in the throat and mouth. Others, with a severe immune defect, may develop *Candida* infections of the eye, kidney, liver or brain, but such cases are very rare.

Those, then, are the hard facts about *Candida*, with which few doctors would disagree. On other points, there is great controversy.

In recent years, *Candida* has come under suspicion as a common cause of diarrhoea, wind and bloating, sometimes with abdominal pain. The main reason for pointing the accusing finger at *Candida* is that these symptoms are sometimes accompanied by itching around the anus and, in women, by recurrent bouts of thrush. Intrigued by this cluster of symptoms, some doctors tried out anti-fungal treatments, consisting of a low-sugar, low-yeast diet, often combined with anti-fungal drugs such as nystatin, taken by mouth for several months. For some people, this treatment has proved very effective in curing their diarrhoea and wind.

This led to the conclusion that *Candida* was definitely a cause of the diarrhoea and wind, an idea that is now being critically reviewed. The main evidence against it is that one cannot detect any more *Candida* in the intestine of people who supposedly have 'candidiasis' than in healthy people. The argument often proposed to counter this is that the *Candida* is, for some reason, undetectable by conventional methods. The idea is that *Candida* might grow in a different form, known as a hyphal form, which resembles a bread mould – long chains of fungus, instead of round, individual cells typical of a yeast. In its hyphal form, so the argument goes, *Candida* clings tight to the gut wall and so escapes detection in the faeces. It is true that *Candida* can switch forms in this way, but there is no evidence that it actually does so in the gut. If it did, it would be almost certain to shed yeast-type cells of *Candida* into the faeces as well, and these would therefore be detected in abnormally high numbers by the usual tests. Doctors who have made intensive studies of the gut flora, such as Dr John Hunter, find this theory increasingly unlikely. 'If there *was* a massive overgrowth of *Candida* in these patients, as there is supposed to be, I'm sure we would have found evidence of it by now. The fact is they have about as much *Candida* in the gut as everyone else.'

Skin-prick tests and intradermal tests for *Candida* have also been tried for patients with supposed candidiasis, and it is true that some show positive reactions – they are making an immune response to *Candida* antigens. But many healthy people also show positive immune reactions to *Candida*, so these tests do not mean very much. And some people who have been diagnosed as having candidiasis do not react to a skin test. In short, *Candida* is beginning to look like a red herring.

But the fact remains that some people *do* recover from diarrhoea and wind when treated with a low-sugar, low-yeast diet. (And, curiously, a number of these patients had previously been eating large quantities of yeast extract.) Nystatin also seems to aid recovery in some of these patients.

It is also true that, for some people at least, there are other symptoms that clear up at the same time. These can include fatigue, poor concentration, irritability, headaches, migraine, aching joints and muscles, hypoglycaemia (low blood sugar), premenstrual problems, irregular periods, sinusitis, urticaria, psoriasis and asthma (both very rarely). How these symptoms might be caused is another matter entirely, and equally controversial, so we will come back to this later.

If not *Candida*, then what? It is rather like the moment in a detective novel when it becomes clear that the jilted fiancée, despite having the motive, the means and the opportunity, *and* being a thoroughly nasty character, is actually innocent. Unfortunately, this is a detective story with no neat ending, as yet. But there are two theories currently on offer – gut fermentation syndrome and gut flora toxins. They are not, strictly speaking, alternative ideas – there are as many similarities between them as there are differences. Only time will tell which is closer to the truth.

Gut fermentation syndrome

This theory holds that there is some imbalance in the gut flora which results in carbohydrates (starches and sugars) being fermented to produce alcohol. Slightly raised levels of alcohol are said to be detectable in the blood, and the symptoms experienced (or some of them at least) are attributed to this alcohol. The symptoms attributed to 'gut fermentation syndrome' are diarrhoea or constipation (or bouts of both), bloating, wind, itching around the anus and genital region, lethargy, poor concentration and memory, inability to think quickly, runny nose or phlegmy cough, sometimes with asthma, recurrent sinusitis, and a craving for sugar. It is not suggested that every patient with 'GFS' has all these symptoms, and no one symptom is always present. The spectrum of symptoms described would take in most cases of supposed candidiasis, but would not cover all the symptoms claimed for *Candida*. Proponents of gut fermentation syndrome suggest that other, associated, problems could explain these – food intolerance, perhaps, or hyperventilation.

The advocates of gut fermentation syndrome do not suggest which microbes in the gut flora might be at fault. Yeasts are a candidate, but not the only ones. They believe that the anti-fungal drug, nystatin, has produced a 'false clue' in this particular mystery. Because it seems to benefit people with diarrhoea, it has created the impression that *Candida* or other yeasts are responsible for that diarrhoea. Nystatin is an anti-fungal drug, and yeasts are fungi – it seemed an obvious connection. But as Dr Keith Eaton, a proponent of 'gut fermentation syndrome', points out, nystatin affects the body in another way, by stabilizing the membranes that line the intestine. This might produce an improvement in symptoms such as diarrhoea even though yeasts had nothing to do with causing the problem.

One related issue should be mentioned here. This is a relatively rare problem, but one which seems to affect Japanese people more than others. Some produce quite large amounts of alcohol from a starchy or sugary meal – enough to become intoxicated. Known as 'auto-brewery syndrome', this disorder is different from the gut fermentation syndrome described here.

Gut flora toxins

This is a theory that has been developed, over many years, by Dr John Hunter of Addenbrooke's Hospital in Cambridge. He believes that, in patients with irritable bowel syndrome, for example, there is an overgrowth of certain microbes in the gut, and a shortage of 'good' microbes. This may result from excessive use of antibiotics, a bad bout of diarrhoea following an infection, radiation treatment or surgery.

But, in Dr Hunter's view, the gut flora disturbance alone is only part of the problem for IBS patients. He suspects that, in addition, they cannot break down the toxins produced by the gut flora as well as they should. So the gut flora produce *more toxins* than in healthy people, *and* the toxins cannot be broken down efficiently. This double defect might produce some of the other symptoms that often accompany IBS, such as headaches and joint pains. (What other doctors have called 'candidiasis' would, in Dr Hunter's view, be cases of IBS.)

As far as Dr Hunter is concerned, alcohol production is not an important aspect of IBS. He believes that the alcohol levels claimed in 'gut fermentation syndrome' are too small to have much effect – or even to be accurately measured.

There is one very interesting aspect of Dr Hunter's theory. He believes that it might be the key to *all* food intolerance, no matter what the symptoms. In his view, one might explain rheumatoid arthritis or migraine in just the same way. Where a patient has a specific reaction to, say, oranges, Dr Hunter believes that the patient's gut flora is guilty of making a particular toxin from something that is found in oranges. Alternatively, oranges might contain a particular vitamin or other nutrient, that allows certain bacteria to grow at the expense of others, because it is something that they especially need. Those bacteria might be ones that produce a particular toxin which the patient cannot break down.

There are only a few documented examples of bacterial toxins that cannot be broken down due to defective enzymes. One is a chemical called p-cresol that seems to play a role in hyperkinetic syndrome in children (see p244). Another possible candidate is a substance produced by an abnormal bacterium which may play a part in Crohn's disease. This substance seems to attract immune cells into the gut, and thus set up a damaging immune reaction. Whether defective enzymes play a part in allowing this substance to survive in the gut is not known.

An unsolved mystery

All this may sound very confusing, with doctors disagreeing about such fundamental matters as whether Disease A and Disease B are the same thing or two entirely different things. If you are feeling puzzled, you may find it useful to read the sections on pp89–91, entitled *Safety in numbers* and *Different doctors, different patients*. They attempt to explain some of the problems involved in identifying diseases, naming them and categorizing them.

You will, however, probably be more interested in getting well than in the intricacies of medical detective stories! If you have a number of the symptoms listed in Table 4, then it may be worth trying a no-sugar no-yeast (NS-NY) diet. Experience shows that this diet can be very helpful for some people, and it will certainly do you no harm to cut out sugar and yeast for a while. The only real inconvenience is that you cannot eat bread, but you can always have soda bread, pitta bread, or chapattis instead (although some pitta breads do contain yeast, so make sure you read the label).

You will probably find it difficult to decide whether to try this diet or the elimination diet first. It is impossible to say which is more likely to work for you. But there is a good argument for first trying the elimination diet (Stages 2 and 3 of the diet are described in Chapter Fourteen), because it produces a much quicker response than the NS-NY diet. If the elimination diet is going to work for you, you will generally know within 10–14 days (see p280). The NS-NY diet may take 4 weeks or more to produce noticeable effects, and they are generally gradual, whereas the elimination diet tends to produce a dramatic 'overnight' improvement, usually after about a week. In general, it would be better to work through the diet described in Chapter Fourteen, then come back to the NS-NY diet later if you have not benefited at all.

Notice, however, that the first stage of the three-stage diet described in Chapter Fourteen excludes all sugar anyway. For some people, this alone is enough – there is no need to exclude fruit, starches and yeast as well. If you get *partially* well at this stage, you could try out the NS-NY diet next, while continuing with the healthy-eating restrictions on coffee, tea etc. If there is no further improvement, you could then go on to Stage 2 of the elimination diet.

Before deciding what to do, please read through the NS-NY diet thoroughly,

GERALD

As a young man, Gerald had suffered a severe bladder infection for which he needed prolonged treatment with antibiotics. Although the infection cleared up, he was left with a mild diarrhoea that proved very persistent. Five or six bowel movements a day were not uncommon. Fortunately, Gerald found an office job, with a national charity, and his symptoms were only a slight inconvenience. But in later years, as he was promoted to more senior posts, he found that he had to travel more and more to oversee fund-raising projects. The symptoms that he had put up with for 20 years now became a real problem. Sometimes he had to leave important meetings hurriedly and rush to the lavatory, which he found extremely embarrassing. His doctor offered him drugs that would control the diarrhoea, but these were only partially effective. Eventually he was referred to a consultant who took a careful case-history and wondered if there might be some connection between the heavy doses of antibiotics he had received as a young man and the continuing diarrhoea. He explained to Gerald that by killing off beneficial bacteria in the gut, antibiotics can open the way for excessive growth by yeasts. Gerald was asked to try a diet containing no sugar or white flour and was given an anti-fungal drug, nystatin. At first there was little change, but after about three weeks his bowel symptoms were much improved. He now has only two or three bowel movements a day, and these are much more predictable and less urgent, which makes travelling easier. A number of activities that were closed to him before – such as camping and sailing – are now a possibility. As a result he gets more exercise and is generally fitter and healthier.

then read Chapter Fourteen carefully too. Plan your diet strategy carefully – it may help to write down what you intend to do. Don't rush at it, or do either of the diets in a half-hearted, indecisive way, swapping from one to the other. You need to be really clear in your mind which diet you are trying out, and what foods you should avoid.

TABLE 4   SYMPTOMS THAT MAY RESPOND TO A NS-NY DIET

Diarrhoea or other bowel disturbances
Wind, bloating, abdominal discomfort or pain
Headache or migraine
Fatigue, poor concentration, irritability, slowness of thought
Joint pains, sometimes with swollen joints
Aching muscles
Urticaria (nettle-rash)
Itchy anus, with the inflammation sometimes spreading to the buttocks
   and thighs
Premenstrual tension and irregular periods
Psoriasis and other skin complaints
Asthma, but only very rarely
Recurrent *Candida* ('thrush') infections in the throat or vagina
Recurrent cystitis, not due to bacterial infection
Recurrent fungal infections of the skin
Craving for sweet foods (this can also be caused by hypoglycaemia, see
   p135)

The no-sugar, no-yeast diet
Step 1
There seems to be some unexplained connection between contraceptive pills
and the condition that has previously been labelled 'candidiasis'. If you are on
the Pill, you should ask your doctor about changing to some other form of
contraception. Women who have been on the Pill may have nutritional
deficiencies (see p270) and you may wish to take a nutritional supplement of
the kind described on p333. It is a good idea to wait for one to three months,
after coming off the Pill, to see what effect this has – for some women, the Pill
itself is the unsuspected source of vague health problems, so the diet may be
unnecessary.

Assuming you continue, the first step should be a sugar-free diet – for some
people this is all that is needed. The foods to avoid are shown in Table 5. If
you are taking any medicines in syrup form, ask your doctor if he or she can
prescribe a sugar-free alternative. Artificial sweeteners can be used if required
(see p337), but it is best to break the 'sweetness addiction' altogether if
possible. Total abstinence from any sweeteners can cure a sweet tooth
permanently – which is much better in the long term. After a few weeks on an
unsweetened diet, it is remarkable how disgusting anything sugary tastes.

Stay on this diet for at least a month. If there is some improvement, persist
for another month or two. If you are no better at all, then go on to Step 2.

Step 2

If the sugar-free diet does not do the trick, the next step is to cut out all fruit for a while. White bread and anything made with white flour (*eg* pastry, pasta) should also be excluded. Wholemeal bread and flour can be eaten instead, as these are broken down more slowly and do not release glucose all at once. But they should only be eaten in small quantities, as should potatoes. The bulk of the diet should be made up of vegetables and high-protein foods, such as meat, fish, eggs and cheese.

Eat plenty of freshly-crushed garlic, as this is thought to combat yeasts in the gut. Fresh herbs and green, leafy vegetables, such as spinach and 'greens', are also recommended as they contain anti-fungal agents. It may also be worth trying a herbal tea, called taheebo or pau d'arco – it is said to have anti-fungal properties, although this has not been verified scientifically. For suppliers, see p336. Eating live yoghurt may also be worthwhile, as it contains some of the 'useful' members of the gut flora, and may help to re-establish a healthy balance among the inhabitants of the gut (see pp199–200).

Giving up fruit may make you concerned about Vitamin C deficiency, but if you eat sufficient quantities of *fresh* vegetables this should not be a problem. Cabbage, broccoli and brussels sprouts are rich in Vitamin C, and potatoes are a valuable source. It is important not to soak potatoes, as this leaches out the vitamin, and not to overcook cabbage and other green vegetables, as heat

ALAN

Alan developed a severe throat infection after swimming in the sea near a polluted stretch of beach. He was treated with antibiotics and his throat healed, but soon afterwards he developed red, itchy bumps all over his body – nettle-rash. He asked the doctor if the two events might be connected but was told this was most unlikely. The nettle-rash got somewhat better in time, but it continued to bother him at regular intervals for the next 20 years. In his forties it grew worse and he decided to see a specialist. When Alan mentioned that he had taken a lot of antibiotics just before the urticaria began, the specialist suggested that he try a diet with no sugar and very little starch. At the same time he was given a course of anti-fungal drugs. The nettle-rash cleared up promptly and has not returned.

LOUISA

Louisa was about 46 when she began to be troubled by unsightly red blotches on her face. She worked as an assistant in a dress shop and it was important that she looked smart. She found that she was having to wear more and more make-up to cover these blemishes. Before deciding on the best treatment, the doctor asked her about her health generally. It emerged that she had suffered from mild diarrhoea and wind for some years, but had not thought it worth bothering the doctor about these minor problems. She had also been feeling very tired, and had some pain and stiffness in her joints, which she thought was 'just her age'. Checking through her notes, the doctor saw that she had been treated for vaginal thrush on several occasions. The doctor had no idea what might be causing the red blotches, but he did have a suspicion that the other symptoms might have a common cause. He put Louisa on a diet which excluded all sugar and most starch. She found this very difficult to keep to, as she had a sweet tooth and loved cakes. But she persisted, and after two months her bowels were functioning normally, she felt far more energetic, and her joint pains had vanished. At about the same time the red blotches on Louisa's face also disappeared.

gradually destroys Vitamin C. Rosehip tea is also an excellent source of this vitamin, as is fresh lemon juice, which is permissible on this diet as it contains little sugar.

Again, you should stay on this diet for at least a month, and longer if you begin to feel partially better. If there is a good improvement on this diet, fruit and other excluded foods can be gradually reintroduced later, but not sugar. If you feel *worse* on this diet, then you may have food intolerance – to eggs or cheese, for example.

Step 3
If there is little or no improvement on the Step 2 diet, then cut out all yeast-containing foods. These are listed in Table 6.

It is sometimes claimed that yeasts in the gut derive nourishment from yeasts in food, but this is not the case. The reason for avoiding yeast is simply that you may be sensitive to it. The distinction is important, because if you are *very* sensitive to yeast, even the smallest amount can make you ill, so scrupulous avoidance is necessary, especially at first.

If there is a partial reponse to this diet, then it is a positive sign, and you should consider going on to Step 4. If there is no reponse at all, it might be a good idea to try an elimination diet instead at this point, if food intolerance is suspected. You can always come back to this diet later.

Step 4

This is a very drastic diet, and should not be started without medical advice. Carbohydrates – the 'starchy' substances in foods – are restricted to 80 gm per day. This effectively means *no* potatoes, bread, flour, rice, breakfast cereals, pasta or other starchy foods, except for one very small portion each day. The incidental carbohydrate in vegetables, nuts and other foods will account for most of your daily allowance. High-carbohydrate vegetables such as sweetcorn, peas, parsnip, lentils and broad beans should be avoided. Nuts can be eaten in moderation, but not cashew nuts as they are rich in carbohydrate. Continue to eat plenty of garlic and fresh, green leafy vegetables.

Keeping the problem at bay

This diet is not a life-long cure – the problem can come back if you revert to your old eating habits. Once you are fully better, and have been so for some time, you can risk the occasional slice of white bread or a sliver of cake. But you should try to eat as little sugar and refined carbohydrate (white flour, pasta etc) as possible. Beware of 'sugar-free' commercial products such as cakes and jams, especially those from healthfood shops – often they are made with fruit-juice concentrate and are just as rich in natural fruit sugars as if they were made with cane or beet sugar. Diabetic products *are* suitable however. If your symptoms start to return, then you must immediately cut out all sugar again.

If you only recovered on Step 3 of the diet, then you are probably sensitive to yeast. In a few cases, this reaction to yeast is permanent, but most people lose their sensitivity after several months of avoiding yeast products. Some people may have to avoid eating yeast every day (see p285).

Some of those who have been successfully treated will still have residual problems due to food intolerance. Although an elimination diet may be needed to sort this out, going straight on to another restricted diet is not a good idea. It is advisable to stay on a normal, varied diet for a while (while still avoiding sugar and white flour, of course). This will give you plenty of vitamins and minerals, to build you up for the elimination diet. In some cases, it may be a good idea to take a nutritional supplement (see p333).

TABLE 5   FOODS CONTAINING SUGAR

White and brown sugar
Honey
Golden syrup
Treacle
Molasses
Maple syrup
Malt
Barley sweetener (macrobiotic sweetener)
Jam, including 'no added sugar' jam
Chutney and pickles
Cakes
Biscuits
Ice-cream
Puddings
Chocolate and other sweets
Fizzy drinks and fruit squash
Any food labelled: corn syrup, dextrose, fructose, glucose, maltose,
    sucrose or sugar
Baked beans, including 'no added sugar' brands
Peanut butter (except sugar-free brands, sold in health food shops)
Some other apparently savoury foods contain sugar – some tinned
    soups for example, and some meat pies
Some medicines, especially syrups and coated tablets
Dried fruits, which are rich in natural sugars, should not be eaten
Anything that tastes sweet should be regarded with suspicion, unless
    designed for diabetics

GIARDIA

Giardia was, until recently, thought to be a harmless member of the gut flora, because it was sometimes found in the intestines of apparently healthy people. Only within the last few years have doctors begun to realize that this microbe can cause disease. It is found throughout the world, and about 5–15 per cent of people are infected. In Britain, these are usually people who have travelled abroad, especially to the tropics, which is where *Giardia* probably originated.

Giardia lives in the gut and produces microscopic hard-walled cysts that pass out of the body with the faeces. These can get into food or water, especially in countries with poor sanitary facilities, and thus infect other people. *Giardia* cysts are resistant to chlorine, at least in the amounts usually used for disinfecting water supplies.

TABLE 6　FOODS CONTAINING YEAST

Main sources of yeast

Bread, including some pitta bread and pizza, but excluding soda bread, matzos and chapattis

Buns and cakes made with yeast *eg* doughnuts

Yeast extract (Marmite, Vegemite etc)

Oxo cubes and most other stock cubes (for non-yeast instant stock see pp312 and 336)

Bovril

Anything labelled 'hydrolysed vegetable protein'

Beer, wine and cider

Vinegar and pickles

Sauerkraut

Vitamin tablets containing B vitamins, unless labelled 'yeast-free'

Secondary sources of yeast

Dried fruit

Over-ripe fruit

Any unpeeled fruit

Commercial fruit juices

Anything labelled 'malt'

Yoghurt, buttermilk and sour cream

Synthetic cream

Soy sauce

Tofu

Any leftover food, unless eaten within 24 hours, or 48 hours if in a refrigerator

Whiskey, vodka, gin, brandy and other spirits

Other sources of fungi which may affect some people

Mushrooms, puffballs, truffles and other edible fungi

Quorn, mycoprotein (meat substitutes derived from fungi)

Cheese, especially Brie and Camembert

Yeasts and moulds in the air

You should stay away from damp houses, greenhouses (unless very dry and clean), compost heaps and rotting leaves. After you have been on the diet for a while, you can test whether such exposure makes you ill.

For most people who become infested with *Giardia* there are no symptoms. Such people are infectious however, and if they are involved in food preparation and are careless about washing their hands, they may be the modern equivalent of 'Typhoid Mary', passing *Giardia* on to others.

Those who do suffer symptoms, when infected by *Giardia*, experience an acute attack of watery diarrhoea, with bloating, abdominal pain, belching and fatigue. This usually clears up of its own accord after a few days – thereafter the person has no symptoms but may remain infectious. However, some patients continue to suffer milder symptoms. Their main problem is that food is not absorbed from the gut properly. This produces loose, frequent stools, often foul-smelling and frothy. There may also be flatulence, pain, nausea, loss of appetite, weakness and weight loss. Children with this disease – and they are the most susceptible group – are often pale and stunted.

There may also be a milder form of the disease, in which there is no diarrhoea as such – discomfort, wind, belching and nausea are the main symptoms in these cases. Urticaria (nettle-rash), joint pains and feverishness may also be present. Not surprisingly, some of these patients are thought to have food intolerance. Indeed, many *do*, because *Giardia* seems to be linked in some way to food sensitivity.

Giardia infection can be diagnosed by looking for the parasite in the stools. It is treated by a short course of drugs, the main one used being metronidazole. This can have some side-effects, such as nausea and vomiting, but only has to be taken for about a week. Unfortunately, it seems to make yeast overgrowth more likely, so anyone taking it would be well advised to adopt a sugar-free diet during the treatment, and for a month or so afterwards.

TREATING A DISTURBED GUT FLORA

In theory, the way to treat a disturbed gut flora is to repopulate the gut with the 'good' bacteria, and so exclude the more damaging bacteria and yeasts. Unfortunately, a reliable treatment of this sort is not widely available yet. At present, the best treatment is to eat live yoghurt, which includes one of the most important bacteria in the gut, *Lactobacillus*. There are also commercial preparations of bacteria which are intended to restore the normal flora of the gut. Some of these have been tested by Dr John Hunter of Addenbrooke's Hospital, who found very few live bacteria in them, making them less useful than live yoghurt.

To ensure that the brand of yoghurt you are buying really is live, add a spoonful to some warm milk that has been heated to boiling point and then allowed to cool. Keep the mixture in a vacuum flask for 6–8 hours. If it has not turned to yoghurt, then the original yoghurt was not live. The best way of ensuring your yoghurt is live is to make your own – starter cultures are available from some healthfood stores, or by post (see p337).

If you cannot eat yoghurt, because of a sensitivity to milk, then commercial preparations of bacteria might be worth considering, but ask to see a bacteriological analysis showing how many *live* bacteria there are per gram (there should be several million) before buying.

Chapter Eleven

FOOD PROBLEMS IN CHILDREN

The other chapters in this book apply equally to adults *and* children, but a special chapter on children's food problems is necessary because there are important medical differences between young patients and older ones. Altering the diet is also far more risky for a child than it is for an adult, so there are more difficult decisions to be made before embarking on an elimination diet. This chapter is intended as a supplement to the earlier ones, for those with a special interest in children's problems. *Parents reading this book with a view to helping their children are strongly advised to read the earlier chapters as well as this one.*

Food allergy and intolerance in children

Food allergy generally begins in childhood, while food intolerance can begin at any time of life. Having said that, there is often no clear distinction between allergy and intolerance (see p9), especially in children. Those with proven allergies, such as asthma or eczema, may show other symptoms that most self-respecting allergists would have nothing to do with – hyperactivity, for example, or muscle aches. If these clear up along with the allergic symptoms when certain foods are withdrawn, then is it allergy or intolerance? To avoid the problem, we will use the term 'food sensitivity', to cover both allergy and intolerance.

Over the past ten years, doctors have begun to recognize just how many different childhood problems can be caused by food sensitivity. Colic, eczema, asthma, persistent runny nose, glue ear, headaches, migraine, and even behavioural problems, have all been traced back to certain foods or food additives. These discoveries have a bittersweet taste for the many mothers who have been told by their doctors that they themselves were at the root of such

---

TABLE 7 SYMPTOMS THAT MAY BE DUE TO FOOD SENSITIVITY IN CHILDREN

The page numbers show where these problems are discussed in detail

Digestive system
Vomiting
Colic, in babies (p203)
Persistent diarrhoea (p210)
Diarrhoea with blood or mucus in the stools (p138)
Poor appetite and failure to grow, in babies
Stomach aches, in older children

Nose, ears and lungs
Rhinitis (runny or congested nose) (p37, p56)
Glue ear (p38)
Asthma (p41, p55)

Skin
Eczema (p45, p58)
Urticaria (hives or nettle-rash) (p44, p60)

Nervous system
Headaches (p125)
Migraine (p96, p126)
Epileptic fits, where these accompany migraine (p134)
Hyperkinetic syndrome (hyperactivity) (p213)

Other symptoms
Aching joints (p122)
Muscle aches (p121)
Rheumatoid arthritis (p124)
Some types of kidney disease (p75)

---

problems – because they were over-anxious, inexperienced, nervy, over-indulgent or whatever. This sort of 'diagnosis' is usually based on minimal evidence and does untold harm to the self-confidence of mothers at a time when they most need help and support. Anxious, inexperienced mothers *can* be the source of their child's mysterious health problems, of course, but there is increasing evidence that it is commonly something in the diet or the environment. There is also evidence that children who show food sensitivity in their early years are more likely to develop other health problems later, often continuing – or reappearing – in their adult lives. Helping these children to adapt to their environment is therefore important, and putting their symptoms down to poor mothering, without any evidence, is irresponsible and potentially damaging.

It is now believed that babies can be sensitized to food even before they are born, because a few food molecules, from food the mother eats, can reach the baby in her womb (see p255). More importantly, food molecules get into the mother's breast milk, and babies that are exclusively breast-fed can be ill because of the sort of food the mother is eating. Although sensitivity to cow's milk is by far the most common problem in babies and children, all sorts of other foods have been implicated. These relatively recent discoveries have meant that food sensitivity can now be recognized and dealt with far more effectively. They have also suggested ways in which parents can reduce the risk of food sensitivity in their children, as explained on pp250–7.

The common features of food sensitivity in children are listed in Table 7. Of these, asthma, eczema and rhinitis (runny or congested nose) are all examples of 'classical allergies' and they are therefore dealt with in Chapter Three. Glue ear, which frequently follows on from rhinitis, is also described there. Treating these conditions is discussed in Chapter Four, although anyone who is interested in investigating the role of food should also read pp221–7 of this chapter. Symptoms that fall outside the allergic camp, and which also affect adults – such as headaches, migraines, nausea, diarrhoea and rheumatoid arthritis – are discussed in Chapter Seven.

COLIC

Colic is a sharp pain in the stomach or intestines of a baby, that causes it to cry uncontrollably. Crying is more usual in the evenings and the baby may draw its legs up as it cries and become very red in the face. Because the attacks are most common in the first ten to twelve weeks of life, the name 'three-month colic' is often used.

The colic controversy

Of course, it is not always easy to tell why a baby is crying – there may be many different causes. Even the question of how much crying is 'natural' is contentious. The following quotations illustrate the widely differing views of this common problem:

'During the first few weeks of life the average baby sleeps a great deal but, when awake, cries lustily and often. . . . It is only from about six weeks of age

TABLE 8   SOME MINOR SYMPTOMS THAT MAY ACCOMPANY COLIC

Frequent regurgitation of food (posseting)
Loose stools
Wind and bloating
Constipation
Poor appetite, stops feeding and screams after a few minutes
Stuffy or runny nose, nose-rubbing
Frequent sneezing, coughing, sniffing or snorting
Noisy breathing
Frequent hiccoughs
Frequent ear infections or colds
Bad breath
Dry, cracked skin, rashes, eczema
Constant scratching or rubbing
Sweatiness, slight fever, or cold hands and feet
Redness around mouth or anus, or on cheeks
Swelling around eyes

(Adapted from *Food for Thought* by Maureen Minchin, with permission)

onwards, when the baby is becoming aware of his or her surroundings, that there are some wakeful periods without crying. . . . There is no reason why the simple milk diet (whether natural or otherwise) of the normal baby should cause tummy ache. If the baby cries uncontrollably for several hours each evening, it is more likely that the cause is so-called 3-month or 10-week *colic* (sharp tummy ache). But, although some doctors consider that the baby has genuine physical pain, others believe that this is an example of the baby reacting to the tensions of the mother at the end of a hard day: and they believe that the crying stops after 10 to 12 weeks because by then the mother has become more competent and confident in her handling of the baby, and has communicated this new calmness to the baby.' (*The Macmillan Guide to Family Health*, edited by Dr Tony Smith).

'We in the West regard infant crying as normal, and in a thousand different ways condition our children to associate babies with bawling. But in societies where infants are exclusively breast-fed from birth and in contact with their non-allergic, non-food-bingeing, non-smoking mothers, "colic" is unknown and infant crying is seen as a sign of distress, which warrants immediate attention. And that is exactly what it sounds like to the new mother, until she is persuaded by others, against every instinct she possesses, that this is "normal" or "naughty" . . . Crying, colic and night-waking are only a tiny portion of the range of symptoms which experienced mothers report as disappearing and reappearing with dietary changes – changes in maternal diet for the breast-feeding mother, or changes in infant diet directly. These symptoms range from minor oddities [See Table 8] to serious problems. In the series of mothers followed up, those who consistently reported the minor symptoms were regarded as neurotic or overprotective. Yet these same mothers found that over months there was often a gradual increase in the severity of symptoms . . . The question should be asked, would the serious symptoms ever have appeared had the mother identified and avoided the dietary allergen responsible? Mothers were almost never taken seriously until the child had gross symptoms . . . Maternal anxiety is an appropriate response to the experience of living with a crying baby – but what physiological mechanism exists to explain the notion that anxiety *causes* colic? In my experience, babies are remarkably placid through all sorts of family rows, so long as they are warm and well fed; while they will infallibly disrupt the most harmonious scene if they have a pain.' (*Food for Thought*, Maureen Minchin.)

JAMIE

Claire's eight-week-old baby, Jamie, was apparently healthy but cried a lot of the time, and seemed to be in pain. As Claire was breast-feeding, her doctor asked about her diet and found that she was a vegetarian. She explained that she had been eating more cheese and drinking an extra pint of milk a day to make sure she got enough protein during pregnancy and breast-feeding. The doctor suggested that she might avoid milk, cheese and butter for a while, to see if this had any effect, and prescribed some tablets to give her extra calcium. He persuaded her to eat a little fish to make up for the missing protein. A couple of days after starting this diet, Jamie's crying was noticeably less and it became easier to get him to sleep each evening. Claire was delighted at the improvement. She tried drinking a glass of milk, to see what would happen, and 24 hours later Jamie, following a feed, suffered, a severe attack of colic. After that, Claire stayed on a milk-free diet for six weeks. She then introduced a little milk and butter into her diet and found that Jamie could now tolerate this.

Is there any scientific evidence for either of these opposing views? The main piece of evidence for the 'tense-mother/crying-baby' idea is that first babies tend to cry more than subsequent ones – doctors infer from this that the mother's inexperience is an important factor. However, there are no data to show that first babies really do cry more – it is just a subjective impression. One study that investigated this idea found that there was little difference between first babies and later ones. Even if a first baby *does* cry more, the link with maternal anxiety is still only a speculative one, and there are other, far more plausible explanations.

The evidence for the second point of view is limited, but certainly stronger than that for the first. A Swedish study of 19 bottle-fed babies with colic found that over 70 per cent improved when changed to formula feeds that did not contain whole cow's-milk protein. The same research team found that cow's milk in the mother's diet could cause colic in breast-fed babies.

Another trial carried out in New Zealand, and widely quoted in the medical literature, apparently failed to find any link between the mother's diet and colic in breast-fed babies. In fact there were several serious flaws in this trial, and its findings have been widely misrepresented anyway. Twenty mothers were involved, and the main focus of the trial was the role of cow's milk in causing colic. The mothers were asked to avoid cow's milk, and were then challenged with it in a disguised form, so that they would not know when they were drinking milk and when they were drinking the 'control' substance. Soya milk was used for this 'control' without any investigation of whether the babies might be sensitive to soya proteins. The mothers were given milk-with-soya to drink for two days or soya only for two days – there was an interval of two, four or six days between the milk challenges. Experience suggests that this may not be long enough to detect changes in the baby's symptoms – although some babies recover within 24 hours of the mother eliminating offending foods from her diet, others can take many days, sometimes as much as two weeks, for their colic to settle down. The whole trial only continued for 12 days.

Interestingly enough, the researchers *did* notice a link between the foods the mother ate and her baby's symptoms. They observed that the colic was worst in those babies whose mothers ate all the commonly implicated foods such as milk, eggs, chocolate, nuts and fish. The fewer foods the mother ate from this list, the less severe was the colic. They concluded that the mother's diet 'may influence the likelihood of infantile colic in breast-fed children, but that the source of the colic cannot be attributed to a single dietary component [*ie* milk]. It may however involve a variety of foodstuffs.' *Despite this clear statement of their findings, this paper is widely quoted as showing that there is no link between colic and maternal diet.*

Other evidence supporting the second point of view comes from a retrospective study of 68 children with proven sensitivity to cow's milk. When the medical history of these children was investigated, it turned out that a very high proportion had persistent screaming and colic as babies. This is only circumstantial evidence for a link between food sensitivity and colic, of course, but it is of interest. And it gives support to the idea that treating the colic is important, because the children in the study all had serious health problems as a result of their sensitivity to milk – problems that might have been avoided if they had been taken off cow's milk at an earlier age.

One aspect of colic is difficult to explain from either viewpoint – the fact that the symptoms tend to disappear or diminish at about three months of age. The traditional explanation is that *all* mothers with colicky babies – regardless of what sort of people they are or what else is happening in their lives – suddenly become more confident and relaxed at this point. This seems implausible, to say the least, but is there an alternative explanation that is compatible with food intolerance? One possibility is that the colic represents an initial 'crisis' reaction as the child is exposed to large amounts of cow's-milk or other foreign proteins. The child later 'adapts' to the problem foods, and the colic apparently clears up, but its sensitivity continues in the form of other, less acute symptoms, such as eczema, asthma or diarrhoea. There is ample evidence from case-histories that this might happen – and the retrospective study described above supports the idea.

Lactose – the sugar found in milk

Before considering what can be done about colic, we need to look at the question of lactose and lactose intolerance. **Lactose** is the main sugar found in all animal milks, including human breast milk (the name means 'milk sugar'). Unlike most sugars, it does not taste sweet – if it did milk would be quite sugary to the taste-buds because it is loaded with lactose.

In order to break down lactose, we have an enzyme (see p18) known as **lactase** (the *-ase* ending denotes an enzyme) in our intestines. Almost all babies have this enzyme, although there are *rare* cases in which the enzyme is entirely lacking – these babies are likely to be detected soon after birth because they are made seriously ill by any sort of milk, cow's or human. Adults tend to lose this enzyme unless they continue taking cow's milk and milk products from the time they are weaned onwards. In China and Southeast Asia, where milk and cheese are not part of the diet, most adults are lactase-deficient, but they can regain the ability to produce lactase if they persist in drinking milk.

If a child or adult lacks the ability to deal with lactose, the sugar passes through into the intestine, where it provides a bonanza for waiting bacteria.

They consume the sugar, giving off gas and toxic products as they grow and multiply. These toxins then cause unpleasant symptoms such as pain and diarrhoea. They may be at the root of colic, which is why lactose intolerance is important here.

Following a bout of diarrhoea – due to an infection or whatever other cause – the digestive processes in our intestines take a little while to get back to normal. During this recovery period, there is often far less lactase produced by the gut lining than there is normally. This is something that happens in both children and adults, and it may cause a continuation of the diarrhoea if milk is consumed after an infection. Formula feeds without lactose are available, and your doctor may be able to prescribe one for you for a time, if your baby has had gastroenteritis and continues to have colic or diarrhoea afterwards. In the case of breast-fed babies, it is probably better, on balance, to continue breast-feeding, even though breast milk contains lactose. In general, children and adults should not be given too much milk to drink if they are recovering from a stomach upset. Yoghurt and cheese (but not cottage cheese) are usually tolerated because they contain far less lactose. Soya milk is lactose-free.

It is also possible that some small babies have insufficient lactase to cope with very large feeds – they can digest small feeds, but if their morning feed is larger than usual, the extra lactose overwhelms their capacity to cope with it. This could explain why some babies only have colic in the evening, when the morning feed reaches the intestines and the bacteria that live there begin to feed on the undigested lactose. This theory has recently been investigated scientifically, and the results suggest that it could well be correct.

In the past, it was often assumed that all babies who could not tolerate milk were lactase-deficient, and this idea is still current in some quarters. It is now known that most children who are sensitive to cow's milk are actually reacting to the proteins it contains. But the diarrhoea produced by this reaction may, in turn, cause lactase deficiency. Doctors refer to this as **secondary lactase deficiency**. There are readily available tests for lactase deficiency, but these do not distinguish between true lactase deficiency (or **primary lactase deficiency**) and secondary lactase deficiency. More complicated tests can distinguish the two, and these show that primary lactase deficiency is actually very rare. So if you are told that your baby is lactase deficient after some routine tests, you should be prepared to question the diagnosis and ask your doctor to help you investigate the possibility of food sensitivity, as described in the following section.

What to do about colic

The first and most important step is to get the baby examined by a doctor, who should check for serious problems such as gastro-oesophageal reflux –

acid passing from the stomach up into the gullet (oesophagus), and thus causing pain – or intestinal obstruction. Assuming that there are no such problems, and that your doctor can suggest no other likely causes for the excessive crying, then it is worth investigating the possible role of food.

Bottle-fed babies

Try giving smaller, more frequent feeds as an initial step – if the baby has slight difficulties with lactose (see above) then this may be the answer. Should this produce no improvement, then follow the measures described on pp221–3.

Breast-fed babies

There are two main possibilities to be considered here: temporary lactose intolerance or other forms of food sensitivity.

If your baby only has colic in the evening, then a temporary deficit in lactase, due to the morning feed being larger than usual, is a possibility (see p208). There are various ways of reducing the amount of milk in the morning feed, and these are worth trying. The simplest approach is to let the baby feed first from one breast only and then from the other – rather than keep switching breasts. This reduces the amount of milk produced overall. If this has no effect, try expressing some milk before the morning feed; refrigerate or freeze it for use later. For advice on how to express milk contact one of the breast-feeding advice groups whose addresses are given on p339. Another method is to give the baby a small amount of boiled water from a bottle before the morning feed, so that it feels full more quickly, or to feed from one breast only – this will tend to reduce your supply of milk overall, so you should only do this if you know your milk is plentiful.

For the baby who does not respond to this, or who has colic at any time of day, food intolerance should be investigated (see pp223–5).

Smoking and babies don't mix!

One significant measure that any mother with a colicky baby should take is to stop smoking and get their partners to stop. Whether you are breast-feeding or bottle-feeding, cigarette smoke will make your baby more prone to colic. In the case of breast-feeding mothers, some of the toxins from the cigarettes that enter the bloodstream are passed into the milk and have a direct effect on the baby's delicate stomach lining.

Prevention of colic

If you are pregnant, or planning to have a baby, there are measures you can take that could well reduce the chances of colic developing. The most important is to make sure that the baby is not given supplementary or 'complementary' feeds while in hospital. It might also be worth avoiding certain foods and drinks while breast-feeding. For more details on this, see pp253–4.

INSOMNIA

A recent report suggests that babies who cannot be persuaded to sleep are suffering a form of food intolerance. A group of these babies were studied, and all were being bottle-fed. When ordinary cow's milk formula was replaced by hydrolysate they began sleeping better, and when they went back onto ordinary formula the insomnia returned. If insomnia is a problem for your baby, ask the doctor if hydrolysate could be prescribed for a while. There are more details about hydrolysates on pp221.

DIARRHOEA IN BABIES AND CHILDREN

Diarrhoea in babies and children can have a great many causes, the most obvious one being infection with bacteria, viruses or other microbes. But if infections and other possible causes (such as cystic fibrosis) have been ruled out by your doctor, then you should consider the possible role of food.

Diarrhoea due to food sensitivity can come on suddenly and acutely, or it may start gradually and slowly get worse. There may be physical damage to the gut wall, which can be checked by taking a tiny sample and examining it under a microscope – this is known as a **biopsy**. However, there can also be diarrhoea due to food without any major damage to the gut. Where there *is* visible damage, this may indicate coeliac disease (see p142) or infant colitis (see p138). The latter is characterized by blood and mucus in the stools. The doctor will wish to eliminate both these possibilities before looking at other forms of food sensitivity.

An acute reaction to food may be difficult to distinguish from a viral infection that produces an attack of gastroenteritis, because the virus cannot always be detected in the baby's stools. Even if there *has* been an infection, this does not rule out the possibility of food sensitivity: diarrhoea of any sort can sensitize the gut so that foods which were previously eaten without trouble now produce symptoms. Drinking milk makes the situation worse, because there is often a transient lactase deficiency (see p208).

Where diarrhoea is due to food sensitivity, in infants and children, the culprit food often turns out to be cow's milk. Where milk sensitivity occurs, problems with other foods may follow, because the structure of the gut wall is altered by the reaction to milk. It becomes more 'leaky', which allows other food molecules through and the body may then react adversely to these as well. Often the reaction to other foods is only temporary – if they are eliminated from the diet for a few months they can be eaten again without difficulty. The reaction to milk tends to be more persistent, but most children who are sensitive to milk as babies can drink it once more by the time they are three or four. For a small number of people, however, the milk sensitivity will be lifelong.

What to do about diarrhoea

Acute attacks of diarrhoea should be taken very seriously indeed, especially in small babies. They can lose so much water from the body that they become seriously ill. In extreme cases they can suffer brain damage or die. The signs of moderate to severe **dehydration** are little urine, which is very dark and smells strongly (or no urine at all), sleepiness, dry sunken eyes, fast breathing and dry mouth. If you see these signs you should get medical help without delay, as the baby needs special treatment to replace the lost water and salts. This treatment may be given by mouth (when it is known as **oral rehydration therapy** or **ORT**) or directly into the bloodstream in more serious cases. In mild cases of dehydration, there are mixtures of salts that can be used for ORT at home. These are marketed under various names, including Rehidrat, Dioralyte and Gluco-lyte, and are available on prescription. Older children and adults can also become dehydrated during severe attacks of diarrhoea, and ORT can be useful for them as well.

Given that the doctor has ruled out infection and other likely causes for the diarrhoea, then food sensitivity should be considered.

As new foods are introduced into a child's diet, there may be temporary bouts of diarrhoea in response to them, although these do not necessarily develop as soon as the new food is eaten. Such transient diarrhoea is sometimes given the name **toddler diarrhoea** and is characterized by loose stools that contain some undigested food. Toddler diarrhoea usually clears up by about two years of age, and the usual medical advice is to leave it untreated. Given what we now know about food sensitivity, this is not necessarily the best advice. There seems to be a general pattern in some children, particularly with illnesses such as colic and eczema, of symptoms disappearing but other symptoms appearing later in their wake. If this is also true of toddler diarrhoea then it might be better, in the long run, to identify the offending foods and avoid them for a while. In one study, six out of 21 children with toddler diarrhoea proved to be food-sensitive. Follow the procedure outlined on p225.

THE HYPERKINETIC SYNDROME

This is a typical day in the life of a hyperactive child, as described by an exhausted mother to Dr Doris Rapp, a paediatrician working in Buffalo, New York: 'In the morning Matthew was stuffy and tired. He was cranky and would get upset over homework not done, cry, call himself stupid, and pester his

TABLE 9   FEATURES OF THE HYPERKINETIC SYNDROME (HYPERACTIVITY)

Overactive, excitable
Unable to keep still, constantly fidgeting
Poor concentration, short attention span, never finishes anything
Sudden mood changes, unpredictable, explosive
Cries easily, has emotional outbursts or temper tantrums
Gets into fights, is aggressive or bullies other children
Cannot cope with being criticized, seems depressed
Talks too fast, or is difficult to understand
Often irritable or unhappy
Easily distracted, impulsive
Quickly becomes frustrated
Clumsy and poorly coordinated
Touches everything and breaks things easily
Unaffectionate to others, has poor self-image
Sleeps badly
Constantly thirsty

sister. When he arrived home from school, he immediately took off shoes and did somersaults throughout the house. He thumped and jumped about the house, or would lie and watch television with his hands and feet tapping and banging away constantly. At dinner he rapped his fork and knife on the plate, picked up and handled things on the table, turned the salt shaker upside down, kicked the table and his sister, and intermittently, throughout the meal, jumped up to do somersaults in the living room. After supper he would try to do his homework. He would get upset because he forgot some books and say he was stupid. He'd write two or three words, rip up the sheet because of an error and do this about five or six times. He'd cry, get upset again, and the next morning either lose or forget his homework. At bedtime he would say that his muscles and belly had ached all day (a problem since his early years) and it would take an hour and a half to get to sleep. He'd roll and toss all night with bad dreams and talking. During the day he talked constantly about anything and would not listen. He never ate more than half a meal, never had an appetite. His nose was usually stuffy.'

The proper name for Matthew's condition is the **hyperkinetic syndrome** – although **hyperactivity** is often used as a diagnostic label, it is actually just one aspect of that syndrome. Other terms used for this collection of symptoms are **minimal brain dysfunction** and **attention deficit disorder**. The symptoms are listed in Table 9.

Estimates of the prevalence of hyperactivity range from 1 per cent to 20 per cent. Boys appear to outnumber girls by about five to one, but it may be that girls with the problem are less overtly hyperactive, and tend to display more subtle symptoms, such as inattention, speech disorders and mood changes, which may not always be identified as hyperkinetic syndrome.

The aggressive, destructive behaviour that is often seen in hyperkinetics usually develops later than the other symptoms, and may be largely a response to feelings of frustration that stem from the other symptoms. Hyperactive children may 'grow out of it' in time, but this takes a long time and their behaviour tends to get worse before it gets better. Their inability to concentrate or order their thoughts means that they generally do not learn much at school, even though they may be quite intelligent. Some have difficulty in writing and spelling. There is evidence of criminality and psychotic behaviour in some hyperkinetics when they reach adulthood, so it is advisable to try to sort out the problem sooner rather than later.

The causes of hyperkinetic syndrome

One of the early theories about the causes of hyperkinetic syndrome put it down to brain damage, but research has failed to find any evidence of this. In fact, the problem seems to be determined genetically, which means that the tendency to hyperkinesis is passed down from parent to child.

One study carried out in Canada showed that 20 per cent of cases could be attributed to true IgE-mediated allergy to food. From the case-histories compiled by allergists treating such children, it seems that most are sensitive to a great variety of things, including pollens, house dust, food additives and household chemicals. So it may be that IgE-mediated allergy plays a role in *more* than 20 per cent of cases, when other types of allergen, besides food, are taken into account.

Hyperkinetic children may also have deficiencies in certain enzymes that break down toxic compounds found in food, or produced by bacteria in the gut. The evidence for this is described on p244. It is quite probable that both IgE *and* enzyme deficiencies are important in causing the symptoms.

The role of food colourings, preservatives and other additives in hyperkinetic syndrome has received a lot of publicity. This idea was first put forward by Dr Ben Feingold of San Francisco, who also suggested that aspirin might be to blame, along with naturally-occurring salicylates (aspirin-like compounds) in fruits and vegetables. His diet excluded all these items and he claimed that 70 per cent of children improved considerably on this regime. Subsequent studies have not endorsed this, but they seem to show that there *is* a more modest level of improvement. For a small percentage of children, the Feingold diet makes a dramatic difference.

It would appear, from more recent studies, that food additives *are* important in a great many children with hyperkinetic syndrome, but that it is unusual to find a child for whom additives are the sole problem. Most also show sensitivity to various commonly eaten foods, pollen, dust, other common allergens and chemicals. The role of natural salicylates seems to be a minor one. When food and other allergens are considered, as well as additives, 50-80 per cent of children respond, although not all of them are completely cured. Sensitivity to unavoidable synthetic chemicals, such as solvents and the contaminants of natural gas, may account for the partial success with some patients.

In one recent study carried out in Britain, an 80 per cent 'cure' rate was found with a group of boys who were both hyperactive and habitual criminals. Ten boys, aged 7 to 17, were chosen for the study, and put on a very restricted diet of lamb, turkey, vegetables and fruit. Six improved dramatically, and two more improved after the third week on the diet. Their hyperactive and aggressive behaviour improved and, for the five who stuck to the diet, criminal behaviour has also stopped so far.

Although Feingold's theory was not entirely right, he was correct to single out food additives for blame – they do seem to play a disproportionate role in hyperactivity, compared to other types of illness such as asthma or eczema. This suggests that enzyme deficiencies may contribute to hyperkinetic syndrome, because such additives need to be detoxified by the body's enzymes. They may also prevent some enzymes from working properly (see p244). The involvement of additives may explain why the incidence of hyperkinetic syndrome seems to have increased dramatically in the last 20 years – a period that has seen the meteoric rise of 'junk food', take-aways and instant-everything. All these convenience foods tend to be rich in colourings, flavourings, preservatives and other additives.

Recognizing hyperkinetic syndrome

The first step for any parent is to decide whether their child's behaviour really is abnormal. As Dr Philip Graham of the Institute of Child Health in London points out: 'All normal children show some degree of aggressiveness, disobedience and antisocial behaviour: all at times show sadness, depression, anxiety and social withdrawal. All are at times unusually active and distractible. What makes a child a cause for concern is the severity and persistence of the problematic behaviour in question.'

Although a child like Matthew clearly shows abnormal behaviour, others with hyperkinetic syndrome may only be mildly affected. In such cases, it may be quite difficult to distinguish hyperkinetic syndrome from 'normal' behaviour – emotional upset and misconduct may be due to family tensions,

DAVID

David was very restless as a baby and slept little. By the time he could toddle he was a constant worry to his mother, because he was 'into everything' and could not be left alone for a minute. Getting him to bed in the evening was almost impossible, and when he was forced to do something he did not want to do he could throw violent tantrums. Like many children, David was fond of sugary foods and liked ice-cream, orange squash, chocolate and crisps. Since he was still only three it was relatively easy to exclude all these items and other common foods, such as milk and eggs, from his diet. On this diet he showed a dramatic improvement. He began to sleep through the night, and became much less active – for the first time he could sit down and watch a television programme through to the end. When he had been on this diet for ten days he was tested with various foods. After eating a small square of chocolate he became very aggressive and rushed around the house frantically banging doors and kicking furniture. Then he became dopey and fell into a deep sleep that lasted for several hours. A similar reaction occurred when he was given sugar, milk and oranges. Avoiding these foods has produced a great improvement in his behaviour.

lack of discipline, an unsettled home life, difficulties at school, or a great variety of other causes. It is very tempting for parents to attribute their child's awful behaviour to some simple external cause when the real problem lies within the family. Conversely, some parents may find lively, childish behaviour disruptive and label it as 'hyperactive' when in fact it is perfectly normal. Parents may not always be the best judge of what is wrong with their child, and it is a good idea to discuss the problem with a sympathetic teacher, doctor or child psychiatrist, keeping an open mind about the possible causes of the problem.

Even if the child is showing hyperkinetic syndrome, the problem may still be emotional rather than dietary, but certain clues point to food or additives as the triggers. Physical symptoms, such as muscle aches, stomach aches, rashes, headaches or bowel problems, usually accompany the mental symptoms in those who are sensitive to something in their diet or environment. (Such symptoms can also be produced psychosomatically however; see p150.) A pale, flushed or blotchy face is another indicator, and an intense thirst is seen in many of these children. In general, it seems that those with atopic symptoms – hay-fever, perennial rhinitis, asthma or urticaria – are far more likely to respond to dietary treatment.

Differences in behaviour between home and school are not uncommon in hyperkinetic children, but they do not really help in deciding whether the problem has dietary origins. The perceptions of parent and teacher are not always the same, for one thing. Parents may be more critical of their child's behaviour than a teacher, or less critical. Or it may be that one environment is over-stimulating for the child – a classroom full of other children, with colourful posters covering all the walls may be so distracting for a mildly hyperkinetic child that he or she behaves far worse than usual. Such children need special teaching in a quieter and less stimulating environment. Children who behave well at school but badly at home may be responding to family tensions, or they may find it easier to accept discipline in the more formal atmosphere of a school.

For some children, however, differences in food and chemical exposure between school and home may explain different behaviour patterns. It is worth investigating what the child eats for school lunch, or how many sweets are consumed at break-time, if school behaviour tends to be worse. For children who show chemical sensitivity, cleaning materials, disinfectants, floor wax, fumes from the heating system, marker pens and other items used in school may be to blame. Conversely, items used around the home, such as perfumes, aerosols and air-fresheners, may make the child more unmanageable than at school. But it makes sense to consider other explanations first, because family problems are far more likely to be the source of trouble than household chemicals.

What to do about hyperkinetic syndrome

Hyperkinetic syndrome can begin in infancy. Babies that sleep little and cry frequently often go on to become hyperkinetic. If there are no obvious reasons for the baby showing this disturbed behaviour, then the role of diet should be considered. Follow the guidelines given on pp221–7.

For older children, there are more complex issues to think over before deciding on a course of action. Restricted diets are socially disruptive and can sometimes be nutritionally inadequate, especially if the child is sensitive to a variety of foods. With mild behavioural symptoms, it may be better to cope with them in other ways, rather than trying a dietary approach. For a child who is very disruptive, however, there is little to lose by trying a diet. Although it might seem impossible to get cooperation from such a child, given his usual behaviour, this should not put you off. If he does respond, the early stages of the diet may produce a remarkable improvement, which makes the subsequent stages a great deal easier for all concerned.

Do not attempt any diet without consulting your family doctor or specialist. If your child is under a child psychiatrist who is totally unsympathetic to dietary ideas, then ask your family doctor to refer you to someone else – an allergist for example, or a more open-minded psychiatrist – who will be prepared to supervise an elimination diet.

The specialist may have their own preferences as regards the diet, but if not, the three-stage diet given in Chapter Fourteen can be used. Once they get to Stage 2, children may need a calcium supplement, to compensate for the lack of milk in the diet, and the doctor can prescribe this. Children who also have asthma should be tested cautiously. *Any child who has had severe allergic reactions in the past should not be tested for foods at home as the reaction can occasionally be life-threatening.*

Drugs used to control behaviour, such as amphetamine derivatives, can be continued during the diet. If there appears to be an improvement in behaviour then you can try delaying the medication, or reducing the amount, but keep an eye on the situation and be prepared to top up the dose if necessary. Drugs used to control specific symptoms such as asthma or hay-fever should not be used routinely during the diet – only use them if they are actually needed. *Needless to say, you should discuss all these points with your doctor before making any changes to the child's medication.*

Although in some children there will be a dramatic response to the diet, in others the reaction may be more subtle. Bad behaviour may seem a lot worse on a day when the washing machine has flooded the kitchen floor than on a day when everything has gone well. To help you assess your child's reaction to the diet objectively, you should keep a score-sheet of symptoms for each day. An example of such a sheet is shown opposite, but the exact symptoms written in the left-hand column will vary for each child. Draw up a score-sheet and get enough photocopies made to last for two or three weeks. Start filling them in at least a week before you embark on the diet, so that you have a 'base-line' from which to judge the effect of the diet. Make sure you sit down and fill the form in every evening, after your child has gone to bed, and try to be objective. You will learn most from the diet if you can time it so that there are not too many parties, outings or other disruptive events, especially during the retesting period.

Always bear in mind that *the diet may not be the answer.* If you pin all your hopes on it, you may see improvements where there are none, and in the long run this could be very damaging to your child. Be careful, also, not to give the child the impression that the diet will 'make everything all right'. He may be so

TABLE 10   SAMPLE SCORE-SHEET FOR A HYPERACTIVE CHILD

Dates: From . . . . To . . . .

Scores: 5 = very bad, much worse than usual
              4 = bad, worse than usual
              3 = about the same as usual
              2 = a little better than usual
              1 = much better than usual
              0 = no sign of this behaviour

	Mon	Tues	Weds	Thurs	Fri	Sat	Sun
Fidgeting							
Aggressive							
Crying							
Overexcited							
Touching everything							
Unable to concentrate							
Aching muscles							
Stomach ache							
Thirsty							
Anxious							
Speech unclear							
Total							

NB *The symptoms shown here are just given as examples. When drawing up your own table, you should include each of your child's symptoms, making the list as long or as short as it needs to be.*

SEAN

Sean, aged 13, was on the point of being expelled from school for his aggressive behaviour, uncontrollable temper and vandalism. Although he was obviously intelligent, he could not concentrate in class and disturbed other pupils. He had been referred to a psychologist, but none of the forms of therapy that had been tried made much difference. Then, by chance, the psychologist discovered that Sean drank cans of cola all through the day, and ate a huge amount of chocolate. Sean admitted to feeling shaky and unwell when he hadn't had a can of cola for several hours.

The psychologist referred Sean to an allergist, who found that the boy also suffered from stomach pains and a constant runny nose. By eliminating cola and chocolate from his diet, Sean recovered from these physical symptoms, and his behaviour improved considerably. He was allowed to stay at school and began to catch up on the education that he had missed. Five years later he is still well, – though he still has to keep off chocolate and cola – and about to go to University. Not all disruptive, aggressive children respond so well to diet, but a significant percentage do.

anxious to please you that he tries extra hard to be good. Psychogenic reactions on food testing (see p155) can occur just as easily in children as in adults, and if knows he is expected to go wild when he tries milk he may well oblige. Throughout the diet, try to keep an open mind about the outcome, and do not put any ideas into the child's head about what might happen.

On the other hand, you do need the child's cooperation, especially if he is old enough to go out and buy sweets or other foods for himself. Rather than forcing the diet on him, you should explain that it might help and ask if he would like to try it. You need to impress on him that it will only work if it is done properly – that there must be absolutely no cheating.

Because food additives are so important in hyperkinetic syndrome, you need to be aware of other ways in which they can be consumed. The colourings in toothpaste are identical to certain food colourings, so white toothpaste should be used. Put any coloured toothpaste well out of reach.

Medicines also contain colorants, often in very large amounts, which is why you should try to discontinue syrups and tablets during the diet (as long as your doctor agrees) or get colouring-free alternatives. Try to stop your child from chewing things, and from licking sticky paper or stamps. Bear in mind that there can be additives in unlabelled food such as bread from a bakery, fish-and-chips, other take-away food and restaurant food, *eg* French fries. For more details on additives, see Appendix VI, p313.

The timing of responses in the diet varies. Most children recover within a week or two on the initial stages of the diet, but others take up to three weeks. Foods should only be tested once there is a noticeable and sustained improvement. If this does not occur, then revert to the normal diet and consider other options. It may be that your child has chemical sensitivities – reading Chapter Nine should help you to assess this possibility. Be prepared to reconsider the likelihood of emotional stresses and strains.

The procedure for testing foods is slightly different for hyperkinetic syndrome. Although a few may take up to a week of daily feeding with the culprit food before they respond, this is probably fairly unusual. The response time for most is between 15 minutes and four hours. Reintroduced foods should be fed in the morning, and again in the afternoon, if there was no reaction, or only a slight reaction, to the first feeding. A normal-sized portion should be eaten, except in children who have asthma or urticaria, where a very small amount should be tried first, in case there is a severe reaction. If, by the morning after, there is no reaction to the food, then it can be incorporated into the diet, and testing begun on a new food. As always, in an elimination diet, it is important not to eat too much of any one food.

Assuming the diet is effective, and you discover what foods or additives cause the problems, then you have to decide on a plan of action. Again, you should discuss this with your doctor. Avoiding the foods in question may be quite difficult, especially at school or with friends, and you may wish to reconsider other options, especially if your child is not affected all that severely or if he reacts to a great many foods. Drugs are one option, and you should discuss the pros and cons of these with your doctor. Another, more controversial form of treatment, is neutralization therapy. Although this is not accepted widely among the medical profession, there are many reports of it being used successfully for the treatment of hyperactive children. For more details see pp296–300.

If you decide on avoidance of the food, bear in mind that the child's sensitivity may disappear in time. The culprit foods should be retested at one- or two-yearly intervals, to see if they still produce the same symptoms.

Although most children remain well as long as they stick to their diet, a few seem to relapse after a few years for no apparent reason. It may be that they have developed new sensitivities to foods, or that they are becoming chemical-sensitive. In general, any child with hyperkinetic syndrome is likely to fare better if their exposure to synthetic chemicals (see pp172 and 258–9) can be minimized. They should also be encouraged to take plenty of exercise and eat a good healthy diet.

INVESTIGATING FOOD SENSITIVITY IN BABIES AND TODDLERS
You should check that your doctor approves of the measures suggested here, and not make any substantial changes to the child's diet, or your own (if breast-feeding), without medical supervision.

Bottle-fed babies
If your baby is being fed with cow's milk or cow's-milk formula feed, and you suspect that this may be the cause of the symptoms, then ask the doctor to prescribe a 'milk-free' formula. These are of three types: **soya-based formula**, such as Wysoy, Nutrilon Soya, Ostersoy, Prosobee or Isomil, **comminuted chicken formula**, and **hydrolysed formula** or **hydrolysate**, such as Pregestimil, Lofenalac or Nutramigen. The hydrolysates are made up of cow's milk, cornstarch and other foods, but treated with digestive enzymes (see p18) so that the milk proteins are partially broken down. This makes them a great deal less allergenic, although they still cause problems in some children who are highly sensitive to cow's milk. For these children there are some new products on the market called whey hydrolysates (*eg* Alfare Nestlé). These are made from the whey of cow's milk – the liquid part that is produced when the milk is curdled or separated. (The other hydrolysates, made from the milk solids, are called casein hydrolysates, as their main protein is casein.) Since whey proteins are less allergenic than casein, these hydrolysates are potentially useful for highly allergic babies, but even they have produced serious problems occasionally.

With hydrolysates generally, there are those designed for *treatment* of an existing allergy and those designed for *preventive* use in bottle-fed babies who are at high risk of developing milk allergy. The ones used for treatment are more highly digested than those used for prevention.

Do not expect instant results, especially if the baby has diarrhoea or colic – it may take up to two weeks for the baby's digestive system to return to normal. If there is no improvement, discuss the situation with the doctor, and consider trying another type of 'milk-free' formula – it may be that one works for your baby while another does not.

In general, there is evidence that children who have developed a sensitivity to cow's milk may become sensitive to soya proteins as well, if they consume them in large quantities. For a young baby who has several more months of formula to come, the hydrolysates are probably a better choice than soya formulas, therefore.

Should the baby recover on one of these alternative formulas, then cow's milk formula should be tested about a month later, to see what effect it has. It may be that the switch to an alternative formula happened to coincide with a spontaneous recovery. Or the sensitivity to cow's-milk could have cleared up thanks to a month of avoidance. Either way, the baby can now return to cow's milk formula.

For babies who seem to react badly to *all* the different formula feeds, the possibility of some other cause, such as an infection, should be reconsidered. If all such causes have been ruled out, and there is strong evidence for food sensitivity being at the root of the problem, then breast milk is the best solution. Enquire about the possibility of donated breast milk from a milk bank – you may be fortunate enough to live in an area where such a bank has been established. Alternatively there is relactation – returning to breast-feeding. This is not possible for everyone, and it is not something to be undertaken lightly, but it may be the only answer for some babies. Help can be obtained from breast-feeding advisory groups (addresses given on p339). Mothers who choose this course of action should not drink cow's milk themselves, nor should they eat butter, cheese, yoghurt or soya.

For the older baby, early weaning may be the answer, although it involves the risk of sensitizing the child to even more foods or – if all the high-risk foods are avoided – failing to give the child an adequate diet. Early weaning is only recommended if the baby is suffering quite badly and you have exhausted all other possibilities. It would not be appropriate, for example, in the case of a colicky baby who was otherwise well and growing normally. If you decide to try early weaning, remember the following points:

1. Certain foods seem to contain more potent allergens than others. Do not give the child eggs, fish, chocolate, wheat, oranges, peanuts or other nuts for at least the first six months, and preferably for the first year of life. If you introduce them before a year old, do not give them every day. Test out beef and chicken cautiously, as these can cross-react with milk and eggs respectively. If they seem to cause no problems, you can include them in the child's diet.

2. Formula feeds commonly contain maize (corn) and tapioca, as well as cow's milk, so your child may have become sensitive to these. Avoid these foods for at least six months and then try them out carefully. Maize comes in many guises, including cornflour, cornflakes, corn oil, corn syrup, sweetcorn, corn-on-the-cob and popcorn. Some medicines contain corn syrup: ask your pharmacist for advice if you are concerned about avoiding all corn products.

3. No food should be eaten in very large quantities, and it is best not to give any one food every day. This means using your imagination and buying some fairly unusual items. Foods such as millet and sweet potatoes make a good basis for baby foods, and if the baby does become sensitive to them, at least they are no trouble to avoid in later years. Appendix V, p307, lists the main 'rare foods' and describes how to prepare them.

4. Do not force the child to eat any food that is obviously disliked. Most children reject new foods the first time they are offered, but if your child clearly finds the food disagreeable, even after trying it three or four times, then don't serve it up again. A dislike of the taste is sometimes an early sign of sensitivity.

5. If a child is not eating eggs, milk or fish, there is a risk of protein being in short supply. Make sure that you include other protein-rich foods, such as lamb, pork and other meats. Beans are a good source of protein, but they are also rather indigestible and cause wind; chickpeas (p311) are less of a problem, and have a milder taste.

6. Your child will probably need a calcium supplement, and the overall diet should be checked by a paediatric nutritionist to see if it contains enough of other minerals, as well as vitamins. Ask your doctor to arrange this for you.

Breast-fed babies

With breast-fed babies who are thought to have food sensitivity, the first step is to check that it is not something *other than* breast milk causing the problem. Think about what else the baby consumes, and if possible eliminate everything except breast milk, including medicines (with your doctor's approval), vitamin drops (which often contain artificial colouring), fruit juices and any solids. If the baby needs to go on taking medicines or vitamins, ask the doctor to prescribe something that does not contain any colouring or other unnecessary ingredients. You may need to give boiled water to compensate for fruit juices or other extra liquids that you have withdrawn.

If this has no effect, the next step is to compile a list of suspect foods from those that you are eating. Keep a record of everything you eat, recording the quantities and times of eating as well. Make a separate record of your baby's symptoms, with the time, duration and intensity. Continue this for a week or two, and compare the two records to see if there are any likely suspects. The time interval between the mother eating the food and the baby suffering symptoms can vary from one day to several days.

Don't make the mistake of thinking that it must be cow's milk, just because this is the food problem that we hear about most often in babies. For the exclusively breast-fed baby, it could be any food. However, babies who have received supplementary bottle-feeds (see p254) *are* more likely to react to cow's milk than anything else. Even if you have never given a bottle-feed yourself it is possible that the baby received one from a nurse while in the maternity ward.

The foods that are most likely to cause problems are those that you always eat in large quantities or 'binged' on during pregnancy, those you have a craving for, and, paradoxically, those that you actively dislike but eat because they 'do you good'. You should also be suspicious of foods that are known to be potent allergens. Apart from milk, these are: eggs, peanuts, other nuts, wheat, chocolate, fish, oranges and other citrus fruits, chicken and beef. If you eat a lot of any of these foods, then add them to your list.

Anything with a drug-like action, such as coffee, tea, wine (especially red wine), beer, spirits or other drugs, is also a prime suspect, especially in the case of colic. Try cutting out all these drug-like items, plus cow's milk, for two weeks and see if the baby improves. Eat extra protein from other sources and take a calcium supplement, which your doctor can prescribe.

If there is no improvement, then you should try eliminating all the other suspect foods that you have listed. Avoid them for two weeks, but substitute other foods that will fulfil your nutritional needs. Remember to cut out all the 'hidden' forms of foods, especially with ubiquitous foods such as milk, eggs and wheat. Read the labels on packaged foods carefully and see p302 for some of the synonyms used, as these can be deceptive. Avoid all restaurant or take-away food during this time as it is difficult to know what you are eating.

If you have cut out more than two or three foods, and your baby gets better, then you will probably wish to test the foods to see which ones were the cause of the trouble – often it will just be one food. Wait until the baby has been well for about a week, and then reintroduce each food in turn, beginning with those least likely to cause trouble, and testing cow's milk last. Eat a normal-sized portion of the food to be tested, every day for a week. If the baby remains well, discontinue that food and go on to test another one, again eating it every day for a week. Make a note of which foods cause symptoms and which do not. When all have been tested, those that produced no symptoms in the baby can become part of your normal diet again.

It is possible that the baby will remain well, and not respond to any of the foods – a brief period of avoidance can sometimes clear up the sensitivity. If this happens, continue with your normal diet, but be careful not to eat too much of any one food.

If cow's milk *does* turn out to be the problem you can try drinking sheep or goat's milk instead, after a few weeks. But keep an eye on the baby's symptoms – it may have problems with these milks too, because of cross-reactivity (see p304) between the proteins. If so, give up all animal milk for a while and try soya milk instead.

Above all, make sure you are getting enough protein, vitamins and minerals, and avoid any drastic changes in your diet. If your list of suspect foods is very extensive, it may be better to split them into two groups and try eliminating each group in turn. Consult your doctor to see if your diet is adequate.

If none of this works, then you could try a full elimination diet as a last resort – but you must ask your doctor first. The elimination diet is fairly stringent, and there is a risk of being undernourished because milk-production makes heavy demands on your body. You should eat plenty of meat and fish while on the diet to ensure you get enough protein, and a vitamin and mineral supplement (see p333) may be necessary. Chapter Fourteen outlines the procedure for the elimination diet – you should have already completed the equivalent of Stage 1, so you can go straight into Stage 2.

If you manage to resolve the baby's problems, but find yourself on a quite restricted diet, then you should retest foods after a month or two. It may be that the baby's sensitivity has cleared up of its own accord, and you can then return to normal eating. If the symptoms recur, go back to the restricted diet.

Older babies and toddlers

For older infants, who are taking some solid food, try cutting out different foods in turn, but replace them with others that are equally nutritious. Begin with the most common offenders: milk, milk products and chocolate, cutting out beef at the same time, as this can sometimes cross-react with milk. If the child is eating any food or drinks containing additives, then these should be avoided as well. Next try eggs and chicken, then nuts and peanuts, then citrus fruits, then fish. Omit each food or set of foods for about two weeks before going on to the next set.

If the child gets better when certain foods are excluded, then they should be reintroduced to check that they were the source of the trouble. Begin with a very small amount and watch carefully for reactions – these can sometimes be severe. Some doctors recommend that no foods should be reintroduced until the child is over a year old, to minimize the risk of future sensitivity. This is probably a good idea, but it means that you may never know if the food you avoided was indeed the guilty party, because the child is likely to have outgrown the sensitivity by the time the food is eaten again.

If these measures are unsuccessful, then it *may* be worth carrying out an elimination diet, as described in Chapter Fourteen. *In no circumstances should you do this without help and advice from your doctor – restricting the diet of small children can be very dangerous.*

JANICE, BEN AND AMY

Janice had suffered a range of health problems for years, including irritable bowel syndrome, migraine, and severe premenstrual tension. She could no longer drive because she had had two car accidents: 'I was just fuzzy in the brain, I couldn't function. I found it difficult to even get out of bed in the morning and get the children to school.' She was then about 35, and had suffered migraines since childhood, but the other problems had only come on in her 30s. Her son Ben developed asthma at 5 years old, and glue ear, producing deafness. Amy, her daughter, developed eczema and glue ear. Janice thought about food intolerance, and, suspecting that it might be the source of her own health problems, went onto a very simple diet of fruit, vegetables, potatoes, milk-free margarine, meat and fish. The improvement was prompt and dramatic. A year later, when both children were quite severely deaf due to glue ear, Janice decided to try the diet out on Ben. 'We had to go back to the doctor a week later for a check-up, and he was amazed. There was almost no trace of asthma, and Ben's hearing was normal. The doctor had to accept that the diet had done the trick. If Ben has to break the diet for some reason, the symptoms always come back.' When Amy too went on the diet, her eczema and glue ear both cleared up. The doctor advised Janice that their food intake be checked by a nutrionist, to make sure that the children, in particular, were getting all the nutrients they needed. 'It's hard work, because I can never use convenience foods, but we are all so healthy that I think it's worth it,' Janice concludes.

In the case of eczema, it may be better to start with a simplified form of the elimination diet. Rather than cutting out a whole range of foods, concentrate on the foods that are known to be problematic in eczema: milk, eggs, beef, chicken, food additives, oranges, lemons and other citrus fruits. These should be avoided during the exclusion phase of the diet (see pp280–5) and then, if the eczema clears up, tested in the normal way during the reintroduction phase (see pp285–7). If there is no response to the exclusion phase, then cut out nuts, fish, wheat, tomatoes, lamb, peanuts and soya as well. Should this produce no results, then you could consider trying Stage 3 of the elimination diet (see p287), if the eczema is bad enough to justify this, and if your doctor agrees.

Staying well

Once you have established a diet on which the child remains well, be careful not to allow too much of any one food. Have your child's food intake checked by a nutritionist – this is something that your family doctor should be able to arrange for you. Incidentally, the most common deficiencies in children on restricted diets are in calcium and iodine. Calcium is most likely to be deficient if there are no dairy products in the diet. It is also found in nuts, seeds, peas, beans, lentils, broccoli and green leafy vegetables, so give your child plenty of these. Or you can get calcium gluconate tablets from the chemist. Iodine may be in short supply if dairy products, meat and grains are not eaten. Other rich sources include fish (particularly sardines, salmon, tuna and haddock), shellfish, pineapple, eggs, peanuts, lettuce, spinach, green peppers and raisins. Some table salts have added iodine – look on the label. Seaweed is an extremely rich source, and can be used as a supplement, but it is important not to eat too much, as *excess* iodine is also damaging.

Most children do grow out of their sensitivities gradually, and it is important not to keep them on a restricted diet any longer than necessary. Retest foods once or twice a year to see if they are still a problem. If the child has ever had a severe reaction, or suffers from asthma, then the retesting must be done very cautiously. Parents who have had one food-sensitive child will want to minimize their chances of having another, and some useful preventive measures are described in Chapter Thirteen.

KEEPING THINGS IN PERSPECTIVE

It is natural to worry about children, especially when they are ill, but worrying too much can be very harmful to them. Children need to feel safe and secure about the world they grow up in, and it is unwise to give them the idea that everything they eat or come into contact with is a potential threat. Parents of allergic children have to walk a tightrope – on the one hand they need to warn their child about things to avoid, but on the other hand they must not make the child over-anxious. Sometimes they must conceal their own fears to avoid alarming the child.

In some families, the question of the child's health becomes entangled with other problems – a tense relationship between husband and wife, for example, or friction with grandparents or other relatives. It is not uncommon for one parent to 'use' the child's illness for their own purposes in these domestic problems. For the child's sake, it is vital to try to keep these issues separate from the question of illness and treatment. If there is disagreement over how seriously ill the child is, or how the illness should be dealt with, try to discuss these matters quietly when the child is not there, and agree on a common approach. Arguing things out in front of the child may give him or her the idea that the illness can be used to manipulate difficult family situations – which can create yet more trouble in the future. Talking the matter over with a sympathetic doctor, teacher or other professional may be helpful.

As children grow older, and start going to school, it is very important that they feel as 'normal' as possible. Anything that makes them different is likely to lead to teasing by other children. So you should try to minimize restrictions about diet and environment as much as possible. If you can keep the home free from allergens and other offending substances, your child's health may be good enough for him or her to tolerate limited exposure at school. This may be less damaging overall than the psychological effects of feeling alienated from normal school life, by constantly having to avoid certain classes or not eat school food. Make sure your child gets enough exercise, so that he or she

STEPHEN

Stephen was a little boy with a constantly runny nose and occasional attacks of 'tummy ache'. He had never been particularly well behaved, but after his parents separated he grew much worse. When a teacher described him as 'hyperactive', his mother, Angela, felt food or food additives might be to blame. So she tried Stephen on an elimination diet. His runny nose cleared up, and he seemed to feel better generally. Angela also thought that his behaviour improved, although the teachers were unsure.

The testing phase of the elimination diet did not go smoothly, because Stephen was uncooperative. As a result – and because any bad behaviour was taken as a positive reaction by Angela – he seemed to be reacting to a lot of the food and additives that were tried out. Angela devised a very restrictive diet on the basis of these tests, and persuaded the school to help in getting Stephen to stick to it. But she was less successful with Stephen's father, Bob, who had Stephen to stay for one weekend every month.

Bob liked to indulge Stephen, since he saw him so little. He let him have all the treats that were forbidden at is fit and not overweight. This will make integration with other children a great deal easier. A well-adjusted, happy child is less likely to be *physically* ill (see Chapter Eight), so it is important to get the balance right.

If the child is allergic to certain foods, and if the reaction is not too severe, then the drug sodium cromoglycate (see p320) may be useful, although it does not work in all cases. The drug can be taken before special events such as birthday parties or Christmas dinner, and allows the child to eat forbidden foods without any symptoms. Unfortunately, it is not usually effective if taken long-term.

Munchausen-by-proxy and Meadow's syndrome

Baron von Munchausen was an eighteenth-century Hanoverian soldier who greatly exaggerated his prowess in war – and his battle-scars. 'Munchausen's syndrome' is the name given to attention-seeking patients who feign illness or deliberately fabricate symptoms. There are instances, fortunately very rare, of

home – chocolate, crisps, fizzy drinks etc. When Stephen returned home, his runny nose had usually returned, and he often behaved very badly. Angela saw both these as an outcome of the broken diet, ignoring the fact that many children whose parents have separated are disturbed after a visit to the 'other' parent, and are difficult and aggressive afterwards. Angela did not want to acknowledge that the break-up of the marriage had affected Stephen badly, because this would have made her feel guilty for not keeping the family together.

She became ever angrier with Bob for not taking the diet seriously, and tried to prevent the monthly visits. She had long wanted to sever all contact with Bob anyway, so the conflict over the diet became a means to this end. Her conviction that food and additives made Stephen hyperactive was now unshakeable, even though he behaved pretty badly most of the time, regardless of what he ate. Angela had a vested interest in her fixed belief, which was now an obstacle to getting to the real root of Stephen's behavioural problems.

mothers simulating illness in their children in order to get medical attention – this is known as 'Munchausen-by-proxy' or 'Meadow's syndrome' after Professor Roy Meadows, who first described two cases in 1977. Doctors are far more aware of this possibility in children than they once were, and any parent attempting to fabricate symptoms is likely to be found out very quickly.

The question of Meadow's syndrome in relation to food sensitivity is a difficult issue. Various doctors have described cases of children whose parents believe them to have food sensitivity, but where no consistent reaction to a food can be shown. If those parents seem over-anxious or over-protective, and have obvious emotional problems of their own, then they have often been labelled as 'Meadow's syndrome'.

Eleven such cases were reported in 1984, in an influential article that has coloured the outlook of many doctors, and led to the belief that Meadow's syndrome is quite common in relation to food sensitivity. However, there were several important differences between the cases described in this article and Meadow's syndrome proper. For one thing, the children involved all had genuine symptoms, and there was no suggestion that the parents had attempted to fabricate any symptoms. Unlike Meadow's syndrome mothers, these women did not seem to relish their child's hospital stay, nor were they willing to subject them to any investigation, however painful and unpleasant. Such differences are important and must raise serious doubts about the conclusions reached – was the label 'Meadow's syndrome' really justified? These parents may have been disturbed or overwrought, but this does not necessarily mean that they were mistaken about their child's illness. The elusive nature of the reactions seen in food intolerance makes it difficult to rule out this diagnosis without very thorough testing, and there seems to have been undue reliance on skin-prick tests in this study, despite the fact that these are unreliable indicators in most cases of food sensitivity. Despite the doubts over this study, the idea of 'Meadow's syndrome' has become a popular one, especially among those doctors who are sceptical of food intolerance generally. This is unfortunate for parents, especially when such a diagnosis is made without proper testing for food sensitivity, and without any firm evidence of fabrication. There undoubtedly *are* cases of parents who exaggerate their child's ills, and who are determined to blame them on some physical cause, when family tensions and emotional problems are actually the true source of the symptoms. *But unless there is gross exaggeration or fabrication of symptoms, these should not be described as Meadow's syndrome.*

From a parent's point-of-view, it is important to be honest about family problems, to yourself, to your partner, and to others. Seeking help from a professional counsellor, when things *begin* to go wrong, may help to avert more serious problems. Try to insulate children from arguments and rows, and to protect them from tense and difficult situations until they are old enough to cope with them. Children are just as susceptible to psychosomatic illness (see p150) as adults are, and sometimes physical symptoms are an expression of their distress. If your child is ill, try to think about that separately from your other problems, and to deal with it as rationally as possible. Be prepared to consider the possibility that it is nothing to do with food. Never exaggerate the child's ill-health to anyone, and resist the temptation to manipulate other people by imposing special diets or other restrictions. Facing up to your own problems, and trying to resolve them, may be the best thing you could do for your child.

It has to be said that the existence of self-help books, such as this one, is regarded as part of the problem by some doctors. Munchausen's syndrome is usually seen amongst those with some medical knowledge, such as failed medical students or nurses. Consequently, some doctors believe that 'ignorance is bliss' – if medical knowledge were more widespread, there would be more cases of Munchausen's and Munchausen-by-proxy. So books that seek to inform the public about illness are simply adding to the problem.

Our own viewpoint is that *genuine* cases of Munchausen's or Meadow's syndrome are very rare because these people are seriously disturbed. If they had not had medical knowledge, their mental problems would have surfaced in some other form. In the same way, many suicides jump from tall buildings, but removing all the tall buildings in the country would not stop people from killing themselves. Presenting the average man or woman in the street with medical knowledge does not turn them into cases of Munchausen's syndrome: if it did, the problem would be far more widespread. On the other hand, lack of knowledge about food sensitivity has led thousands of children to suffer unnecessarily from symptoms such as colic, diarrhoea, asthma, eczema and migraine. Improving their lot is, in our view, far more important.

We hope that parents using this book will read it carefully, try to understand it fully, and use the information responsibly. Above all, they should consult their doctor and make every effort to work with him or her. The human body is very complex, and the human mind even more so – a book such as this can only provide a glimpse of the factors that may be involved in your child's illness. If you feel that the doctor regards you as an overanxious or 'difficult' parent, then try to stay calm and state your case clearly. Remember what Kipling said: 'If you can trust yourself when all men doubt you, but make allowances for their doubting too . . .' It is 'making allowances' that is difficult, but bear in mind that the doctor does see parents who are genuinely harming their children, either mentally or physically, and it is part of his or her job to consider all the possibilities in every case.

Chapter Twelve

WHAT CAUSES FOOD INTOLERANCE?

The simple answer to the question 'what causes food intolerance?' is 'no-one knows'. Which is not to say that no-one has any ideas about the subject – there are ideas and theories in abundance. There is even a certain amount of evidence for some of them. At present, we are at the stage of picking through the ideas, looking at the meagre evidence, and trying to make some sense of it all. Consequently, this chapter is rather like a detective novel with the last page missing. Those who like simple, cut-and-dried explanations would do well to go on to Chapter Thirteen without delay.

One thing is clear. There is no single, straightforward mechanism behind all types of food intolerance. Even in the individual patient, there may be more than one abnormality causing the symptoms. In fact, it is possible that there *has* to be more than one 'fault' for the illness to materialize – in other words, the causes of food intolerance are like straws being added to the proverbial camel's back. One or two 'faults' in the body's functioning, or its environment, are tolerated. It takes several factors working together to produce the actual symptoms of food intolerance. This would explain why every patient is different, in terms of the symptoms they show and the progress of their illness – because each person has a unique combination of circumstances leading up to that illness.

IS THE IMMUNE SYSTEM INVOLVED?

At the beginning of this book, we defined food intolerance as 'any adverse reaction to food, other than false food allergy, in which the involvement of the immune system is unproven because skin-prick tests and other tests for allergy are negative. This does not exclude the possibility of immune reactions being involved in some way, but they are unlikely to be the major factor producing the symptoms'. Because food intolerance has long been thought of as an 'allergy', most research into its causes has centred on the immune system. It is only in the last ten years or so that other possible reasons for intolerance have been investigated.

Despite extensive research, the evidence for immune-system involvement is fairly limited. The general consensus of opinion now is that immune reactions *may* have some role in food intolerance *in some people*, but they are only part of the story – something else must be going wrong as well.

Oral tolerance – how the immune system copes with food

One line of research into food intolerance has investigated what normally happens to food in the healthy person. There is no reason why the immune system should not attack food molecules just as enthusiastically as it attacks invading germs – after all, food is chemically different from our own bodies, and that is exactly how the immune system recognizes unwelcome aliens.

At one time it was thought that the gut wall rigidly excluded all food molecules, but this is not the case (see p21). In fact the body 'learns' not to mount a major immune attack on food. This is done by small areas of the gut wall, known as **Peyer's patches**. These patches, which are part of the immune system, take up small droplets of fluid from the gut, in a process known as **antigen sampling**.

What the Peyer's patch does is to 'examine' the foreign substances it finds in the gut, 'make a decision' about how the body should respond to each of them, and 'communicate' that decision to the rest of the body. They are rather like immigration officials, alerting the body's police force (the rest of the immune system) to the arrival of a suspected criminal (a bacterium or virus). But how does the Peyer's patch distinguish the 'suspected criminals' from the 'innocent holidaymakers' – in other words, harmless food molecules? No-one knows at present, but the smaller size of food molecules and their lack of 'stickiness' is probably important – microbes have a habit of clinging to cell membranes, which is a potential give-away.

Once the Peyer's patch has recognized a given molecule as food, rather than foe, it tells the body to respond to that molecule in a particular way. It produces a type of cell known as a T-suppressor cell, which is specific for that molecule and tones down the immune response to it. T-suppressor cells can also influence the type of antibody produced in response to a particular molecule. Some **isotypes** of antibody (see p25) produce inflammation when they bind to their antigen (in this case, the food molecule). One isotype does not – it is called immunoglobulin A or **IgA**, and it plays an important part in the body's response to food.

When microbes get into the blood from the gut, they are met by IgG and

IgM antibodies. These bind to their antigen (a molecule on the surface of the microbe) and thus form **immune complexes**. Once bound, both IgG and IgM summon the body's defensive forces for an all-out attack, which may cause local damage to the body's own tissues, seen as inflammation. IgA is different – it has a 'softly softly' approach. Although it binds to its target to form immune complexes, it does not provoke inflammation. Circulating immune complexes containing IgA are mopped up by phagocytes or 'eating cells' – the body's garbage-disposal team – without any fuss (see p74).

It will be clear that IgA is the ideal antibody for disposing of food molecules which accidentally make it through to the bloodstream. One effect of the Peyer's patches is to tell the body to form more IgA to food molecules, and less IgG, so that the immune complexes produced are less inflammatory. This process is called **the induction of oral tolerance**.

The idea that this process breaks down in food intolerance is an attractive one. At present, there is some evidence to support it, but not a great deal. It does seem, however, that patients with food intolerance make more IgG to food molecules in the blood, and less IgA. They may also produce some IgE, so that the immune complexes could trigger off mast cells (see p26).

Getting through the gut wall

There is evidence that people with food intolerance have more leaky gut walls than healthy individuals – so they let more undigested food molecules through. This has major health implications which will be considered later, but how does the gut become more leaky in the first place?

Inflammation, produced by immune attack, can make the gut wall more leaky. One source of inflammation is disease – any gut infection that produces diarrhoea may inflame the gut wall. In babies, such infections are often the start of food intolerance.

Alternatively, foods themselves might provoke inflammation of the gut wall, if there is a localized *allergic* response to them. This is not something that most allergists would agree with – they see IgE/mast cell reactions to foods (see p29) as being all-or-nothing affairs which produce immediate and unmistakable symptoms. The idea that there might be a small-scale, localized IgE reaction, whose main effect is to make the gut more permeable, is not widely accepted. The main evidence in its favour is the effect of a drug, sodium cromoglycate, on some patients with food intolerance.

The effects of this drug have mainly been studied in migraine patients. If such patients undertake an elimination diet, a large proportion of them get better (see p129) and can then identify one or more foods which provoke their symptoms. Each time a culprit food is eaten it will provoke a migraine – but not if sodium cromoglycate is given in advance. Sodium cromoglycate is

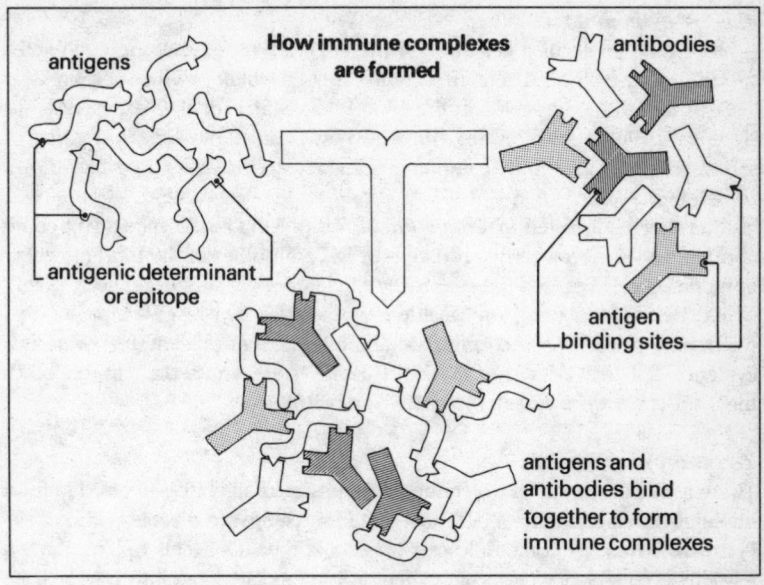

How immune complexes are formed

antigens

antigenic determinant or epitope

antibodies

antigen binding sites

antigens and antibodies bind together to form immune complexes

known to stabilize mast cells and prevent them from releasing their inflammatory mediators. And the drug is not absorbed from the gut in any appreciable quantity. So the logical conclusion is that it prevents reactions to culprit foods by blocking mast-cell reactions in the gut wall. (Unfortunately for those with migraine, sodium cromoglycate is not the 'instant cure' that it might appear to be from these studies – see p320.)

There is a third way in which the gut wall might be made more leaky. We all produce a special type of IgA antibody called secretory IgA or **SIgA**. The production of SIgA is stimulated by the Peyer's patches, and it pours out into the gut, where it binds to its target antigen. By binding to antigens, and locking them into immune complexes, SIgA effectively makes them much bigger. The bigger they are the more difficult it is for them to pass through the gut wall. So SIgA reduces the number of food molecules that cross the gut wall – and the number of microbes, because SIgA is made to these as well. Like IgA in the blood, SIgA does not cause any inflammation.

There is some evidence that people with food intolerance have less SIgA than healthy people. However, there are patients who have *severe* deficiencies of SIgA, and, although they are ill in other ways, they show no more signs of food sensitivity than the population at large. This suggests that SIgA deficiency alone is not enough to cause food intolerance.

The role of immune complexes

If more food molecules get through the gut wall, more immune complexes will form in the blood. There are certain diseases which produce an excessive load of immune complexes in the blood, too many for the 'eating cells' to cope with. This results in **serum sickness**. The unpleasant symptoms of serum sickness are due to immune complexes depositing in small blood vessels (see p75).

It has been suggested that some symptoms of food intolerance might come about in the same way. The reduction of IgA antibodies in the food-molecule immune complexes, and the presence of inflammatory antibodies such as IgE, would be likely to make the problem worse. The two main symptoms that might arise in this way are joint pain and migraine. At present, however, firm evidence for this is lacking. In both cases, there are certain to be other mechanisms at work as well (see p124 and pp130–1).

Too many messengers?

There is one other way in which the immune system might be involved in food intolerance. All immune cells use small messenger molecules, known as **lymphokines**, to communicate with each other. One cell will produce a particular messenger molecule when it is stimulated, and this will make

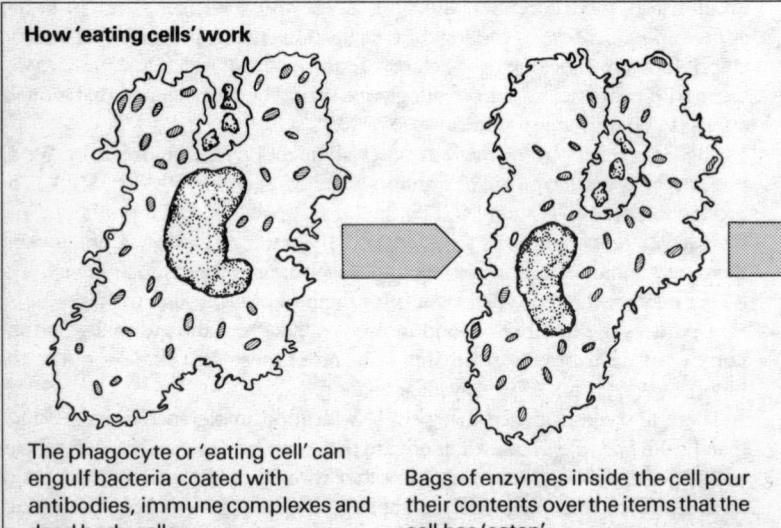

How 'eating cells' work

The phagocyte or 'eating cell' can engulf bacteria coated with antibodies, immune complexes and dead body cells.

Bags of enzymes inside the cell pour their contents over the items that the cell has 'eaten'.

another cell become active, or divide rapidly to produce more cells, or respond in some other way.

One important messenger molecule is **interferon**, whose main job is to combat viral infections. Interferon makes cells resistant to viruses. Some of the less beneficial effects of interferon only came to light when it was used as a medicine. Hepatitis B is a debilitating viral disease that is very difficult to treat. The discovery of interferon led to its use in hepatitis B, because it can stimulate the body to mount a more effective attack against the virus. But the patients who were receiving large doses of interferon suffered from unpleasant side-effects, including severe fatigue, headaches, dizziness, abdominal discomfort, bowel disturbances, nausea and joint pain.

This list of side-effects is remarkably similar to the symptoms of a mysterious and controversial illness that goes by the name of **post-viral syndrome (PVS)**, **chronic fatigue syndrome (CFS)** or **myalgic encephalitis (ME)**. In looking for the causes of this illness, most doctors have concluded that it must be psychosomatic. However, most cases seem to follow on from a viral infection of some sort, and 50 per cent of patients show a high level of antibodies to viral proteins. The parallel with interferon side-effects suggests an alternative explanation to the psychosomatic one – that the immune system has over-reacted to a viral infection and is continuing to produce excessive

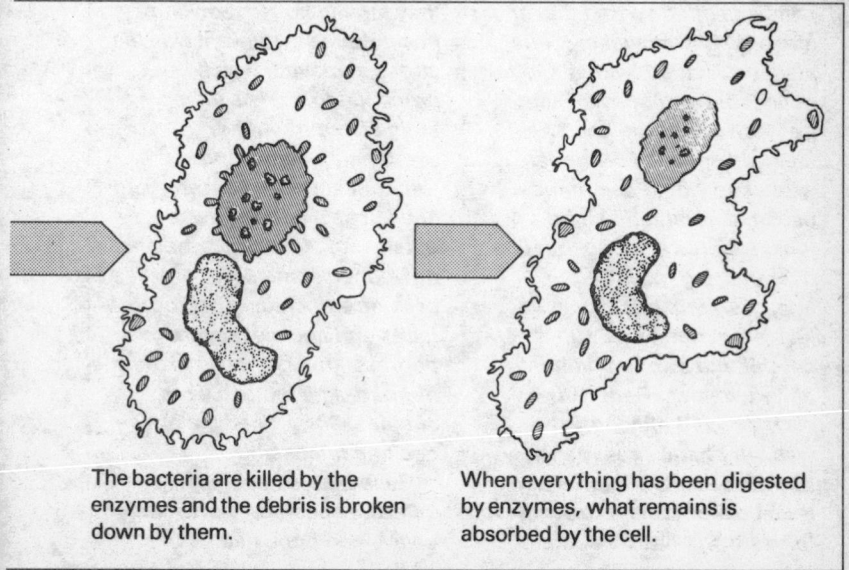

The bacteria are killed by the enzymes and the debris is broken down by them.

When everything has been digested by enzymes, what remains is absorbed by the cell.

amounts of interferon. Alternatively, other lymphokines might be responsible for producing the symptoms – several others have similar effects.

If this is the case – and there is no definitive proof that it is – then interferon might also play a role in food intolerance. Perhaps there is some unknown immune reaction to food which stimulates the body to produce interferon, or other lymphokines, in damaging amounts. It is interesting that many PVS patients have been greatly helped by an elimination diet – it would seem that reactions to food are contributing to their symptoms. Some have also been helped by a no-sugar, no-yeast diet and anti-fungal drugs – see Chapter Ten.

REBECCA

Rebecca began to have problems with severe sore throats when she was in her teens. At the same time she suffered 'swollen glands' (swelling of the lymph nodes) producing painful lumps in her groin, armpits and neck. The pain was often so bad that she had difficulty in walking. She also felt bloated, with a noticeable puffiness around her face and neck, and she suffered spells of dizziness, when she would sometimes pass out. Eventually, her tonsils were removed, but this did not bring much improvement: her throat was less sore, but it was still painful and swollen. In her early twenties, Rebecca married, and although she was very happy with her new husband, her symptoms began to get worse. She frequently felt as if she had flu coming on, with aches and pains, headaches and swollen glands. Severe catarrh, recurrent mouth ulcers and stomach pains were also making life difficult.

All these problems came to a head when she was 25 and they moved house. Looking back, Rebecca thinks it was the stress of moving which precipitated a crisis in her state of health. All her symptoms became more frequent and more severe, and she felt as if her body was 'totally out of control'. She also developed some new problems, including aching joints and bouts of severe depression. She had to give up her part-time job and even simple tasks around the house became impossible.

Rebecca had seen many different specialists over the years, and none had been

Viral infections

Viruses themselves might also play a part in food intolerance. It is known that they can alter our immune responses in subtle ways, and viral infections can certainly spark off true allergic reactions in some people, particularly asthmatics. Some people date their food intolerance to a bout of influenza or other viral infection.

Viruses in the gut could alter the structure of the gut wall, simply by binding to its cells – they might even do this without causing any noticeable signs of infection. Such viruses could make the gut wall more leaky for a while by changing its structure.

---

able to do much for her. But at this point she heard something about 'food allergy' from a friend, and asked her family doctor if he thought this might be worth investigating. The doctor was sceptical, but made an appointment for her to see a specialist, who put her on a strict diet, starting with a three-day fast. Then she went on to a diet of lamb, pears and mineral water. Within a week she felt so much better that she could scarcely believe it. Almost all her symptoms had gone, except for a few aches in her joints. 'I had been ill for so long, I'd forgotten what it was like to be well – it was an amazing feeling,' she recalls.

The long process of testing foods then began. Eventually Rebecca identified the following culprits: most types of additives, wheat, oranges,

lemons, butter, strawberries and alcohol. Eating any of these would produce swollen glands, depression, headache, stomach pains, aching joints and general flu-like symptoms within a few hours. It took her a long time to test all foods and establish a workable diet, but she now enjoys very good health and can eat a variety of foods. She can even tolerate small amounts of wheat and her other culprit foods occasionally, but has to avoid additives.

Cases like Rebecca's are rare but they raise some interesting questions about what causes food intolerance. The swollen lymph nodes suggest that her immune system was affected by her reactions to foods, even though her symptoms were not those one would associate with allergy.

THE EXORPHIN PUZZLE

A good half of patients with food intolerance have cravings for the food or foods that make them ill, and eat such foods to excess. Addictive eating is an aspect of food intolerance that does nothing to improve its medical credibility – yet it cannot be ignored. Within the last few years, a possible mechanism for this strange behaviour has emerged, in the form of chemicals called exorphins. To understand what *exorphins* do (or might do) we must first look at the *endorphins*.

Endorphins – built-in painkillers

Pain is all about survival. We have specialized nerves, known as pain-receptors, to help us avoid damaging ourselves – on sharp objects, for example, or by overextending our joints. But there has to be a way of turning pain off, when it no longer serves a useful purpose. For that reason we have **endorphins** or **natural opioids**.

Endorphins are natural painkillers, released during intense pain, or strenuous exercise, or when some stressful event evokes our 'flight or fight' response (see p151). There are receptors for these molecules on cells in the brain and when the endorphins bind to these, feelings of pain are reduced, and a sensation of well-being ensues. (In fact, there are about four or five different types of endorphin receptor, and they have different effects – although pain-blocking is the main one, there are others as well.)

Morphine, heroin and other **opiates** happen to mimic the endorphins and they bind to the same receptors – hence their use as drugs. They are addictive because they suppress the body's natural ability to produce endorphins – so when they are stopped, the addict suffers agonizing withdrawal symptoms.

Hooked on food?

The endorphins are all **peptides** – short chains made up of amino acids. Proteins also consist of amino acid chains (see p23), but in proteins the chains are much longer. When foods are broken down in the gut, the proteins are split into shorter lengths – in other words, into peptides. By chance, some of those peptides consist of a very similar sequence of amino acid to the natural endorphins. Such peptides are therefore called **exorphins** (*exogenous morphine*-like molecules). In the laboratory, these exorphins have been produced from milk, wheat, maize and barley, using human digestive enzymes. Other foods have yet to be investigated.

Further laboratory experiments show that exorphins can bind to the natural receptors for endorphins – but whether they actually do so in the body is another matter. First they would have to get through the gut wall and into the bloodstream. They would also have to evade protein-cracking enzymes in the liver : endorphins have a special chemical structure at the end of the molecule which prevents such enzymes from attacking them, but exorphins do not.

So can the exorphins have any effect on the body? One experiment suggests that they can. A partially digested sample of wheat protein was fed to human 'guinea-pigs', and produced certain measurable changes in bodily function. The experiment was then repeated, with a drug called naloxone being given before the wheat. This drug is known to block endorphin receptors, and prevents peptides from binding to them. When naloxone was given first, the wheat protein had no effect.

Many more experiments are needed before we can reach any firm conclusions about exorphins, but the results so far suggest that they *might* influence our mood. There is certainly no question of anyone getting 'high' on a glass of milk or a slice of bread – the amounts involved are too small for that – but these foods might induce a sense of comfort and well-being, as food-intolerant patients often say they do. There are also other hormone-like peptides in partial digests of food, which might have other effects on the body.

If foods can produce these peptides, then why do they only affect certain people? It is possible that the leakiness of the gut wall is important here – if more peptides get through, more are likely to get to the receptors before they are broken down by enzymes. Any deficiency in those enzymes would also increase the person's vulnerability to exorphins.

ENZYMES AND FOOD INTOLERANCE

Enzymes make chemical reactions happen, as described on p18. The two main types of enzymes that concern us here are **digestive enzymes** and **detoxification enzymes**.

Digestive enzymes are mostly found in the gut, where they break food down into smaller molecules (see p20). The purpose of digestion is to reduce food molecules to their basic building blocks, which can then be used by the body to construct its own molecules – rather like demolishing an old house and then using the bricks to build something else. There are also some digestive enzymes (mostly protein-splitting enzymes) within the gut wall and in the liver: these complete the digestion of food molecules after they have been absorbed.

Detoxification enzymes are charged with destroying or disarming all the toxins that get into our bodies. Some of these toxins are found in food, where they mostly serve defensive purposes (see p15). Others are produced by the bacteria living in our gut – the **gut flora**. To add to this 'natural' load, there are a variety of synthetic substances that have to be detoxified, including alcohol and nicotine, medicinal drugs, food additives, and pesticide residues in food. Most of the body's detoxification enzymes are found in the liver, but there are also some in other parts of the body, such as the surface of the blood platelets – the tiny 'cells' in the blood that help it to clot.

Detoxification enzymes respond to the body's particular needs – if more toxin is taken in then more of the appropriate enzymes are produced to cope with the added load. An obvious example of this is alcohol – the more we drink, on a regular basis, the more it takes to feel inebriated. Give up alcohol for a few months and a half of shandy is enough to make you tipsy. In effect, the body has become much more sensitive to the effects of alcohol, because the liver has scaled down its production of the necessary detoxification enzymes.

Although this works for alcohol, it is by no means certain that it works for all toxins – with some toxins, the body may only have a limited capacity to cope with them, and increasing the load may not increase the detoxification enzymes. Even with alcohol there is a limit – the task of detoxification eventually becomes too much for the liver, which begins to fail. When this happens, the vital role that the liver normally plays becomes apparent – alcoholics suffer badly from the effects of natural toxins, especially those produced by gut bacteria, which they can no longer detoxify.

Enzyme defects

In some people, certain enzymes are either in short supply, or they fail to work properly because their structure is abnormal. Such people are said to have 'enzyme deficiencies'. Some deficiencies have no obvious effects, because there are other enzymes that can 'cover' for the missing one – the body often has more than one option, especially when it comes to digestion and detoxification. Other deficiencies are far more damaging, because the enzyme is the only one that can do that particular job, and toxic substances build up in the body if it is ineffectual.

Enzyme deficiencies have been known for many years. The more serious ones become noticeable soon after a child is born, or after it is weaned, and can kill or severely disable the child unless treated. The usual treatment is a special diet, which excludes foods that the child cannot deal with. The most widespread enzyme deficiency of this type is phenylketonuria; all babies are tested for this soon after they are born. Another example of a major enzyme deficiency is a shortage of the enzyme lactase, which breaks down the sugar in milk (see p207). Both of these enzyme defects are very rare – phenylketonuria only affects one baby in 12,000. A third type of enzyme deficiency has only been recognized relatively recently, and the frequency is, as yet, unknown. This defect prevents the breakdown of fructose – the sugar found in fruit and in table sugar. Luckily, children born with this deficiency soon develop a strong dislike of anything sweet-tasting, so they remain well as long as they are not forced to eat such foods. Parents should bear in mind that some apparently savoury foods actually contain sugar, and the child's dislike of a food should be their guide. If a child has fructose intolerance, it may be helpful to tell the child's school that they should not be forced to eat any food they actively dislike, as the reaction can be very unpleasant.

In recent years, it has become clear that there may be other, less noticeable, forms of enzyme deficiency. Some of these have come to light when certain patients reacted very badly to particular medicinal drugs – it turned out that they were less able to detoxify them than most people. Special chemical 'probes' have been developed in an effort to detect such patients – these are non-toxic compounds that are processed by the same enzymes, and which can readily be measured. The 'probe' is given to the patient, and the level is later measured (in the blood or urine) to see how thoroughly the drug has been broken down.

When these probes are tried out on people with food intolerance, they produce interesting results. Such people are much more likely to be deficient in *some enzymes* than healthy people are – they do metabolize the drugs, but more slowly. However, there is no single enzyme which is defective in *all* food-intolerant individuals – or if there is, it has yet to be found. With enzyme defects, as with everything else, it looks as if food intolerance is a 'mixed bag'.

One interesting factor to emerge from these experiments concerns patients who are sensitive to man-made chemicals, as well as food (see Chapter Nine). In this group, an even higher percentage are enzyme-deficient than among those with food intolerance alone. For one enzyme, 90 per cent of such patients were deficient, compared with 80 per cent of those with food intolerance, and 20 per cent of the population at large. Interestingly enough, a high proportion of those with food *allergy* – 64 per cent – also showed a deficiency.

The fact that some apparently healthy people are deficient in these same enzymes is revealing. This clearly shows that a single enzyme defect of this type could not be the sole cause of food intolerance. Those who suffer from food intolerance must have other underlying problems as well – perhaps a shortage of another enzyme, or a leaky gut wall, or some other problem entirely. It is tempting to speculate that people with multiple sensitivities (foods and chemicals) are defective for a whole range of enzymes, making them much more susceptible to environmental factors. But at present, there are too few studies of enzyme deficiency to know if this is likely.

Enzymes, colourings and hyperactivity
One discovery about enzyme deficiencies is particularly intriguing, because it may explain the link between hyperactivity in children and food colourings

(see p213). Hyperactive children appear to be deficient in an enzyme known as phenolsulphotransferase-P or **PST-P**. This enzyme detoxifies various compounds, including a substance called **p-cresol** that is produced by bacteria in the gut. No-one has any idea how p-cresol might cause hyperactivity, but it is a phenol, and phenols can be toxic.

What is interesting about PST-P is that it can be **inhibited** by certain food colourings – in other words, the enzyme no longer works if those food colourings are present. If a normal, healthy child eats colouring of this type in moderation, it will not do any apparent harm because that child's PST-P is fully active to begin with. But for a child with defective PST-P, the same amount of colouring could reduce the level of PST-P activity to damaging levels.

It is interesting that a high proportion of patients with migraine, who are affected by dietary triggers such as cheese and chocolate, also have a defect in PST-P. Wine, like some food colourings, appears to inhibit PST-P, and this may contribute to the effects of red wine in triggering migraines. It is likely that enzyme defects play a part in migraine, because migraine sufferers tend to be defective for certain enzymes, but exactly what goes wrong is far from clear. The chemicals that are under suspicion of triggering migraine – tyramine and phenylethylamine (see p128) – are not detoxified by PST-P. Tyramine *is* detoxified by a related enzyme called PST-M, but this is generally not lacking in migraine sufferers. This is a puzzle that can only be sorted out by more research. For more on enzyme defects in migraine, see p129.

BUGS IN THE SYSTEM

Our digestive tract is home to a great many bacteria and other microbes, which do not cause any disease, and are actually important for good health. They are known as **gut flora**. Some doctors believe that the gut flora may becomes 'disturbed', and this might contribute to food intolerance (see Chapter Ten).

A MODERN EPIDEMIC?

Is food intolerance becoming more common? It is impossible to answer this question because there is little agreement on how common food intolerance is today (see p85) and no way of find out how common it was in the past. But the general impression, among doctors who treat food intolerance, is that it *has* become increasingly widespread. There is little hard evidence to support this, apart from a few epidemiological studies. One of these concerns Crohn's disease in Africa. It shows that Crohn's disease – which has been linked with food intolerance (see p118) – is virtually unknown in rural areas, but becomes more common when people move into towns. In Britain, there has been a dramatic rise in the incidence of Crohn's disease since World War II.

CAROL

Carol was an active woman in her fifties, who had a part-time secretarial job and was a voluntary worker at the local hospital. With a large family of children and grandchildren to worry about, she tended to ignore the odd aches and pains that she suffered. But as the years went by these grew worse, and finally began to interfere with her life. She had difficulty getting out of bed in the morning, her joints were so stiff, and it was only by the evening that she really loosened up and could move around normally. As well as joint pain, she began to suffer from diarrhoea and wind, which was worse whenever she drank alcohol. Headaches became more regular until she had them almost every day, and she often had severe pains in her face due to sinusitis. She also suffered repeated thrush infections and an itchy rash between the toes which looked like athlete's foot. Her doctor put Carol on a sugar-free diet and prescribed an anti-fungal drug, nystatin. This made her feel much worse initially, but after a month her bowels were functioning normally, her joints were less stiff and her headaches were less frequent.

Since she was still not completely well, the doctor asked her to try an elimination diet, avoiding cereal grains, dairy products and eggs. Carol was impressed by the change this brought about – she felt much better in herself, less tired and able to be cheerful without making an effort. She also lost some excess weight that she had accumulated. On testing, it turned out to be eggs and wheat that caused her problems. Having improved so much, she was now able to notice the specific effects of certain other foods. For one thing, she noticed that foods containing a lot of additives made her feel tired and unwell, with vague muscle aches. Decorating the house also produced these sort of symptoms, and she found later that solvents, such as white spirit and dry-cleaning fluid, regularly had this effect.

As this case shows, there are often several different factors at work in individual patients. It is not unusual for food intolerance to go hand-in-hand with abnormal gut flora (see Chapter Ten) and sensitivity to synthetic chemicals. How these three problems might interconnect is still unknown.

Rheumatoid arthritis is also steadily increasing, although this is a rise that began in the early nineteenth century.

Crohn's disease is a serious and debilitating illness – most of those with food intolerance have much milder symptoms. Indeed, many people in the early stages of food intolerance may scarcely be aware of being ill: headaches, indigestion, persistent tiredness and occasional diarrhoea are all reported as the early symptoms, by those who later become more seriously ill and then discover they are sensitive to food. Symptoms of this sort are everyday problems that most people tend to accept as part of life. But are they? Or have these things slowly crept up on us all, so that we have scarcely noticed a gradual decline in health? In her autobiographical book *Lark Rise to Candleford*, Flora Thompson recalls life in her native farming village, during the 1880s: 'There were two epidemics of measles during the decade, and two men had accidents in the harvest field and were taken to hospital; but, for years together, the doctor was only seen there when one of the ancients was dying of old age, or some difficult first confinement baffled the skill of the old woman who, as she said, saw the beginning and end of everybody. There was no cripple or mental defective in the hamlet, and, except for a few months when a poor woman was dying of cancer, no invalid. Though food was rough and teeth were neglected, indigestion was unknown, while nervous troubles, there as elsewhere, had yet to be invented.' Contrast this with the general state of health of people today. As Dr Ronald Finn of the Royal Liverpool Hospital observes: 'It is depressingly rare to come across someone who is entirely well.'

Doctors who are involved in treating food intolerance, as Dr Finn is, may not be impartial observers, of course. But others have noticed the same general trend. American psychiatrist, Dr Arthur Barsky, calls it the 'paradox of health'. He points out that in 1900 a man's life expectancy was 47.3 years, now it is almost 75 years, yet we *feel* we are less healthy. In the 1920s only 10 per cent of recognized illnesses could be treated successfully, now the figure is over 50 per cent, but we are all preoccupied with illness. Why should this be? Dr Barsky believes that it is all a question of attitude. One factor, in his view, is our 'heightened awareness of health' due to 'medico-media hype' – in other words, if people knew less about their bodies they would feel better.

An alternative explanation, which psychiatrists such as Dr Barsky seem not to consider, is that people really *are* ill, with vague, long-term symptoms that are not life-threatening, and do not, therefore, reduce their life expectancy. Perhaps such problems have only become widespread within the last 50–100 years – this could explain the 'paradox of health' that Dr Barsky describes. Such illness might simply be due to the increased stress of modern living, but the circumstantial evidence suggests that food intolerance could also be important.

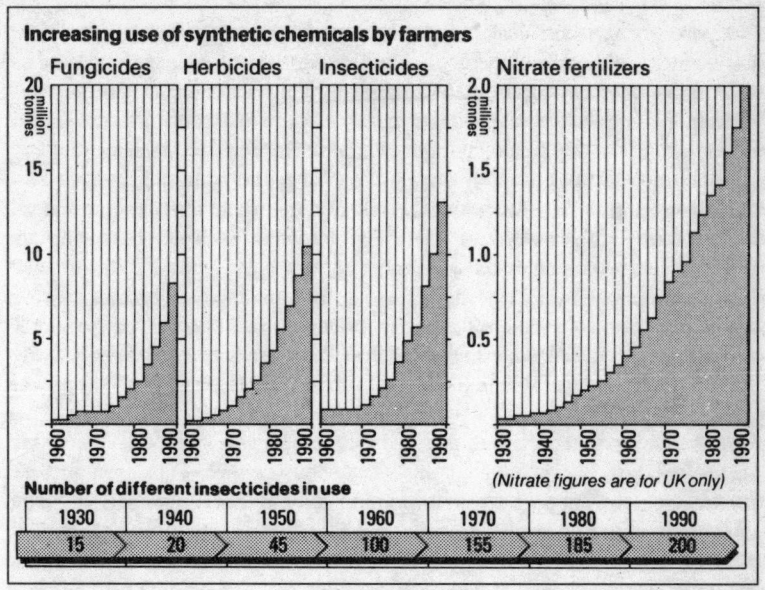

Increasing use of synthetic chemicals by farmers

Number of different insecticides in use						
1930	1940	1950	1960	1970	1980	1990
15	20	45	100	155	185	200

(Nitrate figures are for UK only)

Modern life

A lot of things have changed in the last 50–100 years. Of all the momentous changes that have occurred, is there anything that might have made people more susceptible to food intolerance? On the basis of what we already know about how food intolerance begins, there are several obvious candidates.

Chemical exposure

The main one, in our view, is the increasing exposure to man-made chemicals – food additives, pesticide residues, exhaust fumes, solvents, industrial pollutants and the like. It is known (although only from case-histories) that a single massive exposure to a toxic chemical, such as a pesticide, can bring on a severe form of food intolerance. It is also the case that a small proportion of people with food intolerance are unduly sensitive to everyday chemicals (see Chapter Nine). What is more, if those people can reduce their chemical exposure, they often find they can tolerate the foods to which they are sensitive normally. It seems likely that these people have certain enzyme deficiencies, which make them vulnerable to man-made chemicals *and* intolerant of certain foods – but if the chemical stress can be reduced they are able to cope adequately with those same foodstuffs. Such people would not have been ill if they had lived 50 years or more ago, but they are ill now, because the environment around them has changed.

Environmental chemicals could also be a factor in others with food intolerance – even those who are not overtly sensitive to everyday chemicals. It is possible that chemicals in food and drinking water affect the gut wall, making it more leaky – there might be no obvious effect from the chemicals alone, but they could create the right conditions for food intolerance.

Such chemical exposure might also play a part in true allergy. We have already seen that patients with food allergy are more likely to be enzyme deficient than those with no allergy or intolerance (see p243). And the incidence of certain allergies appears to be increasing – in fact, this is much better documented than the alleged rise in food intolerance, because doctors are agreed on how to diagnose allergic diseases. Eczema is one of the allergic problems that is steadily rising – and it is one that is quite often associated with food sensitivity. Whether chemical exposure is playing a part in this remains to be seen.

Antibiotics

If changes in the gut flora are an important factor in food intolerance, then the use of antibiotics must undoubtedly shoulder some of the blame. The major antibiotics have only been in widespread use since the 1940s, and no-one would deny their major contribution to medicine. Indeed, a short course of antibiotics is unlikely to do anyone much harm. It is prolonged use, or very high doses, that are most likely to affect the gut flora. In some situations the antibiotics are not strictly necessary – in treating acne for example, or in repeated childhood 'infections' that are not really infections at all, but undiagnosed allergies.

Bottle-feeding and early weaning

The change from breast to bottle has been one of the major changes of the past 50 years. Although there is now a reversal of this trend, many babies are still bottle-fed, and many more are given additional, or 'complementary', feeds from a bottle.

Several studies show that babies born into atopic ('allergic') families are less likely to develop food allergies if they are exclusively breast-fed for at least six months (see p253). During the first few months, the immune system is not fully developed, and the 'oral tolerance' mechanism, described above, does not seem to be fully functional. To make matters worse, the baby's gut is excessively leaky to allow protective antibodies from the mother's milk to get through to the bloodstream. These factors conspire to make the baby vulnerable to food allergy.

If food *intolerance* involves some type of immune reaction – even though it is not the major factor involved – bottle-feeding and early weaning could also be a factor in causing food intolerance. So far, there is not much hard evidence for the value of breast-feeding in preventing food intolerance, because very little research has been carried out in this area. But there is good evidence that breast-feeding is helpful in preventing colic.

The Pill
Oral contraceptive tablets – the Pill – have been in widespread use since the 1960s. Some doctors believe that the high incidence of food intolerance in women is related to this, and there are individual case-histories that link the onset of food intolerance with starting the Pill. Unfortunately, there are no studies to show if this reaction is common. One of the difficulties with the Pill is that its ill-effects are usually very much delayed – and even after stopping the Pill there may be lingering effects for months or even years. So the link with the symptoms may be far from obvious.

There are various ways in which the Pill might lead to food intolerance. It appears to have an effect on certain detoxification enzymes in the liver, and this could make women more susceptible to toxins in food, as well as to environmental chemicals. The Pill also seems to affect vitamin and mineral status (see p270) and some nutritional deficiencies may make food intolerance more likely. In the case of migraine, the hormones in the Pill have a direct action on the blood vessels, and are well known as a cause of migraine.

Chapter Thirteen

PREVENTING FOOD SENSITIVITY

There is little doubt that food allergy 'runs in families', and food intolerance may do so as well. But this does not mean that illness is inevitable. It is clear, in food allergy at least, that the environment is important, especially in the first year of life. What a child inherits is a *predisposition* to allergy. The sort of conditions it encounters immediately after birth (and, perhaps, before birth) will decide whether it actually develops allergies. Parents who know that their child is likely to suffer from allergies can take steps to reduce the risk. With food *intolerance*, the case for prevention is less clear-cut. But where one member of the family suffers adverse reactions to food, it is worth considering various simple measures that may help others to escape the same fate.

The allergy risk
The risks of a child developing allergies can be gauged, very roughly, from the health of the parents. If one parent has allergic symptoms, the chances of the child being atopic – predisposed to allergy – is 20–35 per cent. If both parents have allergies, the likelihood rises to 40–60 per cent. Where both parents are affected in the same way – if both have asthma, for example, or both have rhinitis (runny or congested nose) – then the chances are 50–70 per cent.

If neither parent has allergies, but one or both come from families with a history of allergic disease, then there is also an increased risk of the child being affected. However, almost a third of atopics are born into families where no allergic symptoms have ever been noticed. So predicting which babies will be prone to allergies by looking at their families is, at best, an inexact science.

A more accurate prediction can be made by laboratory tests that measure the amount of IgE (see p25) being produced by the child. The level can be measured by taking a sample of blood from the newborn baby, or by

TABLE 11   PREVENTIVE MEASURES FOR ALLERGY

These measures can help to prevent allergies developing in babies born into atopic (allergic) families. See pp250–7 for further details.

Don't eat too much of any one food while pregnant. It may also be worthwhile avoiding foods that are potent allergens (listed below), but there is no firm evidence that this is of benefit during pregnancy. Restricting your diet during breast-feeding is much more important for the baby.

Give up smoking before becoming pregnant. Once the child is born, make sure that no-one smokes in the house.

Breast-feed for the first year if possible. Give nothing but breast milk for the first 4-6 months.

If breast-feeding is not possible, discuss with your doctor the possible alternatives, such as hydrolysate formulas.

While breast-feeding, avoid eating foods that are likely to cause allergic reactions: milk, eggs, peanuts, fish, citrus fruits (oranges, lemons etc), wheat, beef and chicken. To this list, add any food to which a previous child is allergic.

After 4-6 months, introduce some solid foods, but withhold those listed above until 9-12 months.

Introduce these foods gradually, one at a time, so that reactions can be noted. Do not give new foods when the child is ill.

For the first year, have no furred pets, keep dust to a minimum and keep the house free of moulds (see p70–1 for details). If the child has an infection, take special care to keep allergens to a minimum.

Where possible, avoid exposing the baby to air pollution.

Avoid unnecessary surgery during the first year of life.

---

measuring the IgE level in blood from the umbilical cord. A high level indicates that a child has a greater chance of going on to develop allergies. Measuring a group of immune cells called T suppressor cells, *as well as* the level of IgE, provides the best possible test for susceptibility to allergy. If both are high, the likelihood of allergy is over 90 per cent. However, both these tests require very sensitive chemical analysis, and they are unlikely to be available in most hospitals.

If your child happens to be given skin tests or specific IgE tests (RAST tests) at some stage, he or she may show up as having high IgE levels to certain foods. What should you do if the test for a particular food is positive but your child eats the food without apparent ill-effects? You may well be told to ignore it, but in the opinion of many experts this is bad advice. One study of such children has shown that, within seven years, they usually go on to develop allergic reactions.

PREVENTIVE MEASURES FOR FOOD ALLERGY

The aim of the preventive measures described here (and summarized in Table 11) is to reduce the child's exposure to potent allergens, and other factors that can trigger off allergy, during the early phases of life. The measures are relevant to any Type-1 (IgE-mediated) reaction to food, whether that food causes an immediate, violent reaction centred on the mouth and lips, or a much more delayed reaction such as asthma or eczema. In general, however, the former are more difficult to prevent, because the child can become sensitized by such minute amounts of food. In the case of asthma, rhinitis and eczema, a mixture of allergens may produce symptoms: the effect of allergens in food may be exacerbated by inhaled allergens such as pollen, or by allergens touching the skin. For this reason, any preventive measures must include inhalants and contactants as well as foods.

Breast-feeding

A baby's immune system is not fully developed at birth. To protect it against infection in the first few months of life, a mother's milk contains antibodies to commonly found bacteria and viruses, and the baby's gut is 'leaky' to allow these antibodies through into the bloodstream. Because the gut is so permeable, undigested food molecules also get into the blood in far greater quantity than in an older child or adult. At the same time, the control reactions that regulate damaging immune reactions are not yet up-and-running. In particular, the system that prevents the manufacture of IgE to harmless antigens is not fully effective.

Any food that the baby eats or drinks during the first three months of life will be absorbed into the bloodstream in appreciable quantities. Some unknown mechanism prevents a baby from mounting a damaging immune reaction against the proteins in its mother's milk – although there may be cases of babies being allergic to their mother's breast milk, these are extremely rare. Presumably the process by which the baby learns to tolerate the breast-milk proteins happens before birth, while the baby is still in the womb.

A bottle-fed baby, or one that receives solids before three months of age, is exposed to large quantities of 'foreign' proteins entering the bloodstream, and there is ample evidence that these can cause allergic reactions. Even a baby that is never bottle-fed is not entirely safe. Proteins from the mother's food can be absorbed intact from her gut and pass into her breast milk. Although the quantities involved are small, there is little doubt that these can sensitize an atopic child. In fact, the most violent reactions to cow's milk are seen in children who have been sensitized via breast milk, rather than those that have been bottle-fed from birth. This might seem like a good argument for bottle-feeding, on the face of it, but bear in mind that these violent reactions are rare, whereas the less severe but very troublesome symptoms that might result from bottle-feeding are far more widespread.

The advice generally given to parents of high-risk babies is to feed the baby on nothing but breast milk for the first four to six months of life. Weaning should then be conducted at a very gradual pace, with breast-feeding continuing until the child is a year old if possible. If breast milk is still supplying most of the baby's food needs, then the amount of solid food eaten can be much less.

When it comes to introducing new foods, those with low allergenic potential should be given at first, and the foods that most often produce allergic reactions withheld for a time. The main problem foods are eggs, milk, fish, peanuts, wheat, rye, barley, nuts, soya, citrus fruits and chocolate. Beef and chicken should also be kept off the menu, as they share some allergenic proteins with milk and eggs respectively. A working party set up by the World Health Organization has suggested that such allergenic foods should not be given before the child's first birthday, but some doctors feel that avoiding them for six to nine months is adequate.

When they *are* introduced, new foods should be given gradually, one at a time, so that any adverse reactions can be related to particular foods. Infections and bouts of diarrhoea make the child more easily sensitized, so new foods should not be introduced if the child is ill.

Because food molecules pass into breast milk, it is important for the mother to watch what she eats while breast-feeding. She should avoid eggs, cow's milk, peanuts and fish, and should restrict her alcohol intake, especially of red wine. It might also be worth avoiding soya, nuts, citrus fruits and grains (wheat, barley and rye). Calcium gluconate tablets can be prescribed to make up for the lack of calcium in a milk-free diet – or she can try goat's or sheep's milk, in limited quantities. If any previous children are highly allergic to specific foods then these too should be excluded from her diet, and should not be given to the new baby in its first year.

If all these restrictions seem too much to bear, then take a middle road, or allow yourself some days off. *The important thing is to breast feed and to keep it up for as long as possible – six months if you can.* Anything that puts a mother off breast-feeding is a bad idea. Quite clearly, the *best* course is to breast feed *and* keep high-risk foods out of your diet, but there are times when we have to accept that we can only manage 'second best'. If the dietary restrictions become so tiresome that you want to stop breast-feeding after a couple of months, then drop the diet rather than the breast-feeding.

Maternity Wards

Ironically, the most difficult place to ensure that a baby is given nothing but breast milk may be in a maternity ward. The practice of giving supplementary or 'complementary' feeds is still common in some hospitals, and can be very damaging in the first few weeks of life. These feeds contain infant formulas based on cow's milk, which are likely to be allergenic for the susceptible child. At this early stage in life the baby is very vulnerable to sensitization by foreign proteins. One study looked at over 1,700 babies, of whom 1,500 received supplementary feeds and 200 did not. There were 39 cases of cow's milk allergy, and *all* of these were in babies given supplementary feeds.

Giving supplementary feeds can also have more insidious effects that may lead to the baby having to be entirely bottle-fed. Extra feeds from bottles upset the subtle balance of demand-and-supply that is established between a breast-feeding mother and her child. A rubber teat works differently from a real one, and babies that are given bottles do not always suck properly at the breast. Their appetite is also diminished, so they suck less hard, and the mother therefore produces less milk. This sets up a vicious circle, which may end with the mother being told that she 'does not have enough milk' and must therefore bottle-feed.

Where there is a hospital policy of not putting babies to the breast during the night, breast milk can be 'expressed' and stored, to be given from a bottle by a nurse. This method can also be used at home, for times when breast-feeding is not a practical proposition.

Preparing for breast-feeding

The mother who wishes to ensure that her baby is solely breast-fed needs to be prepared in advance. Because breast-feeding is thought of as 'natural' it is often assumed that it 'comes naturally'. Unfortunately this is not true, and many mothers give up because they have not been shown how to breast-feed properly, or because they have sore nipples, or other problems. Advice and help with breast-feeding can be obtained from several organizations whose addresses are listed on p340.

Before going into hospital, enquire about their policy on night feeds and supplementary feeds. Make it very clear to the midwife that you do not wish your baby to have anything but breast milk. Ask whether you will be able to have your baby with you and feed it on demand – this is far more conducive to successful breast-feeding than a system that is ruled by the clock. Another factor in establishing a good working relationship with your baby is starting breast-feeding within four hours of birth. Where a baby or mother is very ill, this may not always be possible, but you should ask that the baby be put to the breast as soon as possible.

If breast-feeding is not possible, for whatever reason, then the mother should not feel guilty about the situation. There *are* alternatives that carry less risk of allergy than standard infant formulas. These are feed mixtures known as hydrolysates (see p221) which are available on prescription.

Formula feeds based on soya (see p221) are sometimes used with children who are known to be sensitive to cow's milk. These tend to be prescribed because they are a great deal cheaper than hydrolysates, and they may be very effective in clearing up symptoms that are due to cow's milk sensitivity. However, there is always the risk that a child will develop allergic reactions to soya proteins, which are themselves noted allergens. This is especially likely if the mother has eaten soya, which she may well have done, since soya flour is increasingly common as a 'hidden' ingredient in many foods. As part of a *prevention* programme, soya-based formulas are not necessarily that much better than standard milk-based formulas – hydrolysates are definitely preferable.

There is little doubt that prolonged breast-feeding and careful weaning are the most important factors in diminishing the risk of *allergy* in newborn babies. There are also good reasons for believing that breast-feeding reduces the likelihood of food *intolerance*, as well as having more general benefits, such as protecting babies from infection. Trying to breast-feed for as long as possible is something that would benefit any child. (A recent study suggested that it led to higher IQ in later years, for example.) As a matter of national health-care policy, the many obstacles and discouragements to breast-feeding should be removed, and the promotion of formula feeds in maternity wards should stop, as the World Health Organization has recommended.

Preventive measures during pregnancy

Although the baby in the womb is nourished by the mother's blood, the blood of mother and baby do not mix. Instead, they both pass through tiny blood vessels (capillaries) in the structure known as the placenta. The capillaries carrying the mother's blood lie directly alongside those carrying the baby's blood, and vital substances such as glucose and oxygen can pass from one to the other through the capillary walls. It used to be thought that larger molecules, such as undigested food proteins, would not be able to get through, but it is now known that they do. Such food molecules could sensitize a high-risk baby even before it is born.

In the light of this discovery, some doctors believe that women whose children are likely to be atopic should restrict their diet during pregnancy. However, the few studies that have attempted to test this idea have produced largely negative results. Given the difficulty of eating a restricted diet during pregnancy it is probably not worth doing so for such uncertain gains. But anyone who is concerned about allergies in their children – having had one severely allergic child already, perhaps – could omit certain foods that are highly allergenic. The list should include cow's milk, eggs, peanuts, fish and wheat, plus any foods to which the earlier child is allergic. It is, of course, essential that you consult your doctor to ensure that you are getting enough nutrients. A calcium supplement will probably be required.

The more of a food that is eaten, the more passes into the bloodstream. So eating huge quantities of one type of food during pregnancy is probably bad for the unborn child who may be predisposed to allergy. There have been no scientific tests to prove this, but not 'bingeing' during pregnancy, or while breast-feeding, would seem to be a sensible preventive measure.

Smoking during pregnancy has been shown to increase the risk of allergy, quite apart from its other damaging effects on the foetus. It is advisable to give up well before conception, and to maintain a smoke-free house once the baby is born – see next section. Putting on excess weight during pregnancy is also a risk factor for allergy in the child.

Pure air

The more allergens a baby is exposed to during the first year of life, the more likely it is to develop allergies. The first three months are much the most crucial. Airborne allergens are just as important as food allergens for the high-risk child, and reducing exposure to the main ones may help your child to escape the miseries of asthma or rhinitis in later years.

The major domestic allergens are house-dust mite, moulds, and particles of animal skin. Suggestions for eliminating these are given on pp69–71. If the child has not shown eczema or any other allergic symptoms by its first birthday, then pets can probably be allowed into the house again, but watch the child for symptoms and bear in mind that these can take some time to develop.

The other major airborne allergen is pollen, which is best avoided by planning the time of birth (if you can!). A baby born between September and February has the best chance of escaping hay-fever, while one born in March or April runs the greatest risk. If one or both parents is a hay-fever sufferer this particular form of family planning may be worthwhile.

Apart from allergens, there are various non-specific irritants that can make allergies more likely. Tobacco smoke is one and industrial air pollution another. A study in Sweden found that asthma and hay-fever were more common in children living near a paper factory than those living in an unindustrialized area. Children whose parents smoked showed more allergic problems, and so did those whose houses were built on badly drained land. The researchers concluded that these houses had more moulds growing in them. The highest risk of asthma and hay-fever was in children who were exposed to the mould allergen and to both forms of pollution – factory fumes and tobacco smoke.

Infections of the throat and chest can sometimes trigger off allergic reactions. Exactly why this should happen is not known, but there is evidence that viruses can have various unexpected effects on immune cells in the area. One effect may be to make IgE production more likely. All babies get colds and coughs, of course, and there is no point in worrying about this too much. But if there is a way of reducing exposure to infections then try to do so. For children with very high IgE levels, keeping them away from crèches and play-groups until three years of age may be advisable – many infections are picked up at such gatherings. There needs to be quite a severe risk of allergy to make this worthwhile however, and the benefits to mother and child of attending such groups will usually outweigh the risk.

Any severe form of stress can also trigger allergies in the susceptible child. Serious illness or surgery during the first year of life is one such stress, and unnecessary surgery is best postponed.

Keeping things in perspective

None of these preventive measures is foolproof, unfortunately. Some children go on to develop allergies, come what may. So a philosophical outlook is essential – do what you can to protect the child from allergens and irritants, but accept that it may sometimes be impossible. Above all, try not to get too anxious. A child needs to see the world as a safe and welcoming place, not one that is fraught with dangers. If your anxiety is obvious it may do a great deal of psychological harm.

Once the child is a year old, the risk of sensitization is far less, and you should be able to sit back and reap the benefits – an allergy-free child. There is no need to continue these stringent preventive measures unless there is a clear need for them – if the child obviously reacts to house dust for example, then you will have to continue being ultra-clean, but if there are no problems then you can allow your standards to slip a little.

If your child develops allergies anyway, then try not to blame yourself or other people – you can never know for sure what went wrong and it is pointless trying. Take comfort from the thought that your child's allergies might have been much worse if you had not gone to so much trouble – in the Swedish study, described above, it was notable that the different risk factors *added up* to give an even greater risk. Your preventive measures must have *subtracted* some aggravating factors and made your child's illness less severe than it might otherwise have been.

PREVENTING FOOD INTOLERANCE

The measures so far described for preventing food allergy are very largely based on scientific trials. Because food intolerance is less well recognized than food allergy, it attracts far less funding for research, and no comparable studies have been carried out. The preventive measures that we suggest here are common-sense ones, based on an understanding of what factors might cause food intolerance. If one member of the family already shows food intolerance, following these guidelines may be worthwhile for those who are presently in good health.

Diet and drugs

Since commonly eaten foods are the most frequent offenders in food intolerance, varying the diet is recommended. In particular, try to avoid eating milk and wheat too often – try to restrict these foods to just one meal a day. Avoid eating large quantities of the other high-risk foods, notably eggs, orange juice and peanuts. Never consume huge quantities of a particular food at one sitting – sausage-eating competitions are not for you.

Try to cut down on the number of cups of tea and coffee you drink each day, and to make them a little weaker. The evils of caffeine are listed on p165, and both drinks contain a variety of other chemical constituents that can irritate the stomach lining or cause changes in the body chemistry.

Avoid anything that increases the permeability of the gut wall: excess alcohol, highly spiced food, raw pineapple and papaya (pawpaw). Certain drugs also make the gut more leaky, notably aspirin and other drugs of a similar type (non-steroidal anti-inflammatory drugs, see p327) – these are used mainly for treating rheumatoid arthritis, osteoarthritis, period pains and headaches. You should only take these if you really need them.

Other factors

One thing that is thought to trigger off food intolerance is a heavy exposure to toxic chemicals. Such exposures are usually accidental and unforseen, of course, but there are some avoidable ones. If a house is to be sprayed with insecticides to eradicate woodworm, or with fungicides for wet or dry rot, then it is advisable to move out for at least a week, to allow time for the fumes to disperse. The company doing the spraying may claim that this is unnecessary, but there are instances of both children and adults being ill after spraying, even though they were not directly exposed to the spray. The fumes travel throughout the house, so even if only one part is being sprayed you should try to find somewhere else to stay for a while. Another hazard that can be very largely avoided is direct exposure to pesticides used on crops. If you see fields being sprayed, keep your distance, especially if they are being sprayed by a plane. The spray can easily drift. If you have a choice, don't buy a house next to a large arable field. Avoid using sprays in your own garden and keep household chemicals to a minimum (see pp179–83).

Finally, the general health measures listed on p300 are recommended to anyone who might be at risk of developing food intolerance. Above all, don't ignore symptoms such as recurrent headaches, regular bouts of indigestion or persistent fatigue. Living on aspirin, antacids, or strong coffee is going to make the problem worse rather than better, and experience suggests that the decline into severe food intolerance is a very gradual one that begins with symptoms of this sort. Treating a mild form of food intolerance – the early stages – is a great deal easier than trying to tackle entrenched symptoms and multiple sensitivities. The longer you leave it the more difficult it may be.

Chapter Fourteen

THE ELIMINATION DIET

The purpose of the elimination diet is to ask your body questions about the foods it has to cope with, and give it a chance to tell you which ones make it ill. In order to hear the answers, you need a period of 'silence' – that is, a period with no symptoms at all. This is why you must exclude all foods that are likely to be causing problems at the outset. Eliminating different foods one by one rarely works because most people are sensitive to more than one food: they must *all* be eliminated at once for the symptoms to disappear – to create the 'silence' which you need. (The main exception to this rule concerns very small children, who are eating a limited number of foods anyway, and are unlikely to be sensitive to a great many of them. See pp221–7 for details of investigating food problems in babies and toddlers.)

All elimination diets fall into two parts. First you avoid any food that might be causing trouble and see if the symptoms clear up – we will call this the **exclusion phase**. If the symptoms do disappear, then foods are reintroduced, one at a time, to discover which ones produce the symptoms. This is referred to here as the **reintroduction phase**.

The elimination diet sounds simple enough, although in practice there can be pitfalls and the results are not always clear-cut. This chapter has been carefully planned to help you avoid as many of those pitfalls as possible, and to give you the clearest possible answers with the least amount of change in your diet. It is very important that you work through it carefully. You should read the whole chapter first, then re-read each section and understand it thoroughly before you begin.

Do not be put off by the constant references to things going wrong. Only a minority of people will encounter problems such as these, but when they do arise, extra advice is needed – which is why the possible pitfalls seem to loom very large in this chapter.

There is no point whatever in doing an elimination diet half-heartedly – it simply won't work. You cannot have a day off it in the middle, unlike a weight-reducing or 'health' diet – it is a **diagnostic diet**, not a treatment in itself. If you stop for a day – or even for one meal – you will not get a clear result.

It is also a mistake to rush into it because things are more likely to go wrong. You may feel impatient to be well again, but try to think ahead. Imagine how you might feel in six months time, if you are only partially better, or little improved, because the elimination diet has not worked out properly. If you had taken it more slowly you might have been fully recovered, and even if it had taken an extra few months, this would have been thoroughly worthwhile because it could mean many years of really good health in the future. Doing the diet again is often very difficult. The process itself can change you – in particular, you *may* acquire new sensitivities to the foods eaten during the exclusion phase, simply because they are eaten more regularly and in greater amounts than before. If you are already sensitive to a wide range of foods, acquiring new sensitivities may prevent you from having a 'second go' at the elimination diet – you need a basic set of foods to which you have no reaction, in order for the diet to work. This is an extreme situation, of course, but it is worth bearing in mind that it can happen. *The important thing is to get the elimination diet right first time.*

Variations on a theme

Although all elimination diets work on the same principle, doctors differ considerably in the sorts of food they allow during the exclusion phase. The objective is to avoid all foods that are likely to cause problems. In essence, this means all foods that are eaten frequently because these are the most likely culprits (see p106). However, the 'safeness' of foods is also taken into consideration – some foods seem less likely to cause problems than others. The question is – how far do you take this? Some patients will be sensitive to 20 or more foods – to get better, they need to avoid almost everything they normally eat. But these patients are a tiny minority. Most patients will be sensitive to between two and five foods. For them, a rigorous exclusion phase is not necessary – they simply need to avoid the most frequent offenders, such as wheat, milk, eggs, citrus fruits, yeast, chocolate and additives. On the whole, the latter group have a much easier task ahead of them in discovering which foods make them ill, so doctors tend to think more about the unfortunate patients with multiple sensitivities. With them in mind, they devise diets that will eliminate most commonly eaten foods, even if this means putting the patients with just a few sensitivities through an unnecessarily arduous regime.

The approach to elimination diet that we recommend is a *flexible* three-stage procedure that provides the best possible diet for each type of patient. This is described on pp275–91 – first we will consider the different types of diet that are commonly used by other doctors.

Different types of elimination diet

The most drastic form of the elimination diet is to fast for the first five days, taking nothing but bottled spring water. This method has several drawbacks. Fasting requires a great deal of will-power and it is bad for anyone who is underweight and in poor health. Even for those who are not underweight, there are major metabolic changes that occur during fasting, as the body begins to break down its fat reserves. These metabolic changes, and others which occur when food is reintroduced, may themselves produce symptoms. For these reasons, we would not recommend fasting except in certain very difficult cases.

One step up from fasting is the **lamb-and-pears diet**, probably the best known type of elimination diet. This is something of an oddity because lamb is quite a common food in Britain. The diet originated in the United States in the early days of clinical ecology – America does not have the steep upland pastures that have made sheep-farming so popular in Great Britain, so lamb is not widely eaten there. While sensitivity to lamb is unusual, it does occur in Britain, so a lamb-and-pears exclusion phase is less appropriate here than on the other side of the Atlantic.

A modified version of the lamb-and-pears diet, used by some doctors, is turkey-and-pears or turkey-rice-and-pears – turkey being less commonly eaten in Britain than lamb. While these diets are useful when someone has a great many sensitivities, they are unnecessarily strict for most people. Again, they require a lot of will-power, and they involve eating huge quantities of two or three foods, which is never a good idea.

The next step up from here is the few-food diet or the rare-food diet. On a **few-food diet** the exclusion phase consists of a dozen or more foods that most people do not eat all that often. The exact foods chosen vary from one doctor to another, but they tend to include things such as parsnips, turnips and carrots which most of us do not eat in great quantity. The allowed foods also vary from patient to patient, because the doctor will ask the patient if any of the foods on the allowed list are eaten often – if they are, these must be excluded too. Most doctors have a second version of their few-food diet, with a different list of allowed foods: patients who do not get better during the first exclusion phase are switched to the second diet, in the hope that they will fare better. Of course, there is always a chance that both lists will include one or two foods which cause symptoms.

The **rare-food diet** is an extension of the few-foods idea, but instead of the patient eating uncommon foods such as turnips or parsnips during the exclusion phase, they are asked to eat exotic items such as yams or buckwheat. Since these items may never (or only rarely) have been eaten before, they are very unlikely to cause any reaction. In a sense the rare-food diet is an improvement on the few-food diet, because if the person fails to get better during the exclusion phase, they are probably not food-sensitive. With the few-food diet there is always some doubt – perhaps they *were* sensitive to parsnips, even though they only ever ate them for Sunday lunch? The drawbacks of the rare-food diet are principally cost – exotic foods are expensive – and the problem of getting such foods for those who do not live in a large city. The foods have to be prepared differently and the taste may take some getting used to, but on the whole they are at least as palatable as turnips! For those with multiple sensitivities who can afford the exotic foods, and have access to them, this type of diet is well worth considering.

The final step takes us to the least rigorous form of elimination diet, in which most fruits, vegetables, fish and meats are allowed, but wheat and other cereals, milk, eggs and other common offenders are excluded. This diet is quite good enough for many people, but those with multiple sensitivities tend to slip through the net because they are still eating some foods which cause symptoms.

One other form of elimination diet should be mentioned here. This uses **elemental diets** during the exclusion phase, rather than any foods. Elemental diets are made from various ordinary foods, but these are treated to break down the food molecules into smaller pieces. They are similar to the hydrolysate formulas used for babies who are sensitive to cow's milk (see p221) but they are designed to be eaten – or rather drunk – by adults. In theory, the molecules that remain in the elemental diet are too small to cause any allergic reactions or other problems. In practice, some people with established food sensitivity do react to them, because the fragments of molecules they contain are too reminiscent of the original molecules. For many people, however, they are very effective.

Various drawbacks are associated with elemental diets. Firstly they taste dreadful. Secondly they are very expensive – the cost of living on them and nothing else is about £20 per day. Although they are available on the National Health, they are classified as 'borderline substances' which means that they can only be prescribed for certain named illnesses – suspected food sensitivity is not one of these. The elemental diet that most doctors prefer to use is Vivonex, and this is only available on prescription. Another form of elemental diet, Elemental 028, is available without prescription, but this contains sugar (sucrose) to which some people are sensitive. Nevertheless, it might be useful as a last resort for someone who is intolerant of a great many foods and has therefore not succeeded with an elimination diet. You should not try out an elemental diet without the help and advice of your doctor.

A three-stage approach

A doctor, whether in private practice or working under the National Health, is obliged to deal with patients quickly and efficiently. If the doctor uses an elimination diet as a diagnostic method, it must be a fairly simple diet that can be given to everyone and does not need a lot of explanation. One advantage of self-help is that the diet can be tailored more closely to the individual patient's needs, and to this end we have devised a three-stage plan that we believe offers the best form of diagnosis for every type of patient.

The plan is outlined briefly in this section, and then described in more detail on pp275–94. You should try each stage of the plan in turn, and only go on to the next stage if you are no better. The vast majority of readers will probably not need to go beyond Stage 1 or 2. The main advantage of this three-stage approach is that it should not involve you in giving up any food unnecessarily, and if you have a simple problem – such as taking too much caffeine – it will lead you to it simply and quickly. There is little point spending a week eating nothing but lamb and pears when all you really needed to do was give up coffee or cut out milk.

Stage 1 of the plan is a one-month 'healthy eating programme'. During this stage, the foods and drinks that have a drug-like action on the body are eliminated, namely coffee, tea, cola-drinks, cocoa, chocolate and all forms of alcohol. The unpleasant (and often unsuspected) effects of caffeine are described on p165. Sugar and sugary foods are also excluded, because these can cause problems in some people, by making their blood-sugar levels go up and down wildly (see p135). Finally, histamine-rich foods (see p83) and all types of additives are excluded, since these are sometimes a source of problems.

If you get better during this first stage then you have got off very lightly, because you have not had to cut out any *foods*, in the strict sense of the word. Even if you do not recover at this stage, there are still substantial advantages. If you are food-sensitive, the withdrawal symptoms that occur when you cut out the offending foods can be pretty grim (see p109). Suddenly cutting out caffeine, alcohol and sugar at the same time is just plain masochistic – it makes much more sense to kick these habits first.

You may also discover that you can feel *partially* better by just eating healthily and avoiding everyday 'drugs'. This information could be useful later, when you have to decide how to cope with your food sensitivities – you will know how much of your illness is due to food and how much is due to other items.

Stage 2 of the programme is a simple form of elimination diet that just excludes the most common offending foods – this is the least rigorous form of exclusion phase. Most people will probably find the answers to their problems here.

Stage 3 of the programme is a more drastic form of elimination diet, designed to detect those with sensitivities to many different foods. The exact form of this exclusion phase can vary to suit individual needs – we suggest either a few-foods diet or a rare-foods diet, or a combination of the two.

Related foods

Before embarking on an elimination diet, some understanding of how foods can **cross-react** with one another is necessary. Foods derived from two related plants (or two related animals) will have similar proteins. They do not have to look like one another to be alike chemically – our own proteins are 99 per cent the same as those of the chimpanzee and the gorilla, our nearest living relatives. In the same way, the potato and the tomato may look quite different, but the plants they come from are closely related.

If you are allergic to one sort of food, you may show a reaction to food from a related source, because the IgE antibodies that bind to the first protein will also bind to a similar related protein. Cross-reactions also seem to occur in food intolerance, although the mechanism is not understood in most of these cases.

Biologists use various methods to work out how closely two animals or plants are related. Having done so, they express these relationships by grouping creatures together in a hierarchical scheme – very closely related creatures belong to the same **species**, related species belong to the same **genus** (plural **genera**), related genera belong to the same **family**, related families belong to the same **order**, and so on. There are often further subdivisions within each level, such as the **subfamily** and the **tribe**, which are subdivisions of the family.

How is this sort of classification scheme relevant to food sensitivity? Practical experience of thousands of patients suggests that they can cross-react to related foods, although they do not always do so. It also seems, from this collected experience, that the **family level** in biological classifications is a useful one in deciding which foods will cross-react – although sometimes one has to look at higher or lower levels to understand the cross-reactions that are seen. For example, all cereals are grasses, and belong to the grass family, Gramineae. Some food-sensitive people react to all cereals – to all members of the family. But others react only to wheat or maize, the two most commonly eaten cereals in the West. Many who react to wheat also react to rye and barley, and sometimes oats. If one looks at the classification of the Gramineae, one finds that wheat, rye, barley and oats all belong to the same subfamily, the Pooidae, and wheat, rye and barley are in the same tribe, the Triticeae. Maize is in a different subfamily, and rice in a different subfamily again, so there is less likely to be a cross-reaction between wheat and these cereals. This nicely explains the observation that wheat-sensitive folk are more likely to tolerate rice than any other commonly eaten cereal.

It has to be said that this is an unusually neat example, and most of the cross-reactions that are seen (or suspected) in patients do not match so well with the biological classification (see p302). For many foods, the use of the family group to predict cross-reactions is more a matter of faith than science, but it is still the most useful guide we have. There are also some unexpected cross-reactions, which do not tally with classification schemes (see pp304–5).

If you have reason to suspect any food before starting on your elimination diet (because you eat it in large amounts, for example), you should check the food-family list (pp306–7) to discover which family it belongs to. All its relatives should be excluded during the first phase of the diet, along with the food itself. But do test these foods later, and do not *expect* a reaction, just because foods are related. While cross-reactions are fairly common with some foods, notably cereals and shellfish, they are very rare with others. For example, tests have shown that most people who are allergic to peanuts are not affected by other legumes such as beans, peas or soya beans. Anticipating a reaction to a food is always a mistake, because it can lead to psychogenic symptoms – those created by the mind. And that could lead you to avoid foods unnecessarily.

The food families may also be useful later, in planning your everyday diet – just as you should not eat too much of any one food, you should not eat too much from any one *food family* either.

PREPARING FOR THE ELIMINATION DIET
Seeing your doctor

The first, and most essential step, is to see your doctor, describe your symptoms fully, and ask for a medical check-up. As explained in Chapter Seven, many of the symptoms of food intolerance can be due to other causes, and some of these may be serious – your doctor can examine you for such problems. Should there be nothing obviously wrong, then the next logical step is to try an elimination diet. Explain to the doctor you want to do so, and ask for advice. He or she may well have reservations about elimination diets, and you will be better prepared if you have read all or most of the book, and understand what is involved. If the doctor feels that you should not alter your diet for medical reasons, you *must* take this advice.

Keeping a record

As soon as you can, start keeping a daily record of your symptoms. This might seem rather unnecessary at this stage, but it will prove very useful later. The main purpose is to give you a detailed picture of how you felt before you began the diet – a base-line to which any later state of health can be compared. It is remarkable how quickly the memory fades – especially the memory of illness. If you only make a partial recovery, as some people do, you may later forget how ghastly you felt at the outset, and begin to think that the improvement is very small. Looking back at your symptom-record is often a startling reminder, and it can help strengthen your resolve to persist with the diet. It is also valuable if friends or relatives start to question the usefulness of what you are doing – you may need to prove to yourself that you really are better.

At the same time, you could also make a record of what you eat. Some people are more conscious of what passes their lips than others, and when you come to plan your diet you need to be aware of what foods you eat very regularly. Keeping a food-diary for a week or two can be quite an eye-opener. It will also get you into the habit of reading ingredients labels and watching out for synonyms (see p302).

Smoking and the Pill

If you smoke, now is the moment to give it up! There is not much point in trying to sort out your health problems while continuing to bombard your body with highly toxic smoke.

The Pill is a more difficult issue, for it is, without doubt, the most effective and convenient form of contraception, and giving it up may not be easy. But it can easily contribute to migraine, headaches, fatigue, and a variety of other symptoms that are also attributed to food intolerance. Some doctors believe that it has more general ill-effects on women's health, and that everyone with suspected food sensitivity or gut flora problems (see p185) should come off the Pill, regardless of what type of symptoms they have.

You may feel perfectly happy with the Pill, because you had no problems when you first began taking it – but as the case-history on p268 shows, this can be quite misleading. Even if you have had short periods (up to six months) off the Pill before, without noting any improvement, it may still be contributing to your symptoms. Nobody knows why the Pill should have these rather odd, insidious effects on some women, but they have been observed often enough to merit being taken seriously.

In general, it makes sense for any woman who is thinking about trying an elimination diet to come off the Pill first, and if migraines are among her symptoms the arguments for it are even stronger. Ideally, she should give the

Pill up for a trial period of three months *before* starting the diet, to see what effect this has, and to regain some sort of equilibrium. For anyone with severe symptoms, waiting three months to begin the elimination diet may not be a very appealing prospect, however. So if you have tried coming off the Pill before, without any obvious benefits, then you could just wait for two or three weeks before starting Stage 1.

EMMA

Emma had first gone on the Pill when she was a student, and had experienced no problems at all. She stayed on the combined Pill throughout her twenties, later changing to the progesterone-only 'mini-Pill', which was considered safer. During her twenties various health problems had developed, notably irritable bowel syndrome and migraines. These problems became much worse in her mid-thirties, which was when Emma first heard about the possible role of food in such illnesses. She discussed the idea of an elimination diet with her doctor, who suggested that she should first come off the Pill, to see what effect this had. Emma stayed off the Pill for two months, but her symptoms continued as before. She then tried an elimination diet, lost all her symptoms and identified milk, chicken and soya as the offending foods. On a diet free of these foods she felt a great deal better, and after a year of this she decided to go back on to the Pill, as other methods of birth control did not suit her. She began taking the mini-Pill again and within two days, to her great surprise, experienced a migraine. This was followed by a migraine the next day and the day after – three migraines in a row, the first she had had for a year. She promptly stopped taking the Pill and they did not recur. In retrospect, she wondered if the Pill had been contributing to her earlier problems, even though stopping it did not alleviate them. As this example shows, taking the Pill for a long period of time can have some rather odd and insidious effects, and stopping it does not always clear the symptoms immediately – they can persist for many months.

There is fairly strong evidence that women who have been on the Pill for some years may be deficient in certain vitamins and minerals. Anyone coming off the Pill should consider taking a nutritional supplement of the type described in the next section.

Nutritional supplements

The question of nutrition is a vexed one at present. The orthodox view is that a balanced diet provides all the nutrients we need, and common sense would suggest that our ample and very varied diet must provide more than enough – rarely have human beings been as well fed as we in the West are today. But there is a new school of thought in nutrition, which maintains that a surprisingly large number of people are deficient in certain vitamins and minerals. The proponents of this view cite many case-histories where patients with long-term health problems have been greatly helped by specific vitamin or mineral supplements.

Is there any possible explanation for this apparent paradox – an overfed people with nutritional deficits? The suggestion is that other factors in our diet and lifestyle can cause these shortages. Some of these factors may be universal, others affect certain individuals only.

At the individual level, our diet varies widely. Although we are better fed, on the whole, some people still eat a very poor diet, rich in sugars and starches, and other highly processed foods, but poor in vitamins and minerals. A recent survey by the London Food Commission found that a third of people buying take-away 'fast food' ate such food *at least once a day*, and for many it was their main meal. Such food provides almost no vegetables, has very low levels of vitamins and is far richer in salt and fat than official guidelines recommend.

Even those who think they are eating healthily may in fact be undernourished. The fashion for wholemeal-everything and added bran is one factor here: bran contains a substance called **phytate** that is known to impair the absorption of iron, zinc, calcium, and possibly magnesium – all essential minerals. The yeasts used in bread-making break down phytates, so ordinary wholemeal bread is not a problem, but unleavened wholemeal bread (*eg* soda bread, chapattis), wholemeal pastry and cakes, bran-containing breakfast cereals and other bran products can block the absorption of these minerals.

Bran can cause serious mineral deficiencies because iron and zinc are often lacking in Western diets. Vegetarians and vegans are particularly liable to iron deficiency (anaemia) since vegetarian food is low in iron anyway. Children under the age of two are also at risk, as are many women, because they lose blood while menstruating and have to make good the lost iron. Drinking tea with meals further reduces the absorption of iron, and is something that all vegetarians should avoid.

Zinc deficiency is more controversial than iron deficiency, and has become something of a fad, but there is fairly good evidence that it may be quite widespread. Vegetarians, pregnant women, elderly people, diabetics, and those on restricted diets are at greatest risk, but almost anyone can be short of zinc. The processing of food may be to blame, since this appears to reduce the zinc content. In addition, virus infections seem to 'use up' some of our stores of zinc.

The second strand of the argument is more contentious and very difficult to test scientifically. It suggests that we need more nutrients than we once did, simply because our bodies have to deal with so many more toxins – pesticide residues in food and water, air pollutants and so on. Although this might seem rather far-fetched, it is not implausible. We protect our bodies against toxins by breaking them down with **enzymes** (see p18). Many vitamins act as **coenzymes** – substances that are needed by specific enzymes to help them do their work. Minerals such as zinc and magnesium are also important for enzyme function. Faced with an extra burden of toxins to destroy, perhaps we do need more vitamins and minerals than our traditional diet provides.

A related issue here is the Pill, which is said to alter the nutritional balance of some women – perhaps the majority of women who take it on a long-term basis. Zinc, magnesium, manganese and iron may be deficient in Pill-takers, while copper is often very high. Vitamin A seems to be stored in excess, while many of the B vitamins are in short supply. Some of the adverse side-effects of the Pill have been linked to these changes in vitamin and mineral status. Simply stopping the Pill does not seem to put these nutritional disorders right – they may persist for three months or more and cause continuing problems.

Doctors who are concerned about possible nutritional defects suggest that *anyone* embarking on an elimination diet should take a nutritional supplement. They argue that many are likely to have deficiencies anyway, especially if they number diarrhoea among their symptoms, and that the restrictions of the elimination diet will only make the situation worse. Such doctors also recommend a *special type* of nutritional supplement to anyone coming off the Pill – and certainly to anyone staying on it. It is quite easy to overdo things with both vitamins and minerals, particularly with the fat-soluble vitamins, A and D, because these are stored by the body if taken in excess – water-soluble vitamins, such as Vitamin C, can be washed out of the body in the urine. So grabbing a handful of ordinary vitamin pills is not the answer – they can be dangerous if the body already has an excess of Vitamin A.

Ideally, anyone who is concerned about their nutritional status should have a full analysis done, so that a supplement can be tailored to their specific needs. Unfortunately, testing itself is a contentious issue. The traditional method of just testing a blood sample is now considered inadequate by many

TABLE 12   SOME SIGNS OF NUTRITIONAL DEFICIENCY

These are some of the physical signs of nutritional deficiencies. Bear in mind that all the signs or symptoms below can be caused by other medical conditions. If you have any of these symptoms you should consult your doctor before taking a nutritional supplement.

Sign or symptom:	Can be caused by deficiencies of:
Cracks at corners of mouth	iron, Vitamins B2 or B6, or folic acid
Recurrent mouth ulcers	iron, folic acid or Vitamin B12
Dry, cracked lips	Vitamin B2
Smooth, sore tongue	iron, Vitamins B2 or B12 or folic acid
Fissured tongue	Vitamin B3
Taste buds at tip of tongue enlarged, red and sore	Vitamins B2 or B6
Bruising or enlargement of veins under tongue	Vitamin C
Red, greasy skin on face, especially sides of nose	Vitamins B2 or B6, zinc or essential fatty acids
Rough, pimply skin on upper arms and thighs	B Vitamins, Vitamin E or essential fatty acids
Red, itchy rash on scrotum or vulva	Vitamin B2, zinc
Dry, rough, cracked or peeling skin	zinc, essential fatty acids
Poor hair growth	iron or zinc
Dandruff	Vitamins B6 or C, zinc or essential fatty acids
Bloodshot, gritty, sensitive eyes	Vitamins A or B2
Poor vision after dark	Vitamin A or zinc
Dry eyes	Vitamin A or essential fatty acids
Brittle or split nails	iron, zinc or essential fatty acids
White spots on nails	zinc
Pale appearance	iron, Vitamin B12 or folic acid

(Adapted from *Nutritional Medicine* by kind permission of the authors, Dr Stephen Davies and Dr Alan Stewart.)

doctors. It appears that some nutrients – zinc for example – can be deficient as a whole, but show normal levels in the blood. The suggestion is that the blood 'needs' the mineral more than other parts of the body, so there are mechanisms that ensure a good supply, scavenging the mineral from other tissues to keep the blood level high. A more extensive method of testing, using hair and sweat samples, as well as blood, often shows up nutritional defects that are not revealed by the blood alone. This form of testing seems to be vindicated by the results in individual cases – correcting the deficiencies shown by hair or sweat tests often does wonders for patients with previously intractable health problems. This is not hard, scientific evidence of course, and some carefully designed trials are needed to test these new approaches to nutrition.

In the meantime, what can be advised? Extensive nutritional testing is only available privately, but for those who can afford it there is little to lose, and useful addresses are given on p340. For anyone coming off the Pill, a special supplement is probably advisable (see p333).

Others who may be concerned about their nutritional status, but cannot afford individual testing, should consult Table 12 and see if they show any signs of deficiency. These are not foolproof signs, however – the same symptoms can be produced by other forms of illness, and there are several deficiencies that do not appear in the table because they produce no clear-cut signs. But if you do show some of these signs, then there is a chance that you are lacking certain nutrients, especially if your diet has not been good. The simplest and cheapest answer is to take a general supplement and one is recommended on p340. This may be slightly more expensive than run-of-the-mill vitamin tablets, but it is far more likely to do you good – and not to do you any harm. It is also free of artificial colours, unlike most commercial preparations which come in lurid shades of red or orange as an indication of their health-giving properties! Avoiding colourings is important if you are embarking on an elimination diet.

One sign that you may notice is white spots on the fingernails. These can be an indication of zinc deficiency, and if you show no other deficiency signs, and generally eat a good diet, then taking a zinc supplement may be all you need to do. Zinc is relatively safe and non-toxic, so a sensible supplement is unlikely to do any harm. For details see p333.

Sort out other problems

The idea of the elimination diet is to create a period of 'silence' in which you can listen to your body answering specific questions. Any sort of background noise is going to confuse you, so you need to eliminate other things that cause symptoms before you start. The three main items to consider are airborne allergens, hyperventilation and chemical sensitivity.

You should suspect airborne allergens if your symptoms include asthma, hay-fever, a year-round runny nose or congested nose (rhinitis), red, watery or itchy eyes, sinusitis, or recurrent 'colds'. Eczema and urticaria may indicate allergens in the air that land on the skin – or things that touch the skin directly. Consult pp67–9 for likely sources of trouble. Avoidance measures are described on pp69–71. Put these into effect for a few months before starting the diet.

Hyperventilation is suggested by dizziness, faintness, tingling in the hands and feet, numbness, spaced-out or confused feelings, shortness of breath and a variety of other symptoms. A full list is given on p163. It appears that hyperventilation often accompanies food intolerance, but it can sometimes be the sole cause of symptoms.

There are no typical symptoms reported for chemical sensitivity, but most people who react generally know that they do, because certain things always make them feel ill – travelling by car, smelling perfume or swimming in chlorinated water, for example. Read Chapter Nine if you are in any doubt. Complete avoidance is difficult, but try to clean up your environment as much as possible (see pp179–83), and wait for about two weeks before starting the elimination diet, so that you can assess the effects of doing this.

If you respond to any of these avoidance measures, however slightly, they should be continued throughout Stages 1, 2 and 3 of the diet.

Planning the diet

Timing is all-important here, as birthdays, Christmas, weddings, family get-togethers and holidays cause immense problems. Ideally, you should plan things so that the diet falls in a quiet period, or postpone celebrations until afterwards. This does not matter quite so much during Stage 1 of the diet, when you can break the rules for one or two meals, if you have to. However, you should keep off alcohol, tea and coffee, and not overdo sugar. During Stages 2 and 3 you cannot do this – *any departure from the diet will confuse the result.* Use the timing guidelines in Table 13 to plan your diet.

Obviously you cannot abandon all social life during these diets, so you have to be flexible. If you are asked out to lunch or dinner, it is not that difficult to take your own food, and you get over the embarrassment fairly quickly. For picnics and days out, cook the foods that you are allowed and take them in plastic boxes. Packed lunches for work, or when travelling, can be prepared in the same way. If you are doing the diet during the winter months, and want hot food, buy a wide-necked thermos flask – they are very useful and not expensive. As an alternative to tea and coffee, take herb tea in a thermos flask or carry some herb teabags – people serving in cafes and restaurants will usually give you some plain hot water if you ask for it, and watching their puzzled expressions can be quite entertaining.

TABLE 13   TIMING GUIDELINES FOR PLANNING THE ELIMINATION DIET

Stage 1 – the 'healthy-eating' diet – should run for at least a month, but it can be continued for as long as you wish. Some flexibility is allowed during this stage – you can have the occasional meal off, but take all forbidden items in moderation, and avoid alcohol, tea and coffee. Stage 1 will go on longer than a month if you improve substantially on this diet – but in this case you will not be proceeding to Stage 2.

If you are going on to Stage 2, you should maintain the 'healthy eating' diet until you are ready to start.

Stage 2 will run for about three weeks if you *don't* respond to the exclusion phase. If you do respond, then it will continue for two to three months. There must be no deviation from the diet during Stage 2.

Stage 3 will run for about three weeks if you *don't* respond to the exclusion phase. If you do respond, then it will continue for two to three months. There must be no deviation from the diet during Stage 3.

You should not start the diet without planning what you are going to eat for the first few days, and buying the things you need. Hunger is a very powerful urge, and unless you have plenty of allowed foods to hand, you may get so famished that you raid the biscuit jar or the bread-bin in a moment of weakness. To avoid such lapses, it is worth cooking up some meals in advance, so that you can have something ready within a few minutes. A freezer, or a fridge with a large ice compartment, is invaluable – you can cook your special meals in bulk and freeze them in individual portions. A supply of allowed 'snacks' in a cupboard is also helpful – see p312 for ideas.

Packaged and tinned foods should be avoided if possible during these diets. You will find that most prepared foods contain excluded items anyway: it may not say 'milk' or 'eggs' on the ingredients label, but it could be there under another name – see p302 for the synonyms used. Even if there are no prohibited ingredients, you are still taking something of a gamble, because you have no idea what sort of processing methods have been used, and how these might affect you. And it is not unknown for labels to omit an ingredient. So it is much better, at this stage, to stick to simple home-prepared foods because you know exactly what has gone into them. Tinned foods should be avoided at first because the lining of the cans, a golden-coloured phenol resin, contaminates the food slightly. Some food-intolerant people are sensitive to this.

From the point of view of food preparation, making two lots of food can be a nuisance, and some people solve the problem by putting the whole family on the diet, at least for the exclusion phase. Doctors using the elimination diet have often observed unexpectedly good results in another family member, as a result of this. There are numerous reports of fatigue, moodiness, headaches, runny noses and other minor problems, that had previously been taken for granted, suddenly clearing up. Sceptics will claim that this could well be psychosomatic, or a result of healthier eating habits, and at present there is no scientific evidence either way. But there is certainly no harm in other adults joining in Stages 1 and 2 of the diet. Children should only be included if they have some identifiable medical or behavioural problem, and consultation with your doctor is essential. Children may need a calcium supplement if milk is excluded.

Stage 3 of the diet is a different matter. It is unlikely that anyone with minor health problems, or no acknowledged health problems, would benefit from it, although a few might do.

STAGE 1 – THE HEALTHY-EATING DIET
This is summarized in Table 14.

Cut out the following foods:
Coffee and tea, including coffee-flavoured cakes etc
Chocolate, cocoa and all chocolate-flavoured items
Coca-cola, Pepsi-cola and other cola drinks
Sugar and any foods containing sugar (see table on p197). Don't worry if you eat a small amount (*eg* in tinned tomato soup) during Stage 1. On Stage 2 and 3 you need to be much more careful.
Saccharin and other artificial sweeteners
All alcoholic drinks, including alcohol-free beers and foods cooked in wine, beer etc. Don't eat too much vinegar or pickled foods – no more than a small portion twice a week.
All colourings, preservatives, antioxidants, flavour enhancers, flavourings, thickeners, emulsifiers, stabilizers and other additives. Anything identified by an E-number: some of these are natural ingredients, but that does not mean they are automatically safe, and at this stage it is easier to just avoid the lot. Read the labels on everything – don't be taken in by 'Natural' or 'Healthy' on the packet. Some unlabelled food contains additives (see p313). Remember

that margarines contain colourings and are highly processed – any food like this should be avoided. So should bacon, ham, corned beef and anything smoked.

Continental sausages and very ripe cheeses – they are often a rich source of histamine.

All take-aways and fast food. Keep restaurant-eating to a minimum, because there are a lot of unexpected additives in such meals.

Anything that makes the gut more permeable: curries and other very spicy foods, raw pineapple and papaya, aspirin and other NSAIDs (see p327).

At the same time, you should try to eat plenty of fresh vegetables and fruits. Green leafy vegetables are particularly important, and salads are valuable. Choose fresh meat or fish rather than pies, sausages or fish-fingers (even if these are additive-free).

If you have been eating bran, gradually cut this out (your bowel may need time to adjust, so don't do it suddenly). A daily intake of vegetables, potatoes, wholemeal bread and fruits should supply all the fibre you need. Try to eat less salt, and avoid highly salted foods such as peanuts and crisps. Keep your diet varied, don't eat too much at one sitting, and don't have huge amounts of a single food.

If you drink a lot of coffee or tea, cut it out gradually or you may get withdrawal symptoms. Avoid painkillers that contain caffeine. Other medicines may contain colourings – ask you doctor to prescribe uncoloured equivalents.

Decaffeinated coffee and tea are not allowed. Herb teas can be used to replace tea and coffee, but not maté (or matté), which contains some caffeine and tannin, nor redbush tea, which shares many chemical constituents with ordinary tea, even though it lacks caffeine. Jasmine tea, gunpowder tea and other 'green teas' are true teas, so these should not be taken.

Stay on this diet for at least a month, unless you feel much better before then.

Possible outcomes

Feeling much worse

You are probably suffering from caffeine withdrawal – or it might be the effects of cutting out alcohol. This is 'cold turkey' – the same sort of withdrawal symptoms that a heroin addict has, though nothing like as bad. You just have to keep going, in the knowledge that it will pass and you will then feel a great deal better than you did before. Not eating sugar might have similar effects until your body gets used to the idea.

It is most unlikely that you will still feel worse after two or three weeks. If you do, think about any other changes that have occurred. Could they be the

---

TABLE 14   THE STAGE 1 DIET

Allowed:

Wholemeal bread
Milk, butter, most types of cheese
Shredded wheat, puffed wheat, and other cereals that have no sugar or
    colouring
Any fresh, unprocessed meat
Any fresh, unprocessed fish
Potatoes
Rice
Beans and lentils
Any vegetables – eat plenty of green leafy vegetables and salads
Any fresh fruit, except pineapple and papaya
Pastry – if homemade
Any unsweetened fruit juice
Herb teas, except maté and redbush

Not allowed:

Alcoholic drinks, including alcohol-free beers and wines
Food cooked in beer, wine etc
Coffee
Tea, including green tea, jasmine tea etc
Cola drinks
Chocolate
Sugar and all sugar-containing foods (see p198)
Artificial sweeteners
Vinegar and pickles (except in small quantities)
Margarine
All food additives
Smoked fish or meat
Bacon and ham
Continental sausages
Very ripe cheeses
Take-away food
Restaurant food (except very occasionally)
Bran
Any very salty food
Aspirin and related drugs (see p327)
Curries and other very spicy food

For further details, see pp275–9.

---

cause? Or were you steadily getting worse anyway? If you're sure it's due to the diet then consider any new foods you are eating, or foods eaten in greater quantity than before. It may be that you are allergic or intolerant to such foods. Consider them suspect and cut them out in the exclusion phase of Stage 2. Alternatively, if you are eating a lot more fruit and vegetables than before, and if you are sensitive to pesticide residues, then this might explain your deterioration. Read Chapter Nine before going on to Stage 2.

Feeling about the same

Proceed to Stage 2. Stay on the healthy-eating diet until you are ready to start.

Feeling partially better

If you are satisfied with your improvement, and don't like the idea of giving up foods, you could stop here. Reintroduce tea, coffee, alcohol etc, to see which was the problem, following the instructions given below.

If you feel you would like to be better still, go on to Stage 2 of the diet. When you have completed Stage 2 (or Stage 3) you can test your reactions to tea, coffee, alcohol etc.

Some people who feel partially better at this stage, may be suffering from gut flora problems. Cutting out sugar could have improved the situation, but to get any further may require a more stringent diet, as described in Chapter Ten. You could either try this diet now, or go on to the Stage 2 diet (described below) and return to the no-sugar, no-yeast diet if this does not work.

Feeling a lot better

Good – you can now test the various things you cut out to see which ones cause your symptoms – see the next section for instructions. Testing can begin as soon as you have been consistently well for a week. If you felt terrible at the start of the diet, then caffeine is the most likely cause. Try a fairly weak cup of coffee or tea for your first test. Bear in mind that there are dozens of other nasties in tea and coffee, besides caffeine – you may be reacting to one of these, in which case you could be sensitive to tea but not coffee, or vice versa.

Reintroduction phase

Reintroduce one item each week, for example:

    week 1 – food containing additives
    week 2 – tea
    week 3 – coffee
    week 4 – beer
    week 5 – white wine

week 6 – red wine
week 7 – spirits
week 8 – chocolate

Take some of the test food or drink every day, starting with a small amount and continuing for a week. If there is a reaction, then stop immediately. Wait until you are better, then go on to the next item. If there is no reaction then give it up again after a week, and test the next item. At the end of the testing period, you can reintroduce all the things that produced no reaction.

If you react to food containing additives, then leave these out again for a while, while you test other items. Then test them again individually – see pp313–15 for details of the different groups of additives. If you react to one member of a group, you may well react to others in that group too.

Try to continue your good eating habits after the diet is finished – don't go back to eating a lot of salt and sugar, or drinking huge quantities of tea, coffee or alcohol (even if these didn't cause any specific symptoms). Keep eating fresh foods, particularly green vegetables, and stay away from junk food.

Once you have established which items cause your symptoms, you will probably need to avoid these entirely for some considerable time, although you might be able to consume a small amount occasionally. Try them out from time to time, to see whether your reaction has abated.

No reactions?

If you still feel better but did not react adversely to anything on testing, then there are various possibilities. One is that you have a genuine intolerance reaction to a component of one of these items, but that the period of abstinence has 'cured' it. This is especially likely with things that are tested towards the end of the reintroduction phase (see p108). If you go back to taking such items every day, then the intolerance may reappear. So if you begin to get your symptoms again, you need to repeat Stage I and test everything in the reverse order this time.

A second possibility is that you may have gut flora problems – see p185. In mild cases, just cutting out sugar can clear the symptoms. If this is the explanation, you will probably begin to notice symptoms again if you start to take significant amounts of sugar or honey again. Obviously, returning to a sugar-free diet is the answer.

STAGE 2 – SIMPLE ELIMINATION DIET

You should have completed at least a month of Stage 1, before starting Stage 2, and you should still be eating the Stage 1 diet. *Continue with all the Stage 1 restrictions during Stage 2.* Do not begin if you have any sort of infection, especially diarrhoea.

Before starting Stage 2, look at the Stage 3 diet and think about how you would do it if you had to. One possible outcome of Stage 2 is that you go straight into Stage 3 – you need to be prepared to do this.

Exclusion phase

This diet is summarized in Table 15.

Cut out the following foods:

Wheat, rye, barley, oats, maize (corn)
Rice, if this is normally part of your diet and you eat it more than once or twice a week
Milk and all milk products, including butter
Eggs
Soya
Oranges, lemons, grapefruit, tangerines, limes and all other citrus fruits
Yeast and yeast extract, including Oxo cubes, other stock cubes, Bovril etc
Mushrooms
Peanuts and any other nuts you eat reasonably often
Beef and chicken
Any food that you eat every day, or eat in large quantities, or have a craving for
Any food that a member of your family reacts to, or which you suspect for any reason
You should still be avoiding all items that were disallowed on Stage 1

As soon as you start the exclusion phase, keep a record of everything you eat, including a rough idea of how much and when. Record your symptoms too and continue this throughout the diet. Be very careful not to eat too much of any one food. Don't have blow-outs – little and often is the best way to eat.

Stay on the exclusion phase of the diet for two weeks or until you feel better – whichever is the sooner. Someone with a serious problem, such as rheumatoid arthritis, may take a little longer to respond, and they should continue for three weeks. Patients with Crohn's disease (who *must* have full medical supervision for such a diet) take about nine days, on average, to respond. They may need to continue the elimination phase for longer than 14 days.

The possible outcomes are dealt with on pp283–5. If you do feel better you should not delay in reintroducing foods – see pp285–7 for instructions.

Some special points about the prohibited foods
Milk
If you are sensitive to milk, you may be able to substitute goat's or sheep milk

---

TABLE 15   THE STAGE 2 DIET

Allowed:

Lamb, turkey, pork, duck, goose, rabbit (all fresh and unprocessed)

Any fresh vegetables

Potatoes

Rice, unless you usually eat this often

Any fresh fruit, other than citrus fruit (oranges, lemons etc), pineapple and papaya

Chickpeas; also beans and lentils (but not if you have bowel symptoms)

Any nuts that you do not normally eat very often

Herb teas, except maté and redbush

Pure vegetable oil

Not allowed:

Bread

Wheat, rye, barley, oats, maize (corn, sweetcorn etc)

Rice, if you eat this regularly

Beef and chicken

Milk, butter, yoghurt and cheese

Margarine

Eggs

Soya

Pineapple and papaya

Oranges, lemons, grapefruit etc

Marmite and other yeast extracts

Oxo cubes, other stock cubes, Bovril etc

Mushrooms

Peanuts

Anything you normally eat every day or crave

Any suspect food

Coffee, chocolate, tea (all varieties), cola drinks

Sugar, any sugar-containing foods, and artificial sweeteners

All additives

All alcoholic drinks, and their derivatives

Vinegar and pickles

Bacon, ham, corned beef and all other smoked or processed meats

Curries and other very spicy foods

Aspirin and related drugs

For further details, see pp279–87.

---

for it once you have completed the diet. But at this stage, it is better to avoid these as well, as there can be cross-reactions. Soya milk is not advisable either at this early stage, as soya is found quite widely in processed foods and meat products, and some people are sensitive to it even though they are unaware of eating it.

You should be avoiding packaged and processed foods anyway, but if you do eat any, be aware that milk may be called by various synonyms on the ingredients label – see p302.

Most margarines contain some milk solids, and should be avoided anyway, as they are highly processed.

Cereals

You can substitute other starchy foods such as sweet potatoes and buckwheat for some of these – see p310. Be careful to distinguish buckwheat from bulgur wheat – the latter is true wheat, but buckwheat comes from an entirely different plant. Millet is a cereal, but few people react to it. You should not eat it at first, but if you find you are unable to eat wheat, you could test it as a potential substitute.

If you are used to eating lots of bread, then you may feel rather empty and it might be tempting to stoke up on potatoes. Try to avoid this temptation, and use some other, less usual foods as fillers sometimes – parsnips or turnips, for example. Acquiring a sensitivity to potatoes is not going to be helpful. Other alternatives to bread and starchy foods are given on pp309–12.

Maize is found in sweetcorn, corn-on-the-cob, cornflour, corn syrup, cornflakes and popcorn; also in the American products known as grits or hominy grits. The Italian dish, polenta, is made with maize. The gum on stamps and envelopes is often made of cornstarch, and highly sensitive people may react to licking these.

Wheat is found in macaroni, spaghetti and other forms of pasta, couscous, semolina, biscuits, cakes and pastry – as well as in bread, most breakfast cereals and most packaged foods. When labels say 'flour' they usually mean wheat flour – or maize.

If you are eliminating rice, then you should also avoid wild rice, since the two are related (though not closely). If you find you are sensitive to rice, then test wild rice later as a potential substitute.

Potato flour, rice flour or arrowroot can be used to thicken sauces and gravies – these are available from healthfood shops and delicatessans. Do not use instant mashed potato as this contains various additives.

Eggs

This means chicken's eggs principally, but there is a strong chance of cross-reaction with other birds' eggs, so it is advisable to avoid all eggs. See p302 for the synonyms that may be used on ingredients labels.

Yeast
Avoiding yeast means not eating Marmite or other types of yeast extract, Bovril, stock cubes, vinegar, and any food containing malt extract or 'hydrolysed protein'. Also avoid over-ripe or mouldy fruit. (Leavened bread and alcoholic drinks are also rich in yeast, but these are not allowed anyway.) Many vitamin tablets are based on yeast, and these should be discontinued – for yeast-free nutritional supplements see p339.

Possible outcomes
Feeling much worse
This often happens during the first few days of the exclusion phase, and it is generally considered a good sign. These 'withdrawal symptoms' are seen in many food-sensitive patients and seem to be caused by suddenly cutting out the offending food. They should pass by the end of the first week, if not before. Don't give up.

Feeling a little worse
This may be a mild version of the withdrawal symptoms, but if it persists after seven days, then it is something else. One possibility is that you were somewhat undernourished to start with and the diet has made things worse. If you think this is likely, go back to the 'healthy eating' diet and take a nutritional supplement – see p333. Stay on this regime for a couple of months to try to recover your general health. Then try the Stage 2 diet again – or move straight on to Stage 3.

Feeling worse, then much better
Once you have felt consistently better for three or four days then you should start the reintroduction phase – see below. Don't delay doing this. Write down exactly how you feel at this point – it may be useful and encouraging to refer back to this later, if you suffer a lot of reactions during food testing.

Feeling much better quite quickly
This can happen, especially in children and young people – they seem to miss out on the withdrawal symptoms. Go on to the reintroduction phase.

Feeling much better, but with one or two lingering symptoms
It looks as if you have cut out your main offending foods, but are still eating something that is a problem. If the lingering symptoms are fairly minor, then

you can proceed to the reintroduction phase. Test the major foods: milk, eggs, wheat, rice etc, and continue eating those that cause no problems. This will help to broaden your diet. Having done this, look through the food diary you kept before the diet and try to identify possible causes for your lingering symptoms – is there anything you used to eat quite frequently and have continued eating throughout the diet? Potatoes, onions, tomatoes, shellfish and fish are likely suspects. Cut all these out and then test them.

If your lingering symptoms are fairly troublesome, or very variable from day to day, then it will not be possible to get clear results from the reintroduction phase. In this case, look back through the food diary you kept before the diet for potential culprits. Cut these out immediately. Should your symptoms clear, then go on to the reintroduction phase immediately. If they don't, then go on to the Stage 3 diet, preferably a rare-food diet.

Before deciding which course of action to take, consider the possibility that it might be something other than food causing the residual symptoms. If you have gut flora problems, for example, the sugar-free, yeast-free diet could have helped considerably, but not removed all your symptoms. Read Chapter Ten again. Or it could be that food was your main problem, but something else is causing the residual symptoms – an airborne allergen or environmental chemical perhaps. If you have not checked out these possibilities, then think about them now. Read pp272–3 again.

Feeling worse, then much better, then worse again

If you go through the withdrawal symptoms, feel greatly improved for a while, but then begin to go downhill again, this is a rather bad sign. It does not happen to many people, but if it does happen to you then you need to think very carefully about the situation.

The most likely explanation is that you are developing a new sensitivity to something allowed on the exclusion phase – probably something you are eating a lot of. Look at your food record for the exclusion phase, and try to work out what this might be – foods you ate plentifully *before* the diet are also suspects. Cut out any such foods and see what happens. Meanwhile make great efforts not to eat too much of any one food. Introducing some rare foods – see pp307–12 – may be the answer, but don't overindulge in these either or you may spoil your chances of doing a rare-food diet later.

If you get better again, and stay better for two or three days, then you can begin the reintroduction phase. Continue to vary your diet as much as possible during this period – if you can, go on to a rotation diet (see p295). If you can't manage a four-day rotation, then three days will be some help at least.

If you are still not well, or if you have unclear results during the reintroduction phase, then the best plan is to go straight on to Stage 3, preferably a rare-food diet. As a last resort, you could try an elemental diet (see p263), but only with medical supervision.

Feeling about the same
You can either go back to the 'healthy eating' diet and think about what to do next, or you can go straight on to Stage 3.

Reintroduction phase
Wait until you have been free of symptoms for two or three days, but don't wait any longer than this. Begin by testing foods that are probably not the cause of any trouble – things you do not eat every day. Choose items that you like – if the foods pass the test, then you can incorporate them into your menus, which will allow you to eat less of the exclusion-phase foods. Throughout the reintroduction phase it is vital that you keep your diet varied and do not eat too much of any one food. In particular, do not eat any one food every day. Continue to record everything you eat, and your symptoms – if something goes wrong, this record will prove invaluable.

Only test one food at a time. Eat a normal-sized portion of the food in question, for lunch and supper. Notice any changes that occur at the time, or later in the evening, or the following day. Most symptoms will show up within this timespan, although bowel symptoms may take longer – they can occur anywhere between four and 48 hours after the food is eaten.

If there is no reaction by the following day, eat two portions of the food again. Should you get no reaction this time then repeat for a third day. If there is still no reaction, then the food can be considered safe, but avoid it again for four days (to offset any possible effect of eating it for three days in succession) before beginning to eat it once more.

If you get a reaction to any food, stop eating it immediately. You may be able to abort the symptoms by taking a mixture of sodium and potassium bicarbonate. It is not known how or why this works, but it appears to do so. However, it is only effective if you are clear of symptoms at the outset – it cannot be used as a general remedy for food-induced illnesses, and in any case, it should not be taken too often. Mix two level teaspoons of sodium bicarbonate (bicarbonate of soda) with one level teaspoon of potassium bicarbonate, dissolve in a small glass of warm water and drink the mixture as rapidly as is comfortable. *Never do this if you have eaten a very large meal as it can be dangerous in such circumstances.* Potassium bicarbonate should be obtainable from your chemist, although it may have to be ordered – if you want to try this remedy, rather than just sweating it out when you get a reaction to a food, then you should buy some in advance. Do not test any more foods until the symptoms have completely subsided.

There are about 16-20 foods to test:

Milk and **cheese** should be tested separately. Test milk first, using fresh milk, not evaporated or dried. If you react to milk you will probably react to cheese and **butter** as well, although some milk-sensitive people can eat butter. Even if you can drink milk, you may react to cheese, because it contains various chemicals produced by bacteria and moulds during the cheese-making process. Some people can tolerate evaporated milk, but not fresh milk. If you react to fresh milk, you could test 'evap' later, but leave at least a week before you do so.

Citrus fruits should be tested with **orange** first, then **lemon**. If you can eat both of these safely then you need not test the others.

Test **yeast** before **mushrooms**. You can either use yeast extract (*eg* Marmite) or yeast vitamin tablets. Or mix half a teaspoon of baker's yeast with water, boil for ten minutes, and drink when cool.

Test **wheat** before other cereals. Do not test it as bread, because this contains various other ingredients as well. Certain breakfast cereals are pure wheat, notably Puffed Wheat and Shredded Wheat, and these are good for testing – they can be moistened with fruit juice if you are not able to have milk. Alternatively, use bulgur wheat, or pasta (checking first for other ingredients), or mix flour into a pancake batter with eggs (assuming you have tested eggs already and they are safe). If using flour, start with wholemeal flour, preferably untreated and organically grown, as you can be sure that it contains no other ingredients. You can test white flour later. Some people are intolerant of the part of the wheatgrain that is lost during the production of white flour, so they only react to wholemeal flour and bread. Others are sensitive to white flour only, probably because of the additives in white flour, or the chemical processes, such as bleaching, that are used in its production.

If you react to wheat, allow at least a week to pass before testing any more cereals – test something else in the meantime. **Rye** can be tested as rye crispbread, but make sure it is pure rye, because some contain wheat bran. (Also bear in mind that some people who react to yeast also react to malt, which is a common ingredient in crispbreads and cereals.) **Oats** can be tested as porridge, and **maize** as sweetcorn or cornflour. **Barley** can be tested by eating pearl barley – boil about two or three tablespoons of it in plain water or home-made stock. It may seem rather pointless testing a food such as barley if you never eat it normally, but you could have become sensitive to it if you drink beer regularly, or if you are sensitive to wheat. Rye, barley and oats are all quite closely related to wheat and cross-reactions are not uncommon.

Other items to be tested are: **eggs**, **beef**, **chicken** and anything else that you decided to avoid, such as **rice** or **peanuts**.

The reintroduction phase should take about seven or eight weeks. If it takes any longer than this, there is a risk of lost sensitivity: the food-intolerant person becomes less reactive after avoiding the culprit food for a time. For some people, it may take many months or years to lose their intolerance, but for others the process can happen within two to three months.

If you have still not tested all foods eight weeks after starting the exclusion phase, then you should reintroduce all those which you have not yet tested. Eat all of them (in normal portions) every day for a week. If, after a week, there is no reaction, then you can consider them all safe. If there *is* a reaction, cut them all out again, and avoid them for five days, or until your symptoms clear up, if this takes longer. Then retest each of those foods in turn, using the same procedure as before.

Once you have tested all foods, and established a diet on which you feel well, you can test the items that you gave up during Stage 1: tea, coffee, alcohol etc. Follow the procedure outlined on pp278–9.

Incomplete testing

If something goes wrong during the testing – you might get influenza for example, or some other infection – then you will have to stop testing foods. All is not lost, but there is no point in trying to test foods beyond three months. If you are unable to test all the excluded foods, then you should go back to the healthy-eating diet for about a month. Eat whatever you like, but if there *are* any foods which gave a positive reaction when tested, then you should continue to avoid these.

Keep a record of your symptoms, and see how you feel at the end of the month. If you are reasonably well, then continue with the healthy-eating diet, avoiding the incriminated foods, and see how you get on. As long as you keep your diet varied, so as not to acquire new sensitivities, you can always go through Stage 2 again later.

If, after a month on the 'healthy eating' diet, some or all of your symptoms have returned, then you should start the exclusion phase of Stage 2 again. Any foods that you previously tested and found safe can be eaten as well, but if your symptoms have not cleared after a week, then you should exclude these foods as well.

Assuming your symptoms clear up, then you can test the excluded foods as described above. If they do not, then you should go on to Stage 3.

STAGE 3 – RIGOROUS ELIMINATION DIET

Only a minority of those reading this book will need to try the Stage 3 diet. They will know they need to do this because they have tried Stage 2 with only partial success – or no success at all. Stage 3 is for those with multiple food sensitivities, which cannot be detected by a simple elimination diet.

The exclusion phase

Stage 3 requires planning, even more so than the previous stages. You must decide for yourself which foods you are going to eat during the exclusion phase, because this diet has to be tailored to your own eating habits. The aim is to come up with a list of at least twelve foods that are nutritious, obtainable, affordable, and which you have never eaten in any quantity, or with any regularity, before. They should include a variety of different items – some fruit, some vegetables, some meat or fish, and some starchy foods if possible, although this is often difficult. The approach we would advocate is a combination of the 'few foods' diet and the 'rare foods diet' (see p263), with the exact mix of foods being chosen to suit your pocket and your palate.

The following foods are suggested:

Vegetables
Celery, fennel and celeriac
Avocado pears
Lettuce
Swede (can be eaten raw, grated, in salads, as well as cooked)
Watercress .
Spinach
Alfalfa sprouts
Okra (also called bhindi, or ladies' fingers)
Asparagus

Meat and fish
Turkey
Duck
Goose
Rabbit
Pheasant or other game
Lamb
Fish (except smoked fish and shellfish)

Fruit
Gooseberries
Blackcurrants
Redcurrants
Bananas
Pears
Kiwi fruit
Mangoes

Pomegranates
Lychees
Passion fruit
Guavas

Starchy foods
Rice
Millet
Buckwheat
Turnips
Parsnips
Yams
Sweet potatoes
Plantains
Wild rice
Tapioca
Sago
Chestnuts
Chickpeas (also a good source of protein)
Pumpkin

Oils
Olive oil
Sunflower oil
Safflower oil
Rapeseed oil
Coconut oil and creamed coconut

Snacks
Pumpkin seeds
Macadamia nuts
Pistachio nuts
Cashew nuts
Brazil nuts
Pine nuts

If there are any foods on this list that you eat more than once a week – or have eaten very regularly at some time in the past – then you should exclude these. Advice on where to obtain exotic foods, and how to cook them, is given on pp307–12. Addresses of stockists, including some who sell by post, are given on pp334–7.

When deciding on your final list, bear the following points in mind:

Avocado pears have a laxative effect on some people. If you have bowel symptoms then you should not include these. If you have never eaten them before, try eating a couple at one sitting before you start Stage 3, to see what effect they have.

Spinach and chickpeas should not be included if you have bowel symptoms. Parsnips should be eaten in limited quantities only, and not too often, as they contain small amounts of a carcinogen.

Plantains are closely related to bananas and should not be included if you regularly eat bananas.

You should only eat sunflower oil if you have not previously eaten much margarine, nor used much sunflower oil (or 'vegetable oil') in cooking. There is some evidence that polyunsaturated oils, such as sunflower oil and safflower oil, are harmful if eaten in large quantities. Since the diet is rather low in calories, it is tempting to make up for this by using a lot of oil in cooking, but this is inadvisable. Olive oil is a monounsaturate rather than a polyunsaturate and is thought to be safer in large quantities – it is probably better for you than other plant oils. Unfortunately, it has a mild laxative effect on some people, so use it in moderation if you have bowel symptoms. If you have not eaten it before, test it out before you start Stage 3 to see if it has any effect.

Other foods that you do not eat often can be included, but not if they are related to frequently-eaten foods. Vegetables such as aubergines and cauliflower are not as 'safe' as they might appear, because they are closely related to staple foods – tomatoes and potatoes, for the aubergine, and cabbage for the cauliflower. Consult p303 before adding any foods to the list. Jerusalem artichokes, lentils, kidney beans and other types of beans should not be eaten, as they all tend to affect the bacteria living in the gut. (Chickpeas are of the bean family, but they are less of a problem in this respect.)

Many nuts are potent allergens. They should be eaten in small quantities and not too often – if you restrict each type of nut to once every four days you should notice any allergic response. Stop eating them immediately if in doubt.

If you are a vegetarian, then you should think carefully before going on this diet, as it will be low in both calories and protein, and will be very limited in scope – which means that you may be eating too much of some foods. If you can allow yourself some fish or meat, at least for a while, then you will probably do better on the diet. Introduce these foods gradually, before starting the exclusion phase, as your body may need time to adjust to the change.

The exclusion phase

This is meant to be a very simple, basic diet, in which you consume nothing but your allowed foods. No herbs, no spices, no flavourings, nothing tinned and no packaged foods of any sort. It is not going to be a gastronomic delight, but the diet does not last long and it may make you well again.

Eat only your allowed foods, remembering to vary your diet, not to eat any one food every day, and not to eat too much of any one food. Drink only bottled or filtered water (see p317). As before, you can drink herb teas, but avoid any that you have consumed regularly before. You should also vary them and not drink more than two or three cups a day – you can become sensitive to anything you eat or drink, and herb teas are no exception. Check the label, avoid those containing orange, lemon or apple extracts.

If, after reading Chapter Nine, you think you may have chemical sensitivity, then you should try to eat only unsprayed food during this diet (as well as following the avoidance measures for synthetic chemicals, pp179–83). Unfortunately, eating 'organic' foods only may be very difficult, since your choice of food is limited anyway, but it is worth choosing organic produce for *some* of the foods, even if you cannot manage it for all of them. Check a variety of sources to see what sort of organic produce is available – the range is widening all the time. Remember that friends' gardens are often the best source of unsprayed fruit and vegetables – ask around to see if you can buy surplus produce. You can test for sensitivity to pesticide residues by comparing your reactions to the same food, sprayed and unsprayed.

Continue the exclusion phase for at least three weeks. If you are not substantially better by then, it is highly unlikely that you have food sensitivity. Keep a record of everything you eat and all your symptoms.

You should also weigh yourself regularly during this diet, especially if you are not overweight at the outset. Anyone who is underweight should not embark on the diet without medical advice. If you find you are losing weight rapidly, then you should discuss the matter with your doctor. Elemental diets can sometimes be useful in these circumstances, as a nutritional supplement.

Possible outcomes: *Feeling much worse*
This often happens during the first few days of the exclusion phase, and it is generally considered a good sign. These 'withdrawal symptoms' are seen in many food-sensitive patients and seem to be caused by suddenly cutting out the offending food. They should pass by the end of the first week.

If you continue to feel worse after about eight days, then it may be that one of the rare or unusual foods you have included in your diet is affecting you. If you are eating buckwheat, cut this out for a few days – it can cause both food allergy and false-food allergy in susceptible people. If this produces no improvement, then cut out all other rare foods at once, and see how you are. Should you continue to have symptoms, go back to the 'healthy eating' diet and reconsider other possibilities: see under *Feeling about the same* below.

Feeling a little worse

This may be a mild version of the withdrawal symptoms, but if it persists after seven days, then it is something else. One possibility is that you were somewhat undernourished to start with and the diet has made things worse. If you think this is likely, go back to the 'healthy eating' diet and take a nutrional supplement – see p330. Stay on this regime for a couple of months to try to recover your general health. Then try the Stage 3 diet again.

Feeling worse, then much better

Once you have felt consistently better for three or four days then you should start the reintroduction phase – see below. Don't delay doing this. Write down exactly how you feel at this point – it may be useful and encouraging to refer back to this later if you suffer a lot of reactions during food testing.

Feeling much better quite quickly

This can happen, especially in children and young people – they seem to miss out on the withdrawal symptoms. Go on to the reintroduction phase.

Feeling much better, but with one or two lingering symptoms

It looks as if you have cut out your main offending foods, but are still eating something that is a problem (assuming that you have ruled out all other problems, such as airborne allergens, hyperventilation and environmental chemicals: see pp272–3). Think again about your previous eating habits – is there anything you used to eat quite frequently and are still eating? Cut all these out.

If your symptoms clear, then go on to the reintroduction phase immediately. If they don't, then the best option is to go on to a full 'rare-food diet', only eating foods that you have never eaten before. See pp307–12 for suitable foods.

If the remaining symptoms are mild, and fairly constant from day to day, then you could go on to the reintroduction phase – you may get some sort of useful result from testing. If you can discover which foods are the main source of trouble, and establish a diet on which you are reasonably well, then you are in a good position to investigate further. It could be that the remaining symptoms are due to some other problem – see below, under *Feeling about the same*, for a list of possibilities.

Feeling worse, then much better, then worse again

If you go through the withdrawal symptoms, feel greatly improved for a while, but then begin to go downhill again, this is a rather bad sign. It does not happen to many people, but if it does happen to you then you need to think very carefully about the situation.

The most likely explanation is that you are developing a new sensitivity to something allowed on the exclusion phase – probably something you are eating a lot of. Look at your food record for the exclusion phase, and try to work out what this might be – foods you ate *before* the diet, rather than entirely novel ones, are obvious suspects. Cut out any such foods and see what happens. Meanwhile make great efforts not to eat too much of any one food.

If you get better again, and stay better for two or three days, then you can begin the reintroduction phase. Continue to vary your diet as much as possible during this period – if you can, go on to a rotation diet (see p295). If you can't manage a four-day rotation, then three days will be some help at least.

If you are still not well, or if you have unclear results during the reintroduction phase, then one possible solution is an elemental diet (see p263), but you should consult your doctor about this and take his advice.

Feeling about the same

It seems unlikely that food sensitivity is your problem. If possible, progress to a full 'rare-food' diet, composed only of foods that are new to you – just to check that none of the foods in the exclusion phase is the source of the trouble. If this has no effect then you should go back to the 'healthy eating' diet and reconsider other possibilities, such as *Giardia* (p196), gut flora problems (Chapter Ten), airborne allergens (pp61–9), hyperventilation (p162), chemical sensitivity (pp168–84), psychosomatic problems (see pp150–2) or nutritional deficiencies (p271).

Reintroduction phase

Wait until you have been free of symptoms for two or three days, but don't wait any longer than this. Begin by testing foods that are probably not the cause of any trouble – things you do not eat very often. Choose items that you like – if the foods pass the test, then you can incorporate them into your menus, which will allow you to eat less of the exclusion-phase foods. Throughout the reintroduction phase it is vital that you keep your diet varied and do not eat too much of any one food. In particular, do not eat any one food every day. Continue to record everything you eat, and your symptoms – if something goes wrong, this record will prove invaluable.

Only test one food at a time. Eat a normal-sized portion of the food in question, preferably with your evening meal. Notice any changes that occur at the time, or later in the evening, or the following day. During the first five weeks of testing, test each food for one day only. (Although eating the food for three days in succession is preferable, it takes so much time that you cannot test enough foods – there are far more to test than on Stage 2). If you think you may have reacted slightly, but are unsure, then test the same food again the next day. After five weeks, your sensitivity may be declining, so you need to test each food more thoroughly, by eating it for three days in succession. If you get no reaction by the fourth day, then the food can be considered safe, but avoid it again for four days (to offset any possible effect of eating it for three days in succession) before beginning to eat it once more.

If you get a reaction to any food, stop eating it immediately. Allow the symptoms to subside before testing any more foods.

The reintroduction phase should take about seven or eight weeks. If it takes any longer than this, there is a risk of lost sensitivity: the food-intolerant person becomes less reactive after avoiding the culprit food for a time. If you are still testing foods eight weeks after starting the exclusion phase, then you need to test the foods more rigorously still. This means eating each reintroduced food every day for a week before declaring it safe.

If there are some foods that you have still not tested after 12 weeks then you have two options. One is to reintroduce all those foods for three to four weeks and see if any symptoms return. If they do, cut all those foods out again, wait until you feel better, then reintroduce them one at a time. Use three-day testing for preference, or one-day testing if you have a lot to get through.

The second option is to reintroduce each of the foods in turn, one per day. If there is no reaction, continue eating the food, but only on a once-every-four-days basis, for about six months. After that time, you should have become much less sensitive and be able to eat all these foods more freely.

If you suspect that you are sensitive to pesticide residues, you should be eating mainly unsprayed food during the exclusion phase of the diet. When you come to test foods, you should test unsprayed versions first, then a sprayed version of the same food, to see the difference. Leave a gap of at least four days between tests – try some other food in the meantime.

No reaction on testing

On either Stage 2 or Stage 3, there is the remote possibility that you will recover on the exclusion phase of the diet, but then show no reactions when foods are tested. It seems that this happens more often with younger patients, but it is unusual even among children.

There are two likely explanations for this outcome. One is that the diet has had a placebo effect (see p153). The other is that the sensitivity has been greatly reduced by simply avoiding the food for a month or two. Further dietary restrictions do not seem to be needed, but it is advisable to keep the diet varied to avoid a recurrence of the problem.

Chapter Fifteen

AFTER THE ELIMINATION DIET – TREATING FOOD INTOLERANCE

The simplest and most effective method of treating food intolerance is to avoid the culprit foods. Assuming that you have successfully identified your culprit foods, by following an elimination diet, the next step is to establish an adequate menu that excludes those foods. Make a list of the foods you cannot eat, and a list of those that you can. Talk to your doctor about your proposed diet, and ask for advice on its nutritional value.

After about six months, you can retest each of the incriminated foods, to see if you still react to them. If you do react, then try again six months later. If not, then you can begin eating them once in every four days. After a year of this, you can increase the frequency cautiously, but you should never go back to eating the food every day, or in large amounts. If symptoms recur, cut out the culprit foods again for a couple of months.

If you are not fully well, even after the elimination diet, then it is worth considering other possibilities – it could be that you have other problems, in addition to food intolerance. Nutritional deficiencies (p271) or chemical sensitivity (p168) are possible candidates. A continuing tendency to diarrhoea and wind may indicate gut-flora disturbances. The only treatment currently available for this is to eat plenty of live yoghurt (see p199).

Rotation diets

For people who acquire new sensitivities easily, eating all foods on a four-day rotation basis may be advisable. This is known as a **rotation diet**. Items from the list of allowed foods are allocated to four separate lists, one for each day of the rotation. Ideally, food relationships should be taken into account, and foods from the same family (*eg* potatoes and tomatoes) should only be eaten on one day in four. This does make the rotation diet quite restrictive, but it

JANET

Janet was 40 years old and had been ill in various ways since she was twelve, with rhinitis, severe migraine, urinary problems and pain in the region of her kidneys. During her thirties she had also developed depression, which had led to two suicide attempts and resulted in electroconvulsive therapy. Over the past six years she had made over 100 visits to her family doctor, spent 63 days in hospital, visited outpatients 49 times and taken 34 courses of drugs.

Janet was then tried on an elimination diet which excluded all commonly eaten foods. This provoked the worst migraine she had ever experienced at first, but then left her feeling a great deal better. On testing, a glass of milk produced sneezing, rhinitis and headache, whereas wheat left her depressed with a severe migraine. Eggs produced a headache, nausea and pain around the kidneys. Eating maize resulted in nausea and fatigue. By avoiding these four foods, Janet has remained very well. In the six years since her treatment she has visited her doctor five times, spent only two days in hospital and not required any drugs – a striking contrast to her previous six years.

may be necessary for some people. See Appendix IV, p302, for information on related foods.

The restrictions imposed by the rotation diet are quite harsh – not only are foods disallowed, but particular foods have to be eaten on particular days. An occasional departure from the regime is acceptable, but even with such allowances, eating away from home is very difficult indeed, and many social events become impossible. Some doctors recommend rotation diets to almost anyone recovering from food sensitivity, but the costs have to be weighed against the benefits. Loneliness and isolation can be as damaging to the health as eating the wrong sort of food.

OTHER METHODS OF TREATING FOOD INTOLERANCE

For anyone with multiple food sensitivities, avoiding all their culprit foods can be very difficult. And it may mean that they eat too much of other foods, with the attendant risk of developing new sensitivities. Even those who are intolerant of just one or two foods may find it difficult to avoid them, especially if they eat away from home a lot. So there have been many attempts to develop alternative methods of treatment.

Given the lack of knowledge about how food intolerance arises, these attempts are largely a 'suck-it-and-see' exercise: trying out treatments and seeing if they work. No treatment has yet been devised which is 100 per cent effective for all patients, and there are some on offer from 'alternative' practitioners that are quite ineffective and even potentially dangerous (*eg* urine therapy). However, there are two methods currently being tried out by some doctors, known as neutralization or desensitization treatments, that are worthy of further investigation.

In some studies, these treatments have performed quite well, but in others they have been less successful. Consequently, such techniques are controversial and many doctors feel that they should not be used until there is more evidence that they work. But given the complex nature of food intolerance, and the evidence suggesting that it is caused in several different ways (see Chapter Twelve), perhaps it is not surprising if a treatment gives varying results – it might be expected to work for some patients and not for others. Our own experience suggests that such methods *are* effective for a proportion of people with food intolerance. But they are probably not worth trying unless there is no reasonable dietary alternative.

These methods have also had some success in treating classical allergies, and in this context they may be very useful. The traditional method of desensitization, once widely used for hay fever and other allergies, cannot now be given by family doctors in Britain. This method involved injecting minute, but gradually increasing, doses of the allergen over a period of many months. There is a risk of collapse, due to anaphylactic shock, with this method, and a few patients have died as a result. Such desensitization treatment can now only be given in hospital, where resuscitation equipment is available.

Other uses claimed for these techniques include desensitization to environmental chemicals, such as exhaust fumes.

Provocation-neutralization technique

This is also known as intradermal neutralization therapy, or the Miller technique, after Dr Joseph Miller of Alabama, who has spent many years developing it and investigating its potential. The treatment can be applied in two ways – either using injections of food extracts under the skin, **subcutaneous injections**, or giving food extract drops under the tongue, **sublingual drops**. In both cases, the doctor establishes a particular dose of the food extract that will 'turn off' or 'neutralize' the symptoms caused by that food.

To test for the correct dose, **intradermal injections**, which put food extracts into the skin, are used. Intradermal injections place food extracts deeper in the skin than skin-prick tests (see p30). A tiny amount of food extract is used – 0.05 millilitres. If the body does not react to this extract it simply produces a small raised area, known as a wheal, which begins to go down soon afterwards. If the body *does* react, then the wheal grows slightly, and takes on a characteristic appearance – it is white, hard and raised, with a sharp edge. This is known as a 'positive wheal' At the same time, the patient may experience symptoms similar to those that are normally produced by the food – this is the 'provocation' part of the test.

The 'neutralization' part of the technique is based on the finding that a particular concentration of the same food extract will put a stop to those symptoms. Such a dose also produces a 'negative wheal' – one that is white, hard and raised, but does not grow larger. It is usually the same size ten minutes after the injection.

The neutralization dose is usually the *strongest* solution that fails to produce a positive wheal, so it is determined by starting with a solution that *does* produce a positive wheal and then working gradually downwards. Using this method, the neutralizing dose can be determined, even though the patient has no symptoms at the time – the wheals alone show when the right dose has been reached.

The fact that the neutralizing dose seems to 'turn off' symptoms which have already begun is truly remarkable, but this has regularly been observed, and many sceptics have been convinced by such a demonstration. How it might work is not known. Dr Miller has speculated that when the neutralizing dose is used, the food extract is 'bound' inside the wheal for a prolonged period, which allows it to exert a particular influence on the immune system. He suggests that it stimulates suppressor cells, which damp down the immune response to the food. This assumes, of course, that an immune reaction is the main cause of food intolerance, which is far from certain. Assuming enzyme deficiencies are at the root of food intolerance, then the neutralizing dose might stimulate the body to produce more detoxification enzymes.

In practical terms, neutralization therapy involves a long session of testing (usually one to three days) with different concentrations of foods – all the foods that have been incriminated by the elimination diet. The extracts are injected into the skin of the upper arm, a process that is only slightly painful. Once neutralizing doses have been determined for each of these foods, a mixture of the extracts is prepared for use. The patient is taught to carry out the subcutaneous injections, which are needed every two days at first, but only twice a week, or even less frequently, once the treatment has been under way for some months. Some people eventually find that they can discontinue the injections without ill-effects.

Sublingual therapy is approached in exactly the same way, the neutralizing dose being determined by a series of injections. But the mixture of extracts for home use is supplied as drops, one of which is placed under the tongue. There is rapid absorption into the bloodstream from this area, and it bypasses the liver, so the extract is not broken down rapidly. The effect of drops is not as long-lasting as that of a subcutaneous injection – the treatment has to be repeated every few hours. However, they are useful for inhalant allergies, or reactions to substances that are only encountered occasionally, because the drops can be used only when needed. Sublingual therapy has been successfully used to treat patients with allergic reactions to house-dust mite and pollen. It is also claimed to be effective for patients sensitive to synthetic chemicals, where industrial alcohol is used instead of an extract, but see p174.

The question of using mixtures of extracts for neutralization is a difficult one. The trials of this technique have all involved solutions containing single food extracts. Yet some practitioners use up to 70 food extracts in a mixture. Whether the method still works under these conditions is uncertain.

There is also concern over the possible dangers of this technique to patients with violent allergic reactions. It is theoretically possible for such a person to suffer anaphylactic shock when injected intradermally with their allergen, and this could be fatal. However, this technique has now been widely used for many years, and no fatal (or even near-fatal) reactions have occurred. Nevertheless, anyone who has experienced immediate and violent allergic reactions to food (or other allergens) should be carefully assessed before such treatment begins.

Finally, it is claimed that the provocation-neutralization method can be used as a diagnostic test, to determine which foods are the culprits and avoid the need for an elimination diet. These claims are rejected by the majority of doctors because they feel the test is too unreliable. Detailed trials show that there are often positive reactions to extracts of foods that do not provoke symptoms when eaten (**false positives**). Occasionally foods that cause symptoms will not produce a positive wheal (**false negatives**).

Enzyme-potentiated desensitization
This method is less widely practised than provocation-neutralization therapy. It depends on the ability of an enzyme, β-glucuronidase, to enhance the desensitizing effect of a food antigen. The food extract is applied to a scrape on the skin, along with the enzyme. Because the extract is not injected into the skin, it is safer for people with violent allergic reactions, and this method has been successfully used to treat a patient with immediate food-allergic reactions involving a range of foods.

In practice, the skin is scratched and the food-extracts-plus-enzyme applied to it in a small plastic cup. Alternatively, it can be given by intradermal injection. The same dose is given to all patients, and a comprehensive mixture of food extracts is generally used – not just those to which the patient is sensitive. This is said to work, and it obviously means that an elimination diet is less important. One drawback of such 'blanket therapy' is that there may be a worsening of the symptoms in the early stages because the patient becomes sensitized to some of the foods in the extract that were not a problem previously. Subsequent treatments apparently cancel out these effects.

An advantage of this technique over neutralization therapy is that the treatments are only needed about once every three months, and the frequency falls to once a year after a time. However, there have been far fewer trials of the method, and it is difficult to say what proportion of patients might be helped by it.

There is a modified form of this treatment in which the mixture of food extracts and enzyme is injected into the skin.

STAYING WELL

Once you have established a workable diet, or other form of treatment, you need to take care of your health generally, so as to guard against becoming ill again. The most important thing is to avoid slipping back into 'food addiction' – if you find yourself eating one sort of food very regularly, take a week off from it and then eat it on a three-day or four-day rotation basis for a while. Continue to eat healthily, with plenty of green vegetables and not too much processed food.

Exercise is very valuable, and does not have to be very strenuous or time-consuming. Walking briskly, running, cycling or swimming for half an hour is adequate. If you can do this two or three times a week you will feel a great deal healthier – every day is even better. Just running upstairs, instead of taking the lift, is beneficial.

Anyone who has had food intolerance should keep their exposure to man-made chemicals to a minimum. Despite the rising level of air pollution and agrochemical use, the worst problems are still to be found in the home, especially the double-glazed, cavity-foam-insulated, aerosol-ridden home. Read Chapter Nine, even if you don't have chemical sensitivities at present, and consider ways of reducing your exposure.

Avoid anything that irritates the gut lining and makes it more permeable: see p258. Look at the general health measures suggested on pp161–2 and follow these if they seem appropriate.

APPENDIX I
Foods that may release sulphur dioxide

Sulphur (or sulfur) dioxide is a gas that can irritate the airways of asthmatics and provoke an asthma attack. Some preservatives give off this gas in small amounts, and it is inhaled during eating. There is no need to avoid these preservatives unless you are sure they trigger off attacks.

Most dried fruits are treated with sulphur dioxide and give off the gas when chewed. *This treatment does not have to be declared on the label.* Dried fruit that has not been treated will usually be labelled 'unsulphured'. *The following preservatives give off sulphur dioxide:*

  Sodium sulphite;
  sodium hydrogen sulphite;
  sodium metabisulphite;
  potassium metabisulphite;
  calcium sulphite.

These preservatives are widely used in wine, beer and cider, and, like other additives used in alcoholic drinks, do not have to be declared on the label. Home-made wine is no exception: Campden tablets, sold to wine-makers, contain potassium metabisulphite.

Fresh sausages may also contain these additives. Cod can be treated with sodium hydrogen sulphite to bleach and preserve it. Although sulphites are not allowed on meat, unscrupulous butchers occasionally add them to old meat to give it a 'fresh' red colour. In all these cases, the greater part of the sulphur dioxide will be driven off by the high temperatures used in cooking.

A fourth 'hidden source' of sulphur dioxide is restaurant, take-away and cafeteria food. French fries used in the catering trade have usually been dipped in a metabisulphite solution and give off significant amounts of sulphur dioxide. Prepared salads, avocado dip, shrimps, prawns and lobster are also likely to have been treated with these preservatives, and sometimes cause problems.

Fruit salad, glacé cherries, fruit juices, fruit pie fillings, dried vegetables and soup, fruit squash, pickled onions, jam, fruit jellies and custard are other possible sources of sulphur dioxide in the catering trade. It is not worthwhile avoiding these foods unless you know they trigger off your asthma attacks.

Packaged foods often contain sulphites and metabisulphites, but these are easier to avoid as they are declared on the label. Look for the names given above, or for the appropriate 'E numbers'. These are E220-E227.

APPENDIX II
Foods containing salicylates

Avoiding foods containing salicylates is unlikely to be of benefit in most cases. But if you show a pronounced reaction to aspirin, yet are still not well after avoiding aspirin, a low-salicylate diet *may* be worth trying. For further information see p57 and p327.

The following foods are high in salicylates:
Most herbs, particularly mint, thyme, tarragon, rosemary, dill, sage, oregano, marjoram and basil. Also celery seed and sesame seed.
Most spices, particularly aniseed, cayenne, cinnamon, cumin, curry powder, fenugreek, mace, mustard, paprika and turmeric.
Most fruits, with the exception of bananas, peeled pears, pomegranates, mangoes and papaya.
Most vegetables, with the exception of cabbage, brussels sprouts, beansprouts, celery, leeks, lettuce and peas. Cucumbers, gherkins, olives and endive are particularly rich in salicylates.
Potato skins, but not potatoes themselves.
Sweetcorn, sweet potatoes.
Almonds, Brazil nuts, macadamia nuts, peanuts, pine nuts, pistachios and walnuts. Also, coconut and water chestnuts.
Coffee, tea, Coca-Cola and peppermint tea.
Fruit juices, most alcoholic drinks (but not gin or vodka), honey, liquorice, peppermints.
Marmite, stock cubes and other yeast-rich products.
Tomato sauce and Worcester sauce.
Many processed foods and instant meals.

The following foods are low in salicylates:
Meat, fish and shellfish.
Milk, cheese and eggs.
Wheat, rye, oats, barley and rice.
Some fruits and vegetables, as listed above.

APPENDIX III
Synonyms for food ingredients

The following synonyms may be used on food labels:

Baking powder	*May contain maize (corn)*
Casein, caseinate	*Milk*
Cereal binder	*Usually wheat*
Cereal filler	*Usually wheat*
Cereal protein	*Usually wheat*
Cereal starch	*Usually wheat or maize (corn)*
Corn meal	*Maize*
Corn starch	*Maize (corn)*
Corn syrup	*Maize*
Dextrose	*A type of sugar, derived from maize*
Edible starch	*Usually wheat or maize (corn)*
Flour	*Usually wheat flour*
Food starch	*Usually wheat or maize (corn)*
Fructose	*A type of sugar*
Glucose syrup	*A type of sugar, usually derived from maize (corn)*
Hydrolysed protein	*Usually yeast*
Hydrolysed vegetable protein	*Usually yeast*
Lactalbumin	*Milk*
Lactose	*Milk sugar*
Leavening	*Yeast*
Lecithin	*Usually egg or soya*
Maltose	*A type of sugar*
Miso	*Soya*
Modified starch	*Usually wheat or maize (corn)*
Ovalbumin	*Egg*
Starch	*Usually wheat or maize (corn)*
Sucrose	*Sugar*
Textured vegetable protein	*Soya*
Tofu	*Soya*
Vegetable gum	*Can be soya or maize (corn)*
Vegetable oil	*Usually a mixture of oils, often including corn (maize) oil*
Vegetable protein	*Usually soya*
Vegetable starch	*Can be soya or maize (corn)*
Whey	*Milk*

In some foods labelled 'no added sugar', apple juice could be considered as a synonym for sugar, because highly concentrated apple juice has been used to sweeten the product.

APPENDIX IV
Related foods

The relevance of food relationships to food sensitivity is explained on p265. Briefly, a person who is sensitive to one plant food (*eg* oranges) may react badly to other foods from related plants (*eg* lemons and grapefruit). The same also goes for foods from animal sources.

In the past, a great deal of emphasis has been placed on 'food families' – by those treating food intolerance. These doctors have automatically looked at the taxonomic *family* of plants and animals to predict when cross-reactions are likely to occur.

But the *family* is just one sort of group in taxonomy – the science of biological classification. A closer look at the cross-reactions shown by patients suggests that the family is not always the most relevant group to consider. Sometimes we need to consider higher or lower levels of classification. *The over-emphasis on food families can create problems.* For example, it can lead food-sensitive people to eat too much of some potentially troublesome foods (*eg* fish), while avoiding many plant foods unnecessarily.

In general, the problem of cross-reactions has probably been exaggerated in the past. The only groups where cross-reactions are at all common are the cereals, shellfish, fish and tree nuts. (Cross-reactions between certain foods and certain pollens are common, however, and these are described on p305.)

TABLE I
Taxonomic groups

A group of very similar individuals makes up a **species**

Related species are grouped together in a **genus** (pl. genera)

Related genera are sometimes grouped together in **tribes and subfamilies**

Related genera (or tribes or subfamilies) are grouped together in a **family**

Related families are grouped together in an **order**

Related orders are grouped together in a **class**

Related classes are grouped together in a **phylum** (pl. phyla)

Related phyla are grouped together in a **kingdom**

The relationships listed below seem to be relevant to food sensitivity. Herbs and spices are only included where they are likely to be eaten in quantity and have the potential to cause a cross-reaction.

PLANT FOODS

1 **Grass family, Gramineae**: wheat, rye, triticale, barley, oats, maize (corn), rice, wild rice, millet, sorghum, bamboo, sugar cane. Some people react to all members of the family, but most are sensitive to wheat and its close relatives, or maize. The subfamilies are more relevant here (see p255). They are:
Pooidae: wheat, rye, barley, oats
Panicoideae: maize, sorghum, sugar cane, bulrush or pearl millet*
Bambusoideae: rice, wild rice
Chloridoideae: finger millet*.
*bulrush or pearl millet is the one commonly sold in Britain

2 **Potato family, Solanaceae**: potato (but not sweet potato), tomato, aubergine, sweet peppers (green, red and yellow peppers), paprika, chilli peppers, tobacco, cape gooseberry.

3 **Bean and pea family, Leguminosae**: peas, haricot beans (kidney beans, whether white-, red-, brown- or black-skinned, also baked beans and flageolets), peanuts, soya beans, lentils, split peas, broad beans, butter beans, mung beans, lima beans, chickpeas, black-eyed peas, carob, runner beans, green beans, snap beans, string beans, mangetout peas. Different kinds of haricot beans and their green forms (snap beans, string beans and green beans, including those sold as a frozen vegetable) are all the same species and should be regarded as the same food. Peanuts belong to a separate tribe from other members of the family, and experience with patients who are allergic to peanut suggests that cross-reactivity with other legumes is generally low, but peanut-sensitive people may react to soya beans. Patients sensitive to soya beans *are* likely to react to a wide range of legumes. Anyone with these sensitivities is usually advised to avoid peanut and soybean oils as well, but this may not be necessary – such oils contain no detectable protein, and tests with allergic individuals showed no reaction to the relevant oil. But there might be a reaction if someone were intolerant of a non-protein component.

4 **Cabbage family, Cruciferae**: Several members of this family are actually part of the same species, which means that they are very closely related indeed. They are: cabbage, cauliflower, brussels sprouts, broccoli, calabrese, 'spring greens', kohlrabi and kale. These should all be regarded as the same food for rotation purposes. Other members of the family are: turnip, oilseed rape, chinese leaves, horseradish, radish, swede, cress, watercress and mustard. Rape-seed oil might cross-react with other cabbage-family foods, but this is relatively unlikely.

5 **Carrot family, Umbelliferae**: carrot, parsnip, celery, celeriac, fennel, parsley, aniseed, caraway, dill, cumin, coriander.

6 **Cucumber family, Cucurbitaceae**: cucumber, melon, watermelon, marrow, courgette (zucchini), squash, pumpkin.

7 **Onion family, Liliaceae**: onion, leek, shallot, garlic, chives, asparagus.

8 **Daisy family, Compositae**: lettuce, chicory, endive, globe artichoke, Jerusalem artichoke, salsify, sunflower, safflower, chamomile. No specific tests have been carried out on sunflower oil or safflower oil, but given the results with peanut and soybean oil (see above), it seems unlikely that they would cross-react with other members of this family.

9 **Spinach family, Chenopodiaceae**: spinach, spinach beet, chard, beetroot, sugar beet.

10 **Walnut family, Juglandaceae**: walnuts, pecans. See also the general section on nuts, p304.

11 **Palm family, Palmaceae**: coconut, dates, sago, palm oil.

12 **Banana family, Musaceae**: banana, plantain, one form of arrowroot (Musa arrowroot).

13 **Mulberry family, Moraceae**: mulberry, fig, hops

14 **Buckwheat family, Polygonaceae**: buckwheat, rhubarb.

15 **Currant family, Saxifragaceae**: blackcurrant, redcurrant, whitecurrant, gooseberry. Note that the 'currants' used in buns and cakes are dried grapes.

16 **Rose family, Rosaceae**: The groups most relevant to cross-reactions are the subfamilies:
Rosoideae: blackberry, raspberry, wineberry, cloudberry, loganberry (all in the same genus, so quite closely related); also strawberry and rosehip
Prunoideae: plum, prune, apricot,

greengage, cherry, peach, nectarine, sloe (all the same genus, so quite closely related); also almond
Maloideae: apple, pear, quince, medlar, loquat.

17 **Citrus family, Rutaceae**: orange, lemon, tangerine, clementine, grapefruit, lime, citron, ugli. These are all members of the same genus, and therefore very closely related, so cross-reactions are likely. Kumquats are also members of the citrus family.

18 **Cashew family, Anacardiaceae**: cashew, pistachio, mango.

19 **Grape family, Vitaceae**: grapes, muscatels, raisins, sultanas, currants (the dried fruits – not blackcurrants or redcurrants).

20 **Bilberry family, Ericaceae**: bilberry (also called blueberry or, locally, whortleberry), cranberry, cowberry.

21 **Mint family, Labiatae**: mint, basil, marjoram, oregano, rosemary, sage, thyme, savory.

22 **Fungi kingdom**: mushrooms, puffballs, truffles, morels, chanterelles, yeast, 'mycoprotein', 'Quorn'.
Also see Table 6 in Chapter Ten.

POULTRY AND EGGS

23 **Pheasant subfamily, Phasianinae**: chicken, pheasant, quail, partridge.

24 **Grouse subfamily, Tetraoninae**: grouse, turkey, guineafowl.

25 **Duck family, Anatidae**: all types of duck and goose.

26 **Pigeon family, Columbidae**: pigeon, squab, dove.

27 **Snipe family, Scolopacidae**: snipe, woodcock.

28 **Eggs**: all birds' eggs are very similar in the proteins they contain, and are best regarded as a single food item.

FISH AND SHELLFISH

29 **Fish**: the family concept is irrelevant when it comes to fish, because all the fish in the main group eaten (the bony fish) share a special type of protein known as a
parvalbumin. The parvalbumins are known to provoke allergic reactions, and they probably account for the fact that many people are sensitive to *all* the types of fish they have tried. It is uncertain whether parvalbumins are found in the other main group of fish, the sharks, rays, skates and dogfish (cartilaginous fish). The two groups are only very distantly related, and it is possible that people sensitive to bony fish could tolerate cartilaginous fish.

30 **Crustaceans, Phylum Crustacea**: crab, lobster, crayfish, shrimp, prawn. A very large group, including many different families. Many patients react to all forms of crustacea, so the family concept does not seem relevant here. There may be some common allergen in all of them, as in fish. *Also see the section on unexpected reactions, below.*

31 **Molluscs, Phylum Mollusca**: mussels, cockles, winkles, oysters, clams, scallops, squid, cuttlefish, octopus, snails (escargots). Again, this is a very broad group, but the family concept does not seem to be relevant here, because people who are sensitive to one type are usually sensitive to them all. *Also see the section on unexpected reactions, below.*

MEAT AND MILK

32 **Cattle family, Bovidae**: cows (beef, veal), sheep (lamb, mutton), goats. The sheep and goats are grouped in one subfamily, the cows in another, so cross-reactions are most likely between lamb/mutton and goat meat. Cross-reactions between the milk of these three species defy the taxonomic groups: those sensitive to cow's milk quite often react to goat's milk but less often to sheep milk. Why this should be is unknown.

33 **Pig family, Suidae**: pig (pork, ham, bacon)

34 **Deer family, Cervidae**: venison

35 **Rabbit family, Leporidae**: rabbit, hare

UNEXPECTED CROSS-REACTIONS

Nuts
These deserve a special note, because it seems that people who are allergic to one type of nut are allergic to others, despite the fact that most nuts are not at all closely related. Apart from those in the walnut family

(10) and the cashew family (18) every nut is an individualist – in all, there are at least eight families of plant that supply us with edible nuts. So why should there be this apparent cross-reaction between them? One can only assume that their common 'way-of-life' requires certain chemical constituents (to prevent rotting for example – most nuts are designed to be carried off and stored by animals). Perhaps the different nuts have evolved similar chemicals for this purpose.

Whether this cross-reaction between different types of nut occurs in food intolerance as well is unknown. One problem here is that both doctors and patients tend to refer to them rather vaguely as 'nuts', instead of specifying which type.

People who are sensitive to peanuts may not be affected by other types of nut, but if they have ever had a serious allergic reaction to peanuts they should try out other nuts with great caution.

Cross-reactions between plant products

Some people with hay-fever find they are affected by foods from the same plant family. In one unusual and alarming case, a boy with mugwort allergy collapsed, and almost died, on drinking a cup of camomile tea. Both mugwort and camomile are members of the daisy family, the Compositae, as is ragweed, a plant with highly allergenic pollen. Sunflowers also belong to this family and their seeds may cause a reaction. When such reactions happen there are usually warning signs, such as tingling of the mouth and lips, which should be heeded immediately (see pp51–3).

A few of those who are allergic to birch pollen cannot eat hazelnuts. This is not particularly surprising, since birch and hazel belong to the same plant family. What is unexpected is the cross-reaction seen between birch pollen and apple – a very high proportion of those with birch hay-fever are allergic to apples. It is thought that this is due to proteins that are widely distributed in plant products. Peaches, pears, plums, cherries and even potatoes are also reported as affecting a few people with birch-pollen allergy. However, apple sensitivity is the most common.

There are other odd cross-reactions between different fruits and vegetables which may be explained in the same way. Ragweed pollen seems to share some antigens with melons and bananas, while mugwort pollen shares antigens with celery. Allergy to celery is particularly dangerous, as it often causes swelling of the throat.

Shellfish

Some people seem to be sensitive to both crustacean shellfish and molluscan shellfish (see above, 30 and 31). Why this should be is a mystery – it is unlikely to be a cross-reaction, in the conventional sense, since the two groups are not at all closely related. Biologically speaking, they are as similar to humans or birds as they are to each other. Again, the use of an imprecise name for both groups – 'shellfish' – is a confusing factor.

For certain people, it may be something other than the shellfish themselves causing the problem. Toxins acquired from their food, or the preservatives that are liberally added to shellfish (see p53) might be to blame. This could explain the apparent cross-reaction.

INDEX OF FOODS
Please read the introduction to this section before using this list.

A number following the food shows the group it belongs to in the list on pp303–4. An 'S' shows that it is the only commonly eaten member of its family. A 'U' shows that it may be involved in some unexpected cross-reactions.

tangerine 17
tapioca (cassava) S
tea S
thyme 21
tobacco 2
tomato 2
triticale 1
truffles 22
turkey 24
turnip 4
ugli 17
veal 32
venison 34
walnuts 10

water chestnut S
watercress 4
watermelon 6, U
wheat 1
whitecurrant 15
whortleberry 20
wild rice 1
wineberry 16
winkles 31
woodcock 27
yam S
yeast 22
zucchini 6

APPENDIX V
Alternatives to commonly eaten foods

For sources of the more unusual foods, and
addresses for mail-order purchases, see
pp334–7. In all recipes, follow *either* the metric
or imperial measurements, not a mixture of
the two.

MILK

Goat's milk can be bought in some
healthfood shops and goat's-milk powder is
available by post. Because supplies are not
covered by the same sort of regulations that
govern cow's-milk production, there is a risk
of infection, and it is a good idea to boil
goat's milk before use, especially if giving it to
children. There are two other drawbacks to
this product: it has a very rank 'goaty' taste
that takes quite a bit of getting used to, and it
often provokes reactions in people who are
already sensitive to cow's milk.

Sheep milk is available in healthfood shops
in some areas. It has a much less powerful
taste than goat's milk and is pleasantly
creamy. Unlike cow's milk, it freezes well, so
you can buy it in frozen form. This milk may
provoke cross-reactions in those sensitive to
cow's milk, but it is less likely to do so than
goat's milk.

Soya milk is made from pulverized soya
beans, and its origin is evident in the flavour.
Most brands have some sugar added. It is
obtainable from most healthfood shops. To
make your own, mix 165 gm (5 oz) of soya
flour to a paste with a few spoonfuls of water,
then slowly add 1 litre (1½ pints) of water,
bring slowly to the boil, stirring continuously,
then simmer for 20 minutes, stirring from time
to time. Add a teaspoonful of honey; store in
the refrigerator. Soya can readily provoke
allergic/intolerant reactions, so it is not
advisable to eat too much of any soya
product. Soya desserts and 'yoghurt' are also
available. Sugar-free forms of soya milk, and
concentrated soya milk, are both available by
post.

Creamed coconut is obtainable from Indian
or West Indian groceries, and some
healthfood shops. It can be used as a
substitute for cream, if mixed with a small
amount of warm water. Or you can just grate
it directly on to fruit salad, chopped bananas
etc.

Ground almonds can also be made into a
cream substitute. Mix it to a paste with water
and a little honey, then add more water until
you get the right consistency.

Cashew nuts (unroasted) can be ground in a blender and mixed with water to form a cream substitute. Add honey and vanilla to taste. Dilute further to make cashew 'milk'.

BUTTER
Margarine is the obvious substitute for butter, but some brands (*eg* Flora) contain small amounts of milk solids. The brands that do not are mainly available from healthfood shops. They include: Granose, Tomor and Vitasieg.

If you hate the taste of margarine, there are other possibilities. One is **tahini**, or ground sesame seeds – quite a strong taste, but a pleasant one. Sesame can readily provoke allergy or intolerance, however, so it should not be eaten too often. **Sunflower spread** is similar. Both are available from healthfood shops.

Another alternative is **clarified butter,** which can be tolerated by most milk-sensitive people. Make it by melting a pack of butter over a gentle heat, allowing it to cool a little and then pouring it carefully into a glass jar. The proteins in the butter will have settled to the bottom of the pan, and are visible as white granules – by pouring very slowly you leave these behind in the pan. Any that do get into the glass jar will settle to the bottom, and since you can see them through the side of the jar you can avoid eating them. Keep clarified butter in the fridge as it is semi-liquid at room temperature. You can also buy this product at Indian groceries under the name **ghee**.

Clarified butter should only be used once you have completed the elimination diet, and know that you have to avoid milk – it should not be used during the elimination diet, as it still contains traces of milk protein and may confuse the result.

In sauces, **creamed coconut** makes an interesting substitute for butter, although it only suits certain foods. Try melting creamed coconut in orange juice over a low heat, adding ground almonds to thicken the mixture, salt and garlic – this gives a delicious rich sauce to accompany pork or chicken.

CHEESE
Goat cheeses and sheep cheeses are available from good delicatessan shops, and healthfood shops. You can also buy them by post. See remarks above on cross-reactivity.

Soya-based 'cheese' spreads are available in some healthfood shops.

Tofu is a more traditional soya product that can act as a substitute for soft cheese. See remarks above about soya.

The following foods are not like cheese in taste, but are useful substitutes for cheese in filling sandwiches or making quick snacks:

Hoummous, if made to a thick consistency, is a very good sandwich-filling or spread. Mash 280 gm (10 oz) of cooked, drained chickpeas with a potato masher, add 5–6 dessertspoons of olive oil, 2–3 dessertspoons of lemon juice, 2 pinches of salt and a clove of garlic, if liked. If you use tinned chickpeas this only takes a few minutes to make. Or you can cook the chickpeas yourself (see p311), to make a larger quantity, and freeze some.

Paté is useful, although most contains preservatives. Making your own is not difficult, especially if you use a blender.

Taramasalata is a Greek dish, made with smoked fish roe, olive oil, lemon juice and garlic. It makes a good sandwich filling, combined with tomatoes, cucumber or watercress. Most taramasalata also contains breadcrumbs and preservatives, and the majority are tinted a bright pink with artificial colourings. Some shops (*eg* Sainsbury's) sell uncoloured taramasalata.

Gjetost (pronounced *yat-turst*) or Norwegian brown cheese is made from milk whey not milk solids. Specialist cheese shops and supermarkets with a cheese counter sometimes sell it. Since most milk-sensitive people are reacting to the protein casein, which forms the milk solids, they may be able to tolerate whey, the liquid part of the milk. This does contain proteins, but different ones, not casein. The thorough cooking of the whey to produce gjetost may also make it less allergenic. Unfortunately gjetost does not taste much like ordinary cheese. It is rather sweet with a nutty, caramelized flavour that seems strange at first, but is delicious once you are used to it. It goes well with wholemeal bread and apples.

EGGS
The eggs of other birds, such as ducks or quail, may be a useful substitute for some people, but they are likely to cross-react with chicken's eggs (see p304) and should be tested alone before being used in recipes. Anyone who has a true allergy to eggs should be *very* cautious about testing other types of eggs.

Nothing can reproduce the taste of eggs, but some other foods can mimic their cooking qualities. In puddings, where they are used to 'set' a liquid, gelatine is a useful substitute. You will have to experiment with each recipe, but one teaspoon of gelatin is roughly equal to one egg. Dissolve the gelatin in water before adding to the other ingredients. In biscuit recipes, one egg can be replaced by 2 tablespoons of water, 1 tablespoon of vegetable oil and ½ teaspoon of baking powder. Commercial egg-replacers and egg-white replacers are also available (see p335 and p336).

WHEAT FLOUR FOR BREAD

If you have an *intolerance* of wheat (rather than food allergy or coeliac disease), it is worth checking that it is *all* types of wheat you must avoid. It may be the proteins in the wheatgerm that affect you, or something in the outer coat of the wheat grain. If this is the case, you will be able to eat white bread and white flour, but should avoid wholemeal bread, granary bread, and any product (eg crackers) with wheatgerm in it.

The proteins in wheat flour – which include gluten – are what makes wheat good for bread-making. Trying to make bread without wheat involves finding a substitute for this protein.

Gluten-free bread is available in some healthfood shops – at a price.

Or you can buy a gluten-free flour and make your own. Those with coeliac disease can get some gluten-free products on prescription.

Gluten-free flours are made from a mixture of different flours, *eg* maize flour, potato flour, soya flour, split pea flour, rice flour, rice bran, carob flour, corn starch and ground almonds. You can improvise with simple mixtures of your own – *eg* one part rice flour, to one part soya or gram flour, to one part potato flour. The mixture must always include at least one type of high-protein flour, such as soya, gram or lentil. Use yeast and make in the ordinary way, but without kneading the bread. It will have a heavier texture than ordinary bread, and may taste better toasted. If you have to avoid yeast as well, it is possible to make soda bread using gluten-free flour. The manufacturers of gluten-free flour usually supply recipes for use with their particular flour mix, and these should be followed for good results.

Bear in mind that most gluten-free mixes contain soya flour or other bean-derived flours. Make sure you are not eating soya and related foods (see p303) too regularly, especially if you are vegetarian – they feature in most commercial meat substitutes, 'vegeburgers' and instant meals.

Rye bread may be a useful substitute for some people, because rye is also rich in protein, though it cannot rival wheat. Because the two are closely related, those who are sensitive to wheat quite often react to rye as well. If you buy rye bread from a local bakery be sure to check that it is 100 per cent rye – speak to the manager, and ask to be notified if they change the composition of the bread. Rye flour often contains some wheat anyway, because wheat grows as a weed in fields of rye.

Rye crispbread can be eaten as long as it is pure rye – some now have wheat bran added.

Oatcakes are available from most good supermarkets, delicatessans and healthfood shops. Oats are preferable to rye since they are less likely to cross-react with wheat. Check the label, as some contain milk or sugar.

Rice cakes and **rice crackers** are available from healthfood shops. The 'cakes' are actually savoury – something like a crispbread, but made from puffed grains of rice. They taste much nicer than they look.

WHEAT FLOUR FOR OTHER USES

Pastry, pancakes and **waffles** can be made with rye flour although the results are heavier than with wheat, partly because rye flour is only available in wholemeal form. Putting the rye flour through a fine sieve first improves the quality by removing the larger pieces of husk from the flour, and adding some baking powder helps too. Pancakes can also be made with maize or barley flour, and taste pleasant although they are slightly rubbery – beat plenty of air into the mixture just before frying to improve the texture. **Buckwheat flour** is fairly protein-rich and makes a good pancake batter, but should be mixed with other flours to dilute the strong taste. Gluten-free mixes for pastry and pancakes can be bought by post and generally give excellent results.

Pasta made with gluten-free flour is obtainable by post. Or you can try **rice noodles**, obtainable in Chinese groceries, or **buckwheat spaghetti**, from healthfood stores.

Soya flour, gram flour and **lentil flour** are rich in protein, as well as carbohydrate. They can be used in baking, combined with other flours (see above under *Gluten-free flours*) and tend to improve the texture of pastry and pancakes.

Rice flour, potato flour, banana flour, chestnut flour, yam flour and other exotic flours are mostly low in protein. They are useful for making puddings and biscuits, or for thickening sauces (see below). Chestnut flour tastes sweet and nutty and is pleasant in shortbread or in a crumble topping for fruit, although it is rather heavy.

CORNFLOUR AND OTHER THICKENERS

Sago flour can be used to thicken soups, sauces and stews, and is obtainable by post. (**Pearl sago** and **pearl tapioca** are obtainable from most large supermarkets and can be made into puddings with milk, or a milk substitute.)

Arrowroot is sold in some delicatessans and is an excellent thickener.

Rice flour, potato flour, barley flour and **rye flour** are sold in some healthfood shops and can all be used as thickeners, although they need to be used with care as they tend to go lumpy more readily than cornflour. Any of the exotic flours listed in the previous section can also be used.

POTATOES

Yams are probably the best potato substitute. They are a large cylindrical white root with a dull brown outer skin. Firmer and more fibrous than potatoes, they are very similar in taste but with an interesting, slightly bitter aftertaste. They are best if prepared like sautéed potatoes – boiled and then fried. You need a sharp knife and a strong hand to peel them and cut them into cubes. Boil for about 20 minutes or until they are tender. If you buy a large piece of yam and boil it, you can then pack the cooked pieces in individual portions and freeze them. You can fry them from frozen in oil – fry slowly over a low heat for best results. Yam can be bought in West Indian groceries, but tends to be rather expensive. Pieces of fried yam dipped in taramasalata are quite delicious.

Sweet potatoes are also found in West Indian and Chinese stores, and occasionally in ordinary greengrocers or supermarkets. There are many different sorts, with flesh ranging from white to deep yellow in colour. Those on sale in Britain usually have a distinctive reddish-purple outer skin. Peel and dice them, keeping them under water as much as possible to prevent discoloration. Alternatively, you can bake them and serve them with butter (if allowed) or slice and deep-fry them. They have a very sweet, slightly sticky flesh which goes well in soups, or with meat casseroles, but is rather cloying on its own.

Serving sweet potatoes with sharp fruit is a good idea, as the acidity offsets their stickiness. Try frying them over a low heat for 20 minutes (after boiling), adding slices of apple and walnuts for the last 5 minutes. This makes a good breakfast dish. Like yams, sweet potatoes can be peeled and boiled in a large batch, then stored in individual portions in the freezer, and fried from frozen.

The Chinese make a soup by boiling sweet potatoes in water or stock until they disintegrate and flavouring the liquid with root ginger. They also make a delicious snack called deep-fried sweet potato balls. To make these, boil some sweet potatoes until soft. Mash them and add rice flour (or wheat flour) to make a stiff dough. Take a small piece of the dough, press it down flat, put a half-teaspoonful of peanut butter (or another nut butter) in the centre and seal the dough around it. Roll in sesame seeds and deep fry in vegetable oil.

PORRIDGE

A hot breakfast cereal based on maize meal can be bought in some healthfood shops. Alternatively, millet can be made into a porridge – see next section.

OTHER SUBSTITUTES FOR TRADITIONAL STARCHY FOODS

Millet can be bought at some healthfood shops – it consists of tiny spherical yellow grains. Measure out half-a-pint of these grains and wash thoroughly before putting them to soak overnight. Throw away the soaking water and replace with a pint of clean water. Add half a teaspoon of salt and bring to the boil. Allow to simmer over a low heat for 20 minutes. The water should all be absorbed at the end of this time.

This porridgey mix can be eaten with milk or a milk-substitute as a breakfast dish. However, it is more appetising if treated as follows:

Prepare and cook half-a-pint of millet (about 225 gm) as above, but use a level teaspoon of salt. While still hot, add half a jar (about 150gm) of sugar-free peanut butter (or another nut butter – see p312), and one level teaspoon of sesame seeds, already toasted (see p312). Mix the ingredients together well, using a potato masher to break up the millet. Take a lump of the mixture – about the size of a small egg – roll it between your palms and squash flat, pressing hard, to make a 'hamburger' shape. It is important to do this while the millet is still warm, as it becomes very uncooperative when cold. These quantities make about 30 burgers.

Fry the 'millet burgers' in oil over a low heat, turning them twice and allowing at least 20 minutes total frying time – this gives the outside a lovely crunchy texture. Use a non-stick pan and plenty of oil or they may stick. The burgers can be made in bulk and frozen unfried; they do not need to be defrosted before being fried. Although making a large batch is fairly time-consuming, it is well worth it as they are both delicious and filling. Four or five make a good meal: eat them for breakfast, with some grated apple, or for lunch, with a salad.

Cooked millet can also be added to soups and casseroles to thicken them. Millet can also be used as a substitute for wheat flour in a cheese soufflé. Make in the usual way, using 115 gm (4 oz) cooked millet, 3 eggs, 55 gm (2 oz) cheese, 140 ml (¼ pint) milk, salt and pepper. Bake for 20 minutes with the soufflé dish in a tray of water.

Sorghum is not widely available, but can be bought by post. Cook in the same way as millet.

Wild rice is only available from a few healthfood shops and delicatessans and is rather expensive. It has long, dark brown grains and a distinctive nutty-earthy taste that goes very well with some foods, notably fish, poultry and stir-fried vegetables. To cook, wash thoroughly, place in a large saucepan, cover with cold salted water, and bring to the boil. Simmer for 45 minutes, then turn off the heat, stir the rice and leave to stand for 15 minutes. Pour off any excess water, but do not rinse. The cooked grains freeze perfectly, and can be defrosted quickly by boiling in water or stock, without becoming glutinous. A mixture of orange or lemon juice and melted butter (if you are allowed these) improves the taste of the rice. For breakfast, defrost some wild rice by boiling in fruit juice, adding dried apricots and nuts.

Maize meal or **cornmeal** can be prepared as *polenta* and used as an accompaniment to stews or casseroles. Combine 115 gm (4 oz) maize meal with a level teaspoon each of salt and mild paprika, and a tiny pinch of cayenne. Mix in ¼ litre (½ pint) of water, adding the water slowly to prevent lumps forming. Steam in a double-boiler – or put a small pan (containing the maize meal) inside a larger one, containing an inch or two of water, to get the same effect as a double boiler. After 30 minutes, turn out into a greased baking dish and bake for 10 to 15 minutes at 170°C, 350°F, gas mark 4. Pour a few spoons of juice from the casserole over the top, and a layer of grated cheese, then put under the grill to brown. This also goes well with fish.

Buckwheat, or *kasha* as it is known in Russia, can be bought in most healthfood shops. It consists of brown triangular grains, whose strong, earthy flavour is something of an acquired taste. Wash the grains thoroughly under the tap, then cook in twice the quantity of salted water. You can make the taste less powerful by pouring off the first lot of water, after it comes to the boil, and replacing it with the same amount of clean salted water. Simmer for about 15 minutes, or until all the water is absorbed and the grains are soft. It needs to be served with a sauce or casserole that has an equally powerful taste – beef and tomatoes with plenty of herbs, for example. Buckwheat spaghetti is also available, but check that it does not contain any wheat. It is not advisable to eat too much buckwheat, as it is often implicated in sensitivity reactions.

Chestnuts are useful as a snack or a breakfast dish. They can also be used to stuff a chicken or turkey, in the traditional manner, and eaten with the poultry as a substitute for potato. Dried chestnuts are the cheapest – they can be found in some healthfood shops, and in Chinese groceries. Soak them overnight, throw away the water and wash them thoroughly. Cook in a pressure cooker, at 15 lbs pressure, for 15 minutes, or boil in the ordinary way for about an hour, until tender all the way through but not disintegrating. You can cook a large quantity and freeze them in individual portions. They can be fried gently in oil to make a light breakfast – serve with grated apple or a salad. Alternatively, you can make chestnuts into a soup, preferably with oranges or some other fruit. For chestnut flour, see p309.

Pumpkin is available from some greengrocers in the autumn. It is sweet and slightly sticky – not unlike sweet potato. Prepare and use it in the same way.

Chickpeas are more floury than other beans, with a less 'beany' taste, and fewer unpleasant after-effects. So they make a good filler if you cannot eat wheat or potatoes. Soak them overnight, pick out any discoloured ones, and cook in a pressure cooker at 15 lb pressure for 20-25 minutes, or in the ordinary way for 1–1½ hours. If you *do* find that they give you wind, try removing the skins – they rub off very easily. Tinned chickpeas are not expensive if you buy supermarket 'own-brands' (*eg* Sainsbury's). Add to soups and casseroles. You can also mash them to make hoummous (see p308). Other **beans** and **lentils** are also useful fillers for those who cannot eat wheat or potatoes.

Pearl barley is sold in most large supermarkets, and in healthfood stores. Add it to stews, casseroles and soups to make them more filling. The barley needs about 1–1½ hours cooking time.

Plantains are obtainable from West Indian groceries and look like very large green bananas. They are starchy and less banana-like in flavour than one might expect. Peel them (quite difficult – needs a sharp knife) and then fry in oil, or boil and mash. They can also be baked in their skins.

Gram-flour pappadams are obtainable in some Indian groceries and can be eaten as an accompaniment to a meal. Check that they do not contain wheat flour. This is a traditional Indian recipe for **gram-flour bread**: mix two cups of gram flour with a small, finely chopped onion, ½ teaspoon cumin seeds, ½ teaspoon salt and a pinch of chilli powder. Rub in 1 tablespoon of clarified butter (see p308). Add a little water – enough to make a stiff doughy mixture. Take small balls of this and press down lightly with your hand on a floured surface. Fry on a griddle or hot plate, turning once.

BAKING POWDER
Most commercial baking powder contains a small amount of wheat flour, and those who are very sensitive to wheat should buy a wheat-free brand or make their own. Combine 60 gm (2 oz) of sodium bicarbonate with 130 gm (4½ oz) of cream of tartar. Add 60 gm (2 oz) of potato flour, rice flour or some other flour which you are allowed. Put through a sieve twice and then store in an airtight jar.

YEAST
The main sources of yeast are bread, stock cubes and Bovril, yeast extract (Marmite, Vegemite etc), and alcoholic drinks.

Soda bread, **pitta bread** and **chapattis** are good substitutes for yeast-leavened bread, although some pitta breads do contain yeast, so check before eating. Soda bread is made using baking powder.

Stock cubes are very difficult to replace, and stews and casseroles do taste rather insipid without them, although your taste-buds adapt to this eventually. If you have the time, you can make your own stock using bones and waste meat, or the remains of a roast chicken for poultry stock. Add some bay leaves or other herbs, and boil for about 20 minutes, in a pressure cooker preferably. Skim off the fat when cold, remove the bones, and then add salt to taste. The stock can be frozen for future use.

When cooking beef casseroles, try frying the beef thoroughly before stewing it, making sure all the juices in the frying pan are subsequently transferred to the casserole. This creates a rich meaty taste, which can be enhanced by adding thoroughly browned onions.

The only 'instant' yeast-free stock is a

vegetable bouillon mix, sold as a powder or a paste. It is obtainable in some healthfood shops or by post. The paste can also be used as a substitute for Marmite.

Toasted sesame seeds (spread them on tinfoil and toast under the grill using a low heat) or toasted sesame-seed oil (available at shops selling macrobiotic food) can also be used to give a stock-like flavour to casseroles, but be careful not to eat too much sesame.

PEANUT BUTTER
Almond butter and **cashew butter** are both delicious. They are sold by some healthfood shops or can be obtained by post. Be careful not to eat too much of either as nuts are frequently implicated as allergens. **Hazelnut butter** is another useful alternative, along with **tahini** (ground sesame seeds) and **sunflower spread**.

CHOCOLATE
Carob makes a reasonable substitute. Healthfood shops stock various carob products, and you can also buy carob powder for cake-making.

COFFEE AND TEA
Redbush or **roolbosch** tea tastes very similar to the real thing. It contains no caffeine and little tannin, but may still provoke symptoms in people who are sensitive to tea. Caffeine-free coffee substitutes abound, including **dandelion coffee** based on the roasted root, and Barleycup and Pioneer which are both based on roasted barley and chicory. Any coffee substitute may irritate the stomach lining of those who are already sensitive to coffee. **Herb teas** are much less likely to cause problems.

SNACKS
Pumpkin seeds and **sunflower seeds** make an excellent snack, and both are sold by most healthfood shops. Such shops also sell most kinds of nut, including some of the more unusual varieties, such as **cashews, pistachios, Brazil nuts** and **pecans** – these can be useful for keeping the diet varied. **Macadamia nuts** are very filling, although rather expensive – they are only sold in large supermarkets as a 'cocktail nut'. **Potato crisps** without additives can be bought at healthfood stores, and make a good snack. **Maize chips**, also without additives, and **popping corn** are useful for those not sensitive to maize. **Dried fruit, desiccated coconut** and **roasted chickpeas** (sold in most Indian groceries) are other useful snack items.

FRUIT AND VEGETABLES

Some people who are allergic to a type of fruit find they can eat the same fruit if it has been canned, cooked or even just frozen and defrosted. The allergens would appear to be modified by these processes, but the modification does not help everyone. The same is true of some allergies to vegetables that are eaten either raw or cooked, such as tomatoes.

Indian and West Indian grocery stores sell many exotic fruits that can be substituted for common ones. Some of the larger supermarkets also stock a wide range of unusual fruits, such as **mangoes**, **pawpaws**, **star fruit** and **lychees**. These can be useful during the first phase of an elimination diet, although they tend to be expensive.

APPENDIX VI
Synthetic chemicals in food and water

This appendix summarizes the main groups of synthetic chemicals to be found in our food and drinking water. The general comments on safety and toxicity refer to the 'average' healthy person, rather than someone who is unduly sensitive to one or more synthetic chemicals.

FOOD ADDITIVES

About 3,500 additives are in use, but not all of these are synthetic compounds. Some are natural products, or synthetic versions of natural chemicals, although this may not mean that they are things we would normally eat. On average, each person in Britain eats 4.5 kg (10–11 lb) dry weight of additives each year. This is ten times the amount used 30 years ago, but only half the amount eaten by the average American. Those who eat a lot of packaged, processed or take-away foods may eat twice the average amount or more. Children, in particular, have a very high intake because many of the manufactured foods that appeal to them are rich in additives.

Most foods and drinks have to be labelled, with all additives (apart from flavourings) listed. Certain items are exempt: wine, beer and other alcoholic drinks, and any food or drink served in cafes and restaurants. Food that is sold unwrapped does not have to be labelled either, including bread, cheese, paté and similar foods, sausages, bacon, cakes and confectionery. All these are likely to contain additives. Dried fruit is usually treated with sulphur dioxide, but this may not appear on the label – fruit that has not been treated is usually labelled 'unsulphured' (see also p301).

Even with labelled food, manufacturers only have to list those additives which they themselves have put in – for example a packet of crisps may be labelled 'potatoes, vegetable oil and salt' but the oil may have contained an antioxidant, such as BHT. Because the crisp manufacturer bought the oil with BHT already added, he does not have to include it on the label.

Another source of 'hidden additives' is medicinal drugs. They may contain colours, preservatives and anti-oxidants. These do not have to be declared on the label, and some people have reacted adversely to the additives in drugs, particularly the colourings. Azo-dyes (see p315) are among the most troublesome additives, in terms of the numbers of cases of sensitivity reported, yet these are widely used in medicines, particularly in syrups given to children.

Food additives include:

Preservatives, E200-297. These prevent bacteria and fungi from decaying the food. Over 40 are approved for use in Britain, and the amount that can be used is limited by law. Those most dangerous to health are the nitrates and nitrites (E249–252) which have been used for hundreds of years to make bacon and ham – they are potentially carcinogenic. Because of the long tradition of use, and the fact that the characteristic flavour of bacon cannot be produced in any other way, these preservatives are difficult to outlaw.

Preservatives are used in almost all wines (but see p336). One group of preservatives, the benzoates (E210-219) sometimes seem to cause sensitivity problems in people who are also sensitive to aspirin and/or tartrazine (E102). The sulphites, metabisulphites and sulphur dioxide (E220-227) can trigger off asthmatic attacks (see p301) because they have an irritant effect on the airways.

Antioxidants, E300-321. These stop fats and oils from going rancid. These are restricted to certain foods and the amount used is limited by law. Those most likely to cause health problems are BHA and BHT, (E320 and 321). One study showed BHT to cause behaviour disorders in animals.

Emulsifiers, stabilizers and thickeners, (E322-495). These improve texture. The amount that can be used is not limited, but they are restricted to certain foods. Several of those permitted in Britain are banned by the EEC because they are potential carcinogens – these include E430, E433 and E435.

Colourings, E100–180. These include both natural colourings and synthetic ones. Some of the 'natural' colours are extracted from grass, nettles and other plants, or produced by a chemical process. There is a new trend towards colours produced by fungal cells or plant cells in culture – because these too can be labelled 'natural', even though we would not consider eating the items from which they are derived. Such colours are being sought as a replacement for the synthetic colours known as azo-dyes, which have caused much concern. Azo-dyes include colours such as tartrazine, sunset yellow and amaranth – a complete list is given at the end of this section. Eighteen of these artificial colours are permitted in Britain – of these, eleven are banned in the United States, and six are not approved by the EEC, because they are suspected of being carcinogens. Two of the 'natural' colours – caramel (E150) and vegetable carbon black (E153) – are also

potential carcinogens (some forms of caramel appear to be safe but not others – most of it is now made by chemical processes). Carbon black is banned in the United States. Apart from their potentially carcinogenic effect, many of the azo-dyes have been reported as causing sensitivity reactions, especially in children.

Flavour enhancers, E620–E635. The most important of these is monosodium glutamate, or MSG, and its relatives, E620-623. Eating large amounts of MSG is said to produce a set of symptoms known as 'Chinese restaurant syndrome' – the symptoms described for this condition vary considerably: 'tightness, pain and tingling in the front of the chest, radiating to the arms, often associated with palpitations and faintness' according to one authority, but 'flushing, sweating, loss of coordination, headache and hypotension [low blood pressure]' according to another. Some studies have failed to confirm the existence of a reaction, but it has been suggested that the *source* from which the MSG is manufactured is important. There are reports of MSG triggering attacks in some asthmatics.

Flavourings. These do not have to be listed on food labels, unlike the other additives. There are over 3,000 of these, they do not have E-numbers, and most have never been properly tested for safety. However, they are used in extremely small quantities, and are assumed to be non-harmful for this reason. Although this may be true for the majority, there are doubts over some flavourings, particularly a group known as the allyl alcohols which are potent toxins. The average person only receives small amounts of these, but anyone eating large amounts of sweets, crisps and soft drinks would get a much higher dose.

Testing additives
New additives are all tested very thoroughly, although there are rarely tests on humans – rats, mice, bacteria and human cells cultured in a test tube are the main subjects used for testing. There are quite a few reports of illness among food-workers handling certain additives, which raises the question of whether humans might react differently from these test animals. There has also been some concern about how well tests are carried out. A commercial laboratory in America, which was reponsible for over 30 per cent of the world's safety testing, was found to have been fabricating its data for many years. Although the laboratory was closed down, many of the additives that were passed as safe on the basis of its tests are still in use.

Concern has also been expressed over the possibility of 'cocktail effects' – the unknown impact of eating two or more additives together. A single meal can contain as many as 60 different additives, yet, surprisingly, the effect of additives in combination is *never* taken into account when setting safety standards. Very few tests have been carried out in this area, because of lack of resources. One test, in which two preservatives were tested together, showed that they had a much greater effect in combination than when eaten separately. A public health specialist, writing in a book on additives published by the European Commission, comments: 'It is not scaremongering to say that the possibility cannot be ruled out of two substances, both harmless by themselves, interacting to yield a product which is toxic.'

The azo-dyes

Tartrazine	E102	*Banned in Austria and Norway*
Quinoline yellow	E104	*Banned in Australia, Japan, Norway and the USA*
Yellow 2G	107	*Not approved by EC*, and used only in Britain. Also banned in Austria, Japan, Norway, Sweden, Switzerland and the USA*
Sunset yellow FCF/orange yellow S	E110	*Banned in Finland and Norway*
Carmoisine/ azorubine	E122	*Banned in Japan, Norway, Sweden and the USA*
Amaranth	E123	*Banned in France and Italy (except in caviar), Norway and the USA*
Ponceau 4R/ cochineal red A	E124	*Banned in Norway and the USA*
Erythrosine BS	E127	*Banned in Norway and the USA*
Red 2G	128	*Not approved by the EC, and used only in Britain. Also banned in Australia, Austria, Canada, Finland, Japan, Norway, Sweden and the USA.*
Allura red AC	129	*Not approved by the EC*
Patent blue V	E131	
Indigo carmine/ indigotine	E132	*Banned in Norway*
Brilliant blue FCF	133	*Not approved by EC, but permitted in some countries, including Britain. Banned in Austria, Norway, Sweden and Switzerland*
Green S/acid brilliant green S/ lissamine green	E142	*Banned in Canada, Finland, Japan, Norway, Sweden and the USA*
Brilliant black PN	E151	*Banned in Canada, Finland, Japan, Norway and the USA*
Brown FK	154	*Not approved by EC and only used in Britain and Ireland. Also banned by Austria, Australia, Canada, Finland, Japan, Norway, Sweden and the USA*
Chocolate brown HT	155	*Not approved by EC, and not permitted in several member countries. Also banned in Australia, Austria, Norway, Sweden and the USA*
Pigment rubine/ lithol rubine BK	E180	*Only used for colouring the rind of Edam cheese*

*Those not approved by the EC do not have an 'E' before their identification numbers.

PESTICIDES

There are three main types of pesticide used on food crops: **insecticides** to kill insect pests, **fungicides** to kill fungal diseases, and **herbicides** to kill weeds. There are over 420 pesticides that can legally be used in Britain, and others are known to be used illegally. The vast majority of these pesticides leave residues on the crops, but there are time limits between when the crop is last sprayed and when it is harvested – this allows time for the residue to break down. Unfortunately, there is no legal requirement on growers to observe the safe period between the last spraying and the harvest – and no official means of checking if they do so. Health and Safety Officers only visit farms once every 11 years, on average, due to shortage of manpower.

The only checks that take place are routine tests of foods for pesticide residues. Until recently, there was no legal limit on the amount of pesticides in food, although there were guidelines, and food above the recommended levels could be seized and destroyed. In July 1988, maximum residue limits (MRLs) came into force for cereals, and in January 1989 MRLs for fruit and vegetables were introduced. These limits have only been introduced by the British government because EC legislation required them, and they do not cover post-harvest fungicides, such as those sprayed on to stored potatoes (see p181).

The main burden of testing foods falls on local authority Environmental Health Officers, who are able to test for about 20 pesticides –

only 5 per cent of those in use. Although the 20 they test for are those most widely used, this is still rather worrying, since there are about 400 pesticides whose misuse would go unnoticed. When foods are found with excess pesticide levels, they are simply destroyed – no effort is made to trace the source of the food or prevent further misuse of pesticides.

Pesticides are also monitored annually by the Total Diet Study, which considers a larger number of pesticides – over a hundred in recent years. Samples are taken that correspond to the national average diet, all the foods are combined and the mixture is tested for pesticide residues. Unfortunately, only about 25 samples are taken, representing a minute fraction of the total food eaten annually in Britain – the chances of missing high residues on certain crops is enormous. And the Total Diet Study is still only looking at a quarter of all the pesticides available for use.

When pesticides are banned in the West, the companies producing them often try to increase their sales to Third World countries, where safety regulations are less stringent – or non-existent. So imported foods may contain residues of pesticides that are banned in Britain. Despite this, there are no special provisions for testing imported foods – these are subjected to the same tests as home-grown produce. *Paradoxically, pesticides that are banned in Britain are not tested for at all.* In America, where testing is rather more thorough, high pesticide residues have been found on imported food, including dangerous pesticides that have been banned in the USA. In many Third World countries, there are regular reports of pesticides being used very carelessly, or safety measures being ignored entirely. Deaths among farmworkers in Third World countries, due to pesticide misuse, are believed to be very high.

Pesticide residues and health
Could the minute amounts of pesticide that we eat with our food be injurious to health? The answer to this question really depends on how dangerous those pesticides are – and this is something that cannot easily be answered. All new pesticides are tested very rigorously, and the risk posed by eating small amounts is assessed. Unfortunately, many of the pesticides that are widely used today were developed before adequate testing procedures were introduced, and there is concern that some of these may be toxic or carcinogenic, even in minute doses. A government programme is under way to retest such pesticides, but there are only four scientists involved in the testing, and at the present rate of progress it will be at least 50 years before all those now in use have been properly tested.

Even with the newer pesticides, there is some cause for concern. Some were tested by the discredited commercial laboratory mentioned on p314, in connection with food additives. Despite the doubts that this casts over their safety, these are still in use. More seriously, pesticides are never tested in combination, for any possible 'cocktail effects'. Such effects are not unlikely. It is known that some insecticides affect the liver, for example, making it less able to detoxify other chemicals. The safety data on pesticides, like that on food additives, are not open to public inspection because they are covered by the Official Secrets Act.

After many years of assuring the public that pesticide residues were insignificant and harmless, the Ministry of Agriculture has recently admitted that there are serious problems. A confidential report, leaked to the press in August 1988 states 'consumers may be exposed to higher dosages of these chemicals than has hitherto been suspected. These residues could present a health hazard to man and it is plainly desirable that appropriate statutory controls are enacted to limit human exposure to pesticide residues from food'. The report adds that even the 'inert substances' used to dilute the active ingredients of pesticides may be damaging to health.

In addition to pesticide residues, some foods contain hormones and antibiotics that are routinely fed to farm animals. Meat, poultry, milk, cheese and eggs are the main sources of these chemicals, but fish from fish farms may also contain some antibiotics. Some individuals are allergic to minute amounts of certain antibiotics, and they may react to traces of antibiotic in food (see p53).

WATER POLLUTION
The level of pollutants in drinking water has been steadily rising in recent years. Pollutants run off the land into rivers or seep down through the soil into groundwater. Various purification measures are taken before the water reaches our taps, but these are never 100 per cent effective.

Agriculture makes the major contribution to water pollution. Nitrates, used as fertilizers, run off from the fields, and in several parts of Britain, tap-water regularly exceeds the EC limit on nitrates. Although nitrates have received a lot of publicity, they are not as worrying as some of the other water pollutants. There are no clear signs that the nitrate levels found in drinking water are damaging to health, except in newborn babies. As far as chemical-sensitive patients are concerned, nitrates are unlikely to be a problem.

Small amounts of pesticides also get into the water supply from farm use. In addition, there have been accidents in which large amounts of highly toxic pesticides, such as dieldrin (now banned for agricultural use), have been emptied into drains or soakaways close to boreholes, causing major pollution of the groundwater below. Most water authorities do not systematically monitor drinking water for pesticides.

Oil from spillages may find its way into drinking water, but usually this is only in minute amounts. Organic solvents (see p172) also turn up in water supplies – a study by Imperial College, London, found the solvent trichloroethylene in 36 per cent of the 168 groundwater samples they tested. The level was higher than the limit set by the World Health Organization in 10 per cent of the samples, and in one it was seven times the WHO limit. Other solvents are also found in groundwaters, usually as a result of factories discharging their waste solvents into drains or ditches. Very few of the water authorities systematically check their supplies for solvents or other industrial pollutants, and serious incidents of pollution may easily go undetected. Some of the chemicals used for purification also leave a residue in the water, but this is unlikely to be harmful as long as the correct amounts are being used.

Chlorine is added to water to kill bacteria and viruses that might otherwise cause disease. Unfortunately, chlorine readily reacts with certain organic molecules to produce chlorinated hydrocarbons. (The organic molecules may themselves be pollutants, or they may be produced by large amounts of waterweed, growing and then rotting down in reservoirs.) Some of these chlorinated hydrocarbons are carcinogenic, and they have occasionally turned up in drinking water.

For details of water filtration systems that can remove some of these pollutants, see p318.

OTHER SYNTHETIC CHEMICALS THAT CAN CONTAMINATE FOOD

A variety of other synthetic chemicals may find their way into our food, including detergent from unrinsed crockery, droplets from aerosol sprays, and plasticizers from cling-film and some other soft plastics. These plasticizers are used to give such items their flexibility, but they are soluble in oil and fat, and will migrate into the food if used to wrap fatty foods such as cheese or paté. In general, little is known about the safety of these substances, but there are unconfirmed reports that plasticizers can accumulate in the eye, leading to a form of blindness known as 'macular eye disease'. Some insecticidal strips, which are not safe for use near food (eg Vapona), are often hung in the kitchens of cafés and pubs.

APPENDIX VII
Bottled water and water filters

BOTTLED WATER

There is some confusion about the meaning of 'mineral water' which complicates the issue of bottled water. All tap-water, and any water from a spring or well, contains some mineral salts (calcium, magnesium, sodium, iron etc) dissolved in it. The composition of the water is affected by the sort of rock it percolates through, and some spring waters contain large amounts of minerals. At one time, it was believed that these waters had health-giving properties and they were marketed as 'mineral waters'. (In fact, mineral-rich water is of little benefit to health, and some can be injurious to those with kidney problems.) Today's bottled waters often come from the same springs and tend to be sold under the name 'mineral water' because this denotes that they are high-quality waters from a natural source. However, the most richly mineral-laden waters are not marketed, and those that are on sale are generally low in minerals – so they would not cause any health problems. A few brands are rich in sodium (eg Badois, Ramlosa) and should be avoided by those on low-sodium diets.

The main reason for buying bottled water now is not what it contains, but what it doesn't contain. To a large extent it is free of the contaminants now found in most tap-water. Bottled waters are not treated with chlorine and, for the most part, contain far fewer nitrates. (Perrier is an exception. A Consumer's Association survey showed that its nitrate content was almost as high as the maximum level permitted for tap water by the EEC, and twice as high as other mineral waters.) Because of the locations of the springs, bottled mineral water is unlikely to be contaminated by pesticides, industrial solvents and other pollutants. Bottled waters taste much better than most tap water, and are generally more palatable than filtered water as well.

Because they are not chlorinated, bottled waters can foster large numbers of bacteria. Tests have shown very high levels in some brands. However, these are not harmful types of bacteria. Sparkling mineral water resists bacterial growth better than still water.

The price for still bottled water is about 90p to £1.30 per gallon. Sparkling mineral waters can cost up to £2.70. This makes bottled water very expensive, compared to filtered water, for long-term use.

WATER FILTERS

There are two main methods of removing

contaminants from water: activated carbon filters and reverse osmosis.

Activated carbon filters

Activated carbon is a highly reactive surface which attracts substances such as chlorine, chloroform, carbon tetrachloride, trichloroethylene, phenols, DDT, other pesticides, PCBs and dioxins. These and other organic molecules found in tap water (see p316) stick to the carbon leaving the water much less contaminated.

There are various forms of activated carbon, granular activated carbon or GAC being one of the most effective. The amount and quality of activated carbon in a filter determines how efficient it is at removing pollutants. Plumbed-in filters contain far more activated carbon than jug filters.

A major problem with these filters is that they are an ideal breeding ground for bacteria, including harmful forms. To combat bacterial growth, most such filters are now impregnated with silver. There have been alarming reports of silver leaching out into the water, and this can happen with some filters. But new production methods, such as bonding the silver to the carbon at high temperatues, can overcome this problem.

Reverse osmosis

This form of filtration is only available in plumbed-in units. It uses a membrane with microscopic holes in it that only water molecules can get through. Tap water is held in one chamber and water molecules slowly seep out into the other. It removes the vast majority of organic pollutants (but see below), *and* takes out fluoride, lead, aluminium and other metals, unlike the activated carbon filters.

Unfortunately the process is very slow (even the best filters only produce 5 gallons a day) and uses up large amounts of tap water to produce a relatively small amount of filtered water (up to 10 gallons per filtered gallon). Many of the natural minerals in the water are removed at the same time, leaving a product with an indifferent taste. Without minerals, water loses its characteristic flavour, and since we probably need certain amounts of minerals in our water, this highly purified water may not even be very healthy.

More worryingly, a few molecules can get through the membrane along with the water, including some chlorinated compounds which are known to be injurious. These tend to *concentrate* in the filtered water, making the original problem worse. This difficulty is easily overcome, however, by combining the reverse osmosis unit with an activated carbon filter. Systems of this type produce a water of very high purity, which may be needed by

some patients with severe chemical sensitivities. However, the problem of low mineral content has still to be overcome, and anyone drinking this sort of water constantly may need a mineral supplement. Expense and slow filtering speed are the other main drawbacks to this type of system.

Some doctors report that patients with extreme sensitivity to chemicals react to water that has been in contact with plastic, because minute quantities of material leach out of the plastic into the water. This is unlikely to be true except for a tiny minority of highly sensitive patients. Where such problems are suspected, reverse osmosis units in non-leaching plastic or stainless steel housing are a possible solution. The former are available in Britain, but stainless steel units are only sold in the USA, and the cost of importing one is likely to be very high. Check that plastics really are the source of the problem before pursuing this option. Drinking mineral water in glass bottles for a while should provide a good test. If you are still having problems on this type of water, write to the manufacturer to check that the water is not stored in plastic before bottling. Always bear in mind that it could be something other than water causing your symptoms.

Choosing a filter

There are two major problems in choosing a filter. Firstly, it is impossible to tell if the product is working properly, without chemical analyses, although if it has a serious defect, a smell of chlorine in the filtered water might be noticeable. Secondly, there are no British Standards for domestic water filters at present. As a customer, you therefore need to be well informed about what you are buying. Some of the filters at present on the market actually remove very few contaminants from the water supply. Others may work well at first, but their performance drops off sharply – long before they have filtered the number of gallons claimed by the manufacturer.

The only country to apply consumer standards to domestic water filters is the USA, where the Environmental Protection Agency requires filters impregnated with silver to be registered and sets a limit on how much silver can leach into the water. In Britain, the Water Research Centre operates an approval scheme for some aspects of water filters, but not for their overall performance. It seems likely that the approval scheme in Britain will be improved in the next few years.

The vast majority of water filters bought in Britain are of the jug type. The advantage of these is that the initial outlay is very low (£10–15). The cost per gallon is between 12 pence and 30 pence, which is cheaper than bottled water, although the taste of the water is not as good.

The prime objective of the jug filters is to improve the taste and appearance of water, and to remove hardness (calcium carbonate or 'chalk') so that kettles do not become lined with scale. They contain an activated carbon filter to remove chlorine and another component, an ion exchange resin, which takes out the calcium carbonate. The latter component also removes lead and some other metals. Calcium carbonate is not injurious to health and cannot cause sensitivity reactions, so it is the kettle that benefits rather than the drinker.

The activated carbon also takes out some organic pollutants such as chloroform and trichloroethylene, but the majority of jug filters are not really designed for this task. They contain a relatively small amount of activated carbon and cannot remove all organic contaminants. In fact, most of the manufacturers do not claim that they can, but many people who buy these filters have an exaggerated idea of their abilities.

For people whose main problem is sensitivity to chlorine, and who cannot afford a plumbed-in filter, a jug filter would be a good choice.

Most jug filters contain silver to prevent bacterial growth, but even if silver is present it is important not to leave water standing in the jug for more than a day, as there can be a build-up of bacteria. These are not usually harmful species, but it is wise to be careful. The top part of the jug should be cleaned out once a week. Jug filters without silver cannot be recommended. To discover if the filters do contain silver, you will probably have to write to the manufacturer.

In areas with hard water, the filter may not last as long as the manufacturer claims. However, the activated carbon element should go on working after the ion-exchange resin is saturated with calcium carbonate. So you should continue to get chlorine removal, even if the kettle furs up slightly.

Plumbed-in filters using activated carbon are intended to remove much more from the water than jug filters. They contain far more carbon, and it is generally of a higher quality. Most of these filters do not contain ion-exchange resins, so they do not remove hardness from the water, nor do they take out metals such as lead. But for anyone whose main problem is chemical sensitivity, they are a good choice. (Lead is only really a problem in areas with soft water.)

A high quality filter of this type will cost between £100 and £200, but the filter should last for several years. The actual running costs work out at between 3 pence and 5 pence per gallon, quite a lot cheaper than the jug filters. (Reverse osmosis units usually cost £300 or more. Once this outlay has been made, the running cost, in terms of replacing filters and membranes, is about 3 or 4 pence per gallon.)

Needless to say, the better filters are more expensive, but a high price is not an unfailing guide to quality, so you need to ask some searching questions:

Does it contain silver? (If not, then it is probably dangerous.)

Is the filter registered with the EPA? What is the registration number? If not EPA-registered, then you should ask what quantity of silver leaches into the filtered water. (Ask to see test figures. They should be less than .05 parts per million, which might be expressed as 50 parts per billion, 50 micrograms per litre or 50 g per litre.)

What percentage removal of chlorine, chlorinated organic chemicals, pesticides and organic solvents does it give? Ask to see test results. (Should be more than 95 per cent for each of these groups. The tests should have been carried out by an independent laboratory.)

How many gallons will the filter process?

What percentage removal can be expected when it is nearing the end of its life? (This is a crucial question – the manufacturer may say the filter is good for 5,000 gallons, but if it is only removing 30 per cent of contaminants after 4,000 gallons you may as well drink tap water. Good filters should still be removing 90 per cent or more at the end of their useful life.)

How much does a replacement filter cost?

Given these figures, you can work out the cost per gallon. Ask whether they are working in British gallons or US gallons, as this will make a difference. (1 British gallon = 1.2 US gallons, so 5,000 US gallons is only 4,160 British gallons.) Bear in mind that the cheapest price per gallon may not be the best in terms of water quality.

The same sort of questions should be asked if you are choosing a filter that combines activated carbon with reverse osmosis (see p318). If they do not include silver, ask about bacteriological control. Filters that work by reverse osmosis alone are not recommended.

None of the above systems remove harmful bacteria, and they are only suitable for use with tap water that has already been chlorinated or otherwise treated by the water authority. *All water used for baby feeds should be boiled before use, including bottled or filtered water.*

For people who can obtain water directly, from a borehole or spring, there are large-scale devices that kill bacteria as well as removing pollutants and sediment. These are known as water purification systems and are much more expensive, but the water obtained should be of very high quality.

Firms supplying filters direct to the public include:
Aqua Brite
Station Farmhouse
Thuxton
Norfolk NR9 4QJ
Telephone 0362 850320
Supplies the Aqua Brite range of activated carbon filters, manufactured in the USA by Amsoil and EPA-registered. The unit fits under the sink and the filter needs changing about every two years.

Aqueous Solutions
25 Cherington Road
Bristol BS10 5BL
Telephone 0272 629957
Distributes another American-made range of filters, called NSA Water Filters. These are also EPA-registered. Some fit under the kitchen sink, others are 'counter-top' designs. The filters need changing about every three years.

Jug filters can be bought from most health-food shops, and from some chemists and department stores. They are also available by mail-order (see p337).

In Australia, water filters can be bought through the Allergy Aid Centre (p337).

Water-softeners for eczema
In hard-water districts, children with eczema may suffer less skin irritation if the water used for washing and bathing is softened. Plumbed-in water-softeners are available which take out most of the calcium carbonate (limescale or chalk) from the water.

APPENDIX VIII
Medicinal Drugs

This appendix covers the drugs commonly used in allergy, and in some of the other conditions discussed in this book. Where food plays a part in such an illness, it may often be a question of deciding whether to alter the diet or control the symptoms with drugs. Almost all drugs have some side-effects and the decision to use them involves weighing their good effects against their bad ones. This is a decision which only a qualified doctor can make. The information given here is intended to help patients understand the basis for such decisions, and participate in them where this is appropriate.

Drugs are referred to in two ways – by their proper name (or generic name), and by the trade names given them by the manufacturers. The same drug may be marketed under a number of different trade names if it is produced by different manufacturers. Some medicines contain a mixture of two or more drugs. Drugs are described here under their generic names, which are given in italics, *eg salbutamol*. The trade names are shown with a capital letter *eg* Ventolin.

This list of drugs is reasonably comprehensive, but bear in mind that new drugs are introduced all the time. So a medicine you are prescribed may not be mentioned here if it is fairly new on the market.

1 MAST-CELL STABILIZERS
These drugs have the effect of stabilizing mast cells so that they do not release histamine and other mediators. The main one used is *sodium cromoglycate*. It is only effective if it reaches the mast cell before the allergen. So it can be used to prevent the symptoms of allergy, as long as the patient remembers to take the drug when they are feeling well, *before* they encounter the allergen.

The drug is given in inhalers (Intal) as a preventive treatment for **asthma**. The time from when treatment starts to when the good effects become noticeable is variable – from a few days to several weeks. The drug must be taken continuously to be effective. In some people, it can cause irritation of the throat, coughing or, more rarely, an asthmatic attack. In rare cases there may be a true allergic reaction to the drug. In general, however, *sodium cromoglycate* is remarkably free of side-effects.

Although the main effect of *sodium cromoglycate* is to stabilize mast cells, it appears to make the bronchi less reactive in other ways as well. Thus, it is used for exercise-induced asthma. Its long-term effect is to make the bronchi less sensitive, which is beneficial.

A related drug, *nedocromil sodium* (Tilade), is sometimes prescribed instead of *sodium cromoglycate* for asthma. It acts in much the same way, but is a more powerful drug, and is not prescribed for children. Sometimes *sodium cromoglycate* is combined with other drugs, as in Intal Compound, which contains *isoprenaline* (Section 4A).

In cases of **food allergy**, taking *sodium cromoglycate* by mouth (Nalcrom) can block the allergic reaction. But it is only used where the symptoms are not of the immediate-and-violent kind. Thus, it might be prescribed for patients with food-induced symptoms, such as diarrhoea, asthma, rhinitis, eczema or chronic urticaria, but not for those who suffer swelling of the mouth and tongue on eating a particular food. In such cases, the slight risk of the drug not working has to be considered, because of the serious consequences of such a failure.

Sodium cromoglycate appears to block mast cell degranulation in the gut wall, which prevents the gut wall becoming inflamed and thus makes it less permeable to food molecules.

To be effective, *sodium cromoglycate* (taken by mouth) must be taken 10 or 15 minutes before the food is eaten. The beneficial effects of the drug may not appear for several days. Occasionally, the drug may make the symptoms worse, for reasons that are not yet understood, and sometimes it has no effect, or only partially controls the symptoms. Sometimes patients experience side-effects such as headaches, urticaria, diarrhoea or vomiting.

Because of doubts about its effectiveness if used long-term, simply taking *sodium cromoglycate* is not the best way to deal with food allergy. Its main use is in patients with reactions to a very wide range of foods, who find it difficult to avoid them all. Even though they are taking the drug, such patients must usually restrict their intake of the main offending foods as well. Babies who react to a wide range of foods on weaning have been helped by *sodium cromoglycate*.

This drug can also be useful in giving food-allergic people a 'day off' from their restricted diet. Children may be given it for Christmas or birthdays, to allow them to eat normally for a day. *Sodium cromoglycate* is also used in **hay-fever** and other forms of **allergic rhinitis** (Rynacrom Resiston-one) and in **allergic conjunctivitis** (Opticrom). It can cause stinging when applied, but this wears off quickly and again there are no serious side-

effects. The drug must be used regularly and consistently for the good effects to be maintained. In Rynacrom Compound, *sodium cromoglycate* is combined with xylo-metazoline, a sympathomimetic (Section 3).

2 DRUGS THAT COUNTERACT HISTAMINE

Histamine is one of the mediators released by mast cells when they degranulate (see p25). It is also released by various other cells in the body, since it acts as a local messenger substance, conveying instructions to neighbouring cells.

The main effects of histamine are to make smooth muscles (in the bronchi, gut, bladder etc) contract, to make the small blood vessels enlarge, and to make the capillaries (tiny blood vessels) become more leaky. These last two effects cause a drop in blood pressure. Locally, the increased leakiness of the capillaries contributes to inflammation.

Antihistamines (more correctly referred to as 'histamine H1-receptor antagonists') block the effects of histamine. They do this by binding to the H1 receptors on cells. Histamine normally binds to these receptors triggering off a reaction by the cell. So by blocking the receptors, antihistamines prevent histamine from affecting those cells.

There are a wide range of antihistamines available today (see Section 2A). Most of these are rather unspecific and can also bind to the receptors for other messenger substances, such as adrenaline (p151) and serotonin (p128). They tend to cause drowsiness through blocking messengers such as adrenaline, and they can also cause dizziness, nervousness, tremors, stomach upsets, dry mouth, blurred vision and impotence. These side-effects are not damaging in the long term, although they can be inconvenient. Some patients develop a tolerance of these drugs after a while, and the side-effects diminish. So, if an antihistamine controls the allergic symptoms well, but causes side-effects, it is worth persisting with it for a while. Sometimes the sedative effects of antihistamines can be advantageous, as in children with urticaria who tend to scratch at night.

More specific drugs, which show a stronger preference for histamine receptors, have now been introduced. *Astemizole* (Hismanal, Pollon-eze) and *terfenadine* (Triludan, Seldane) are the main ones. These can have some side-effects but should not cause as many problems as the other antihistamines. If you are taking β-blockers for a heart condition, ask your doctor's advice before taking *terfenadine*.

Antihistamines, taken by mouth, are useful in **hay-fever** and **perennial rhinitis**, where there are symptoms in both the nose and eyes, together with itching in the mouth or ears. Where there are only symptoms in the nose, a *sodium cromoglycate* or corticosteroid spray may be more appropriate, as these have fewer side-effects. Some medicines contain antihistamines combined with sympathomimetics (see Section 3).

Antihistamines are also effective in some cases of chronic **urticaria**, including cold-induced urticaria. They are not effective in asthma, because other mediators, besides histamine, play a major role in producing the symptoms.

2A *Antihistamines*
acrivastine (Semprex)
astemizole (Hismanal, Pollon-eze)
brompheniramine (Dimotane)
cetirizine (Zirtek)
chlorpheniramine (Piriton, Haymine)
clemastine (Tavegil)
dimethindene (Fenostil)
diphenylpyraline (Histryl Spansule)
hydroxyzine (Atarax)
loratidine (Clarityn)
mebhydrolin (Fabahistin)
mequitazine (Primalan)
oxatomide (Tinset)
phenindamine (Thephorin)
pheniramine (Daneral)
promethazine (Phenergan)
terfenadine (Triludan, Seldane)
trimeprazine (Vallergan)
triprolidine (Actidil, Pro-Actidil)

Ketotifen (Zaditen) acts both as an antihistamine and a mast-cell stabilizer (Section 1), and is used to prevent asthma attacks. Its side-effects are similar to those of most antihistamines.

Azatadine (Optimine) and *cyproheptadine* (Periactin) act both as antihistamines and serotonin antagonists (Section 12A). They are used for allergic rhinitis and urticaria.

3 SYMPATHOMIMETICS
These are drugs which mimic the effects of naturally produced adrenaline, the messenger of the sympathetic nervous system (see p150), which produces the 'flight or fight' reaction. Sympathomimetics have various effects, but one local effect is to make small blood vessels (capillaries) contract. Thus, they have an opposing effect to histamine. This is exploited in some nasal sprays for **hay-fever** and **perennial rhinitis**. The drugs concerned are *phenylephrine* (Fenox), *oxymetazoline* (Afrazine) and *xylometazoline* (Otrivine).

These sprays make the capillaries in the nose contract providing immediate relief from congestion, but if used for more than two weeks they can have adverse effects. The blood vessels become 'hooked' on the drug so that when the spray is discontinued they

react by expanding, causing congestion again. These sprays are for short-term use only.

Some sprays combine sympathomimetics with antihistamines (*eg* Otrivine-Antistin). Others combine sympathomimetics with antihistamines and antibiotics (Vibrocil) or with corticosteroids and antibiotics (Dexa-Rhinaspray). Sprays containing antibiotics are only used where there are signs of infection as well as allergy.

Sympathomimetics such as *pseudoephedrine* and *ephedrine* are sometimes combined with antihistamines in medicines taken by mouth, such as Haymine (*ephedrine* and *chlorpheniramine*) and Sudafed Plus (*pseudoephedrine* and *triprolidine*).

When taken by mouth, the sympathomimetic helps to overcome the main side-effect of the antihistamine, drowsiness. (See p167 for side-effects.)

4 BRONCHODILATORS
These are drugs which make the bronchial muscles relax, and are therefore useful in **asthma**. There are three types of bronchodilators: β2-adrenoceptor agonists, xanthines and anticholinergics.

4A *β2-adrenoceptor agonists*
Antagonists are drugs such as antihistamines (section 2) which bind to receptors and block the effect of the natural messenger (*eg* histamine) that normally binds to the receptor. Agonists have the opposite effect. They bind to receptors and stimulate the cell, in the same way that the natural messenger would – in other words, they mimic the effects of that natural messenger.

The β2-adrenoceptor agonists mimic the effects of adrenaline (see p150) on the bronchial muscles, by binding to receptors for adrenaline. These are called β2 adrenoceptors, hence the name of the drugs. They include *salbutamol* (Ventolin, Ventodisks, Volmax, Maxivent, Rimasal, Salbulin, Salbuvent, Asmaven, Aerolin-Auto), *terbutaline* (Bricanyl, Monovent), *fenoterol* (Berotec), *pirbuterol* (Exirel), *reproterol* (Bronchodil), *rimiterol* (Pulmadil), *salmeterol* (Serevent). Sometimes such drugs are combined with corticosteroids (see below), as in Ventide, which contains *salbutamol*.

Of all the bronchodilators, these drugs have the most specific effects on the bronchi. They are now preferred to *isoprenaline* (Medihaler-Iso) which has a less specific effect, and tends to combine with adrenaline receptors in the heart muscles as well as those in the bronchi, sometimes causing irregular heartbeat, flushing and headaches. *Isoprenaline* is combined with a sympathomimetic, *phenylephrine* (Section 3) in Medihaler-Duo.

Isoetharine is another non-specific β-agonist. It is combined with *phenylephrine* (Section 3) in Bronchilator. *Orciprenaline* (Alupent) is a drug of the same type that is partially selective for bronchial muscles, and has similar side-effects.

Side-effects *can* also occur with the specific β2-adrenoceptor agonists, such as *salbutamol*, although they are generally less of a problem. They include tremor, nervous tension, headache, flushing and dry mouth. Taking the drugs from an inhaler reduces the side-effects by targeting the drug on the bronchi – this allows a much lower dose to be used than if the drugs were taken by mouth.

The effects of these drugs lasts for up to six hours, and the timing of doses should be geared to the patient's needs. Learning how to operate the inhaler properly is very important, as the drug can be ineffective if the inhaler is misused. Disk inhalers (Ventodisks) are easier to operate than conventional inhalers.

Even if they are used at quite high doses over long periods of time there seem to be no serious ill-effects with these drugs. On the other hand, they do not reduce the sensitivity of the bronchi, as *sodium cromoglycate* does (Section 1), so once they are discontinued their beneficial effects cease. A combination of the two drugs is sometimes used.

4B *Xanthines*
These are naturally occurring substances that are chemically similar to caffeine. They include *theophylline* (Biophylline, Labophylline, Lasma, Nuelin, Pecram, Pro-Vent, Sabidal, Slo-Phyllin, Theo-Dur, Uniphyllin Continus), *aminophylline* (Phyllocontin Continus) and *choline theophyllinate* (Choledyl). They make the bronchial muscles relax, but affect the heart muscles as well. The dose must be exactly right, as there is only a small difference between the dose that will relax the bronchi and one which will cause irregular heartbeat. Other possible side-effects include headache, nausea, stomach upsets, depression, aching limbs and insomnia. Smoking and drinking will affect the dose needed, as will viral infections or taking other drugs. So it is important that patients taking these drugs have close medical supervision. As long as the dose is correct, they are suitable for long-term use, since there are no serious side-effects.

These drugs are usually taken by mouth. They can also be given as suppositories, inserted before going to bed, for those who suffer from early-morning attacks of asthma. They make the bronchial muscles relax by working *inside* the cells, whereas the β2 agonists (see p322) work *outside* the cell. The two different types of drugs therefore have complementary effects, and using both can be helpful for some patients.

Theophylline is combined with a sympathomimetic, *ephedrine* (Section 3), in Franol and Tedral.

4C *Anti-cholinergics*
The main drugs in this group are *ipratropium* (Atrovent) and *oxitropium* (Oxivent) which are taken by inhalation. Side-effects are rare except at high doses. They include dry mouth, difficulty in passing urine and constipation. Other anti-cholinergics include *butethamate* and *atropine*. Anti-cholinergics help to reduce the amount of mucus present in the airways as well as relaxing the muscles, and may be useful where asthma and bronchitis occur together.

Sympathomimetics (Section 3), such as *adrenaline* and *ephedrine*, are sometimes combined with anticholinergics in inhalers. *Atropine* is combined with *adrenaline* and a muscle relaxant in Brovon. *Butethamate* is combined with *ephedrine* in CAM, which is taken by mouth. *Ipratropium* is combined with the bronchodilator *fenoterol* (Section 4A) in Duovent.

4D *Other bronchodilators*
Sympathomimetics (see Section 3 above) were once the main drugs used for bronchodilation, but they are much less specific for the bronchial muscles than the drugs described above. They produce side-effects more easily than modern bronchodilators and are much less used now. They include *adrenaline*, *ephedrine* and *phenylephrine*. Typical side-effects include nervousness, anxiety, tremor, irregular heartbeat and dry mouth.

5 CORTICOSTEROIDS
These drugs mimic the action of the hormones produced by the outer layer (cortex) of the adrenal glands, a pair of small glands that sit on top of the kidneys. The main hormone produced is *hydrocortisone* (*cortisol*), which has a variety of effects on the body. It controls the amount of sodium and potassium ('salts') that the kidney allows to pass into the urine, and releases glucose into the blood. *Hydrocortisone* also moves protein out of the muscles and bones, and influences the way fat is deposited. Finally it suppresses inflammation. In the case of asthma, it does so by damping down late-phase reactions (see p42), but in other inflammatory conditions the mechanism of action is probably more complex. This effect on inflammation makes corticosteroids useful

in the treatment of allergic reactions, and in other diseases – such as rheumatoid arthritis, Crohn's disease and ulcerative colitis – where inflammation plays a major role.

Because corticorsteroids have so many different functions in the body, there are various unpleasant side-effects from using them as drugs. These effects mainly occur when the drugs are taken by mouth. Long-term use of these drugs at high doses can result in Cushing's Syndrome, characterized by deposits of fat around the face ('moon face'), and on the shoulders and abdomen, water retention producing puffiness, bruising, acne, muscle wasting and weakening of the bones leading to easy breakage. In children, there is also stunted growth. All these changes are due to the effects of corticosteroids on other body processes, as described above. Some of the effects are reversible, if corticosteroids are withdrawn, but there can also be permanent damage.

In using corticosteroids to suppress allergic reactions, the trick is to persuade the drug to damp down inflammation, without carrying out any of its other actions. This has been achieved, to a large extent, by modifying *hydrocortisone* and the other adrenal hormones chemically. Chemical tinkering with the *hydrocortisone* molecule has produced drugs such as *prednisolone*. This suppresses inflammation but has very little effect on the excretion of salt by the kidneys, so it will not cause water retention.

Unfortunately, these are not the only bad effects of corticosteroids. Because they suppress inflammation, which is a valuable part of the body's fight against disease, they tend to make infections more likely. Viruses and fungi, in particular, are likely to flourish.

If corticosteroids are taken over a long period of time, the adrenal glands' natural activity is suppressed. Stopping the drug leaves the body without corticosteroids which can lead to collapse in the worst cases. This means that corticosteroids taken by mouth should never be stopped abruptly if they have been taken for more than a few weeks. The glands must be given time to recover their natural level of activity, by gradually reducing the dosage. Even after as little as two weeks, corticosteroids should be withdrawn gradually, by halving the dose each day, to avoid a flare-up of the original problem.

In general, applying corticosteroids locally (*ie* where they are needed) is preferable to taking them by mouth or injecting them, because it reduces the dose needed and thus minimizes side-effects. This means applying the drug in creams or ointments for eczema, inhaling it for asthma, or injecting it directly into an affected joint for rheumatoid arthritis. Some of the drug still gets into the

bloodstream however – for example, it can be absorbed through the skin. Children with eczema who are smothered in high-dose corticosteroid cream by their parents can develop Cushing's Syndrome, although this is now very rare as doctors are more aware of the dangers.

Corticosteroids are valuable weapons in the fight against many diseases, but must always be used with some caution. The doctor's instructions, as regards the amount and timing of the dose, must be followed exactly.

Corticosteroids are often used in chronic **asthma**, if the problem of bronchoconstriction is being worsened by inflammation of the membranes lining the bronchi and the production of mucus. In such cases, bronchodilators (see Section 4) may be effective most of the time, but exercise or cold air brings on an asthma attack. Corticosteroids can be given by inhaler, in these circumstances, and this allows a very low dose to be used. Little is absorbed into the bloodstream, so it is safe to use corticosteroids in this way for many years if necessary. The main drugs used are *beclomethasone* (Becotide, Becloforte, Becodisks), and *budesonide* (Pulmicort). In general, if the asthma is known to be provoked by an allergen, it is a good idea to try out *sodium cromoglycate* inhalers before giving corticosteroids, as this drug alone may be effective.

The only common side-effect of corticosteroid inhalers is *Candida* (thrush) infections in the throat, due to suppression of the immune response there. This can be reduced by washing the mouth out with warm water after each inhalation. If infections do develop, they can be controlled with anti-fungal lozenges.

Acute attacks of asthma are often dealt with by giving a short course of corticosteroid tablets. Such treatment suppresses inflammation in the bronchi within a few days, but is continued for about three weeks, followed by gradual withdrawal. This allows the bronchi to settle down and become less sensitive. Stopping the course of treatment before three weeks can result in a flare-up of asthma again, shortly afterwards.

For some asthmatics, controlling their attacks may require treatment with three or even four different types of drugs – *sodium cromoglycate*, a β2 agonist, a xanthine and a corticosteroid inhaler. By using several different drugs, good control of the symptoms can be achieved without the need for high doses of any one drug.

In **hay-fever** and **perennial rhinitis**, corticosteroid sprays or drops are sometimes used. The drugs used include *beclomethasone* (Beconase), *betamethasone* (Betnesol, Vista-

Methasone), *budesonide* (Rhinocort) and *flunisolide* (Syntaris). In general, these are very effective. Relatively little corticosteroid is absorbed, and there seem to be few side-effects, but over-use should be avoided. A *sodium cromoglycate* spray would be preferable if it controls the symptoms well. Students who suffer from bad hay-fever are sometimes given corticosteroid tablets to help them get through important examinations, but this is only done in exceptional cirumstances.

Some doctors use short courses of corticosteroid tablets for patients with chronic **urticaria**, to allow the irritation to settle down before other treatments are tried. In very severe cases of **rheumatoid arthritis**, corticosteroid tablets are sometimes used (see Section 5). A corticosteroid injection into an affected joint can reduce inflammation for some time.

In **eczema**, corticosteroid creams or ointments are used when other forms of treatment (see Section 6) have failed. The creams, ointments and other preparations are classified into four groups: mildly potent, moderately potent, potent and very potent. In general, only preparations in the first two groups are prescribed for children, since there is a risk of stunting and other side-effects when corticosteroids are absorbed into the bloodstream (see p324). Even in adults, the potent and very potent preparations are generally only used for a few weeks, to control an acute outbreak of skin irritation; a less potent preparation is then substituted.

The amount absorbed depends on certain other factors, besides the potency of the cream or ointment. More will be absorbed from the face and genitals, and creams should be used sparingly in these areas. Damaged skin will also absorb more.

If corticosteroids have been applied to the skin for more than a few weeks, treatment should not end abruptly, or there may be a flare-up of the eczema. The cream should be withdrawn gradually, a little less being applied each day. The corticosteroid cream can be used alternately with an emollient (see Section 6) to ease withdrawal.

In general, treatment with mildly potent corticosteroid preparations can be continued for as long as necessary. Provided there is good medical supervision, such treatment can safely continue for several years if needed.

The corticosteroids most commonly used in creams and ointments for eczema is *hydrocortisone*. (See also Section 5A.)

Creams and ointments used for eczema often contain other drugs, besides the corticosteroid. Some include antibiotics and/or anti-fungal drugs (*eg* Terra-Cotril-Nystatin), to treat secondary infections. Others contain substances that help to reduce itching, soothe the skin, or restore its water content.

Preparations containing a mixture of coal-tar (which reduces itching) and hydrocortisone (*eg* Carbo-Cort) are often very effective, the coal-tar helping to make the hydrocortisone effective, even at a low dosage.

5A *Corticosteroids used in creams and ointments for eczema*
alclometasone, beclomethasone, betamethasone, clobetasol, clobetasone, diflucortolone, desoxymethasone, desonide, fluocinolone, flurandrenolone, fluocortolone, fluclorolone, halcinonide, hydrocortisone, methylprednisolone, triamcinolone

5B *Trade names of corticosteroid preparations used in eczema*

Group 1
  Mildly potent
Cobadex
Dioderm
Efcortelan
HC 45
Hydrocortistab
Hydrocortisyl
Lanacort
Mildison Lipocream
Modrasone
Synalar Cream 1:10

Group 2
  Mildly potent, with anti-bacterial/anti-fungal drugs added
Barquinol
Daktacort
Econacort
Framycort
Fucidin H
Gentisone HC
Gregoderm
Hydroderm
Neo-Medrone
Nystaform-HC
Quinocort, Quinoderm
Terra-Cortril
Terra-Cortril-Nystatin
Timodine
Tri-Cicatrin
Vioform-hydrocortisone

Group 3
  Mildly potent, with drugs added to reduce itching or moisturise skin
Carbo-Cort
Epifoam
Eurax-Hydrocortisone
Hydrocal
Sential
Tarcortin

Group 4
  Moderately potent
Eumovate
Haelan, Haelan X
Stiedex LP
Synalar 1:4
Ultradil
Ultralanum plain

Group 5
  Moderately potent with anti-bacterial/
  anti-fungal drugs added
Haelan C
Stiedex LP N
Trimovate

Group 6
  Moderately potent, with drugs added to
  reduce itching or moisturize the skin
Alphaderm
Calmurid HC

Group 7
  Potent
Adcortyl
Betnovate, Betnovate RD
Diprosone
Ledercort
Locoid, Locoid Lipocream
Metosyn
Nerisone
Preferid
Propaderm
Stiedex
Synalar
Synalar Gel
Topilar
Tridesilon

Group 8
  Potent, with anti-bacterial/anti-fungal
  drugs added
Adcortyl with Graneodin
Aureocort
Betnovate C, Betnovate N
Fucibet
Locoid C
Lotriderm
Nystadermal
Peveryl TC
Propaderm A
Synalar C, Synalar N
Tri-Adcortyl

Group 9
  Potent, with drugs added to restore skin
  texture
Diprosalic

Group 10
  Very potent
Dermovate
Halciderm
Nerisone Forte

Group 11
  Very potent, with anti-bacterial/anti-fungal
  drugs added
Dermovate NN

6 EMOLLIENTS AND RELATED TREATMENTS

An emollient is a substance that soothes the skin and restores water to it, thus damping down the symptoms of **eczema**. White soft paraffin, glycerin and lanolin are commonly used. Most emollients and similar preparations contain several different ingredients. Urea is sometimes added to the cream or ointment because it helps the skin to bind water, but it may sting slightly and has a urine-like smell. Emollients may be applied directly to the skin or added to the bath, and some can be used instead of soap.

Crepe bandages soaked in calamine lotion, or bandages soaked in saline, are also used in eczema, to relieve the itching and prevent scratching.

Drugs which reduce itching (anti-pruritics) such as *crotamiton* (Eurax) or *antazoline* (R.B.C.) may also be used. Non-steroidal anti-inflammatory drugs (see Section 7) such as *bufexamac* (Parfenac) are sometimes helpful.

Soothing treatments of this type are generally tried as a first step, where the eczema is not severe. They are free of side-effects, although a small minority of patients may become sensitized to lanolin, so that lanolin-containing creams cannot be used thereafter.

6A *Trade names of emollients and other soothing treatments used for eczema*
Alcoderm
Alpha Keri
Aquadrate
Aveeno
Balmandol
Balneum
Calmurid
Cream E45
Dermacare
Diprobase
Diprobath
Eczederm
Emulsiderm
Epogam
Eurax
Humiderm
Hydromol
Keri
Lacticare
Lipobase
Locobase
Miol
Nutraplus
Oilatum Emollient
Parfenac

R.B.C.
Siopel
Sprilon
Sudocrem
Thovaline
Ultrabase
Unguentum-Merck

7 NON-STEROIDAL ANTI-INFLAMMATORY DRUGS (NSAIDs)

These are drugs which suppress inflammation but are not corticosteroids (see Section 5). They work by reducing the quantities of prostaglandins (p28) produced by the body. Their main use is in **rheumatoid arthritis**, where they can reduce the pain and swelling in the joints.

The NSAID that everyone knows is *aspirin*, which belongs to a group of drugs called *salicylates*. There are many other NSAIDs, and they are very varied chemically, the only common factor being their effect on prostaglandin synthesis.

Because prostaglandins do a variety of different jobs in the body, a drug that interferes with their production is likely to have side-effects. In particular, prostaglandins play an important role in the stomach, and NSAIDs tend to cause stomach upsets, or more serious damage to the stomach lining. *Aspirin* is the worst offender in this respect. Various modified forms of *aspirin* have been introduced in an effort to reduce its side-effects on the stomach. But these may still affect the stomach, and should not be taken by anyone who has ever had a stomach ulcer. *Aspirin*-containing drugs are listed in the next section.

Prostaglandins also play an important role in the kidney, and some NSAIDs affect kidney function causing water retention (oedema). Long-term use of NSAIDs, without proper supervision, can lead to kidney damage, but this is rare.

Some people appear to be particularly sensitive to *aspirin* (see p57) and may suffer from asthma or urticaria as a result. Some of these people react in a similar way to other NSAIDs, and some may be affected by *paracetamol* as well. There are other painkillers, available on prescription, that are suitable for such patients.

7A *Drugs used for rheumatoid arthritis containing aspirin and other salicylates*
aloxiprin (Palaprin)
aspirin (Anadin, Aspro-Clear, Caprin, Claradin, Nu-Seals, Paynocil, Disprin, Solmin)
benorylate (Benoral)
diflunisal (Dolobid)
salsalate (Disalcid)
choline magnesium trisalicylate (Trilisate)

7B *Propionic acid derivatives*
Another important group of NSAIDs are the propionic acid derivatives. These do not reduce inflammation quite as well as aspirin, but they are effective pain-killers and cause far fewer problems in the stomach than aspirin. However, some patients may suffer from stomach upsets or rashes, and some of the drugs can also cause headaches, drowsiness and other minor problems. These drugs are generally used for mild forms of **rheumatoid arthritis**, where the inflammation is not very great. Some are available as gels which are applied directly to the affected area. They include:

ibuprofen (Apsifen, Brufen, Ebufac, Fenbid Spansule, Ibulere, Ibugel, Lidifen, Motrin, Nurofen, Paxofen, Proflex)
felbinac (Traxam gel)
fenbufen (Lederfen)
fenoprofen (Fenopron, Progesic)
flurbiprofen (Froben)
ketoprofen (Alrheumat, Orudis, Oruvail, Oruvail gel)
naproxen (Laraflex, Naprosyn, Nycopren, Synflex)
tiaprofenic acid (Surgam)

Naproxen combined with *misoprostol*, a prostaglandin (Napratec), is used when protection from stomach upset is necessary.

Mefenamic acid (Ponstan) is a similar drug whose main value is in relieving pain. It can cause diarrhoea or rashes, and is not generally given to elderly patients.

7C *Other NSAIDs*
The remaining NSAIDs have a powerful anti-inflammatory action, on a par with aspirin. They can all produce side-effects in susceptible individuals, but are reasonably safe for long-term use. Some are available as gels, which are applied directly to the affected area.

Indomethacin (Artracin, Flexin Continus, Imbrilon, Indocid, Indolar, Indomod) is a powerful anti-inflammatory drug that has been in use for many years. It is useful for morning stiffness because it goes on acting for a long time, and a dose taken the night before will make getting up easier. This drug can cause stomach upsets, headaches or dizziness, in which case another drug will usually be tried. When taken for a long period of time it can also affect the eyes, and it is important to have regular check-ups. Anyone who is allergic to aspirin may react to this drug too.

Sulindac (Clinoril) is a similar drug, with less anti-inflammatory effect than *indomethacin* but fewer side-effects. It sometimes causes stomach upsets, rashes, dizziness or ringing in the ears. Occasionally more serious side-effects occur which should be reported to the doctor. Other NSAIDs that are similar to *indomethacin* are *etodolac* (Lodine), *diclofenac* (Rhumalgan, Volraman, Voltarol, Voltarol gel application) and *tolmetin* (Tolectin)

Piroxicam (Feldene, Feldene gel application, Larapam) and *tenoxicam* (Mobiflex) are NSAIDs with strong anti-inflammatory effects. They have the advantage of only needing to be taken once a day. These drugs can sometimes cause stomach upsets, water retention, ringing in the ears, headaches or other side-effects.

Azapropazone (Rheumox) is another powerful anti-inflammatory. It can sometimes cause side-effects in the form of stomach upsets, headache, water retention and rashes (the skin may become more sensitive to sunlight). As with other drugs of this type, anyone taking them on a long-term basis should have regular check-ups.

8 MORE POWERFUL DRUGS USED IN RHEUMATOID ARTHRITIS

These drugs are used where NSAIDs (see Section 7) have been tried, and have failed to control the symptoms. Most have some effect on the immune response within the joint. They have the advantage of checking the progress of joint destruction caused by rheumatoid arthritis, whereas NSAIDs simply suppress the immediate effects. On the other hand, they are powerful drugs which are more likely to cause side-effects. Once they are started, they will probably have to be taken for many years. For this reason, doctors delay using them until they are sure they are necessary. If taking such drugs, it is very important to have regular medical supervision and report any side-effects to the doctor.

The drugs commonly used are:
penicillamine (Distamine, Pendramine)
gold salts (Myocrisin, Ridaura)
sulphasalazine (Salazopyrin)
hydroxychloroquine (Plaquenil).

In severe cases of rheumatoid arthritis, that do not respond to other treatments, drugs which have a general suppressive effect on the immune system may sometimes be used. The main one is *azathioprine* (Azamune, Imuran, Berkaprine, Immunoprin). These drugs make the body less able to fight infections, and at high doses they could make patients more susceptible to cancer. Corticosteroids (see Section 5) are sometimes used where none of the above treatments are effective.

9 PAIN-KILLERS

(Trade names are not given in this section, as the common pain-killers are used in a great number of different preparations. The ingredients are shown on the packet for those bought without a prescription.)

These are drugs that can block pain sensations. Our main interest in them is in connection with **headache** and **migraine**.

Aspirin and other salicylates (see Section 7A) reduce pain and damp down inflammation. They also have some effects on the blood platelets (see p128), and this may help to abort a migraine attack. Regular, prolonged use of salicylates can irritate the stomach lining and have other adverse effects, so this should be avoided.

Paracetamol reduces pain but has very little anti-inflammatory effect. It has no ill-effects on the stomach, and as long as the maximum dose is strictly observed it is a very safe drug. However, it should not be taken long-term at the maximum dosage, nor should it be taken by anyone who has kidney or liver disease. There are rare instances of paracetamol causing skin rashes.

Ibuprofen and related drugs (see Section 7B) are effective pain-killers and have fewer ill-effects on the stomach than aspirin, although they can cause problems for some people.

Codeine is a very mild opiate (a morphine-like drug) used in some migraine preparations. It is fairly safe but can cause constipation.

Caffeine is added to some pain-killers to speed up absorption and improve the effectiveness of the drug. Caffeine can also produce headaches (see p166), so heavy use of this type of pain-killer is not advisable.

10 DRUGS THAT REDUCE NAUSEA AND VOMITING

Migraine remedies often contain a drug to reduce nausea and vomiting (anti-emetics), as well as a pain-killer. One problem in migraine, is that absorption from the stomach is much reduced once an attack starts, so that pain-killers taken by mouth have little effect. Anti-emetics can improve the absorption of the pain-killer, so they are useful for migraines, even if nausea is not a symptom. The main drugs used (see Section 10A) are *buclizine*, *cyclizine* and *metoclopramide*. These are safe drugs with few side effects.

Because of the problem of non-absorption, it is very important to take migraine treatments as soon as an attack begins – or in advance, for those patients who have advance warning of their attacks, in the form of visual disturbances, mood changes etc.

10A *Composition of migraine preparations containing pain-killers and other drugs*

Midrid – *paracetamol*, plus a sedative, and a sympathomimetic (see Section 3)

Migraleve – *paracetamol*, *codeine* and
buclizine (anti-emetic) in the pink tablets;
paracetamol and *codeine* in the yellow tablets
Migravess – *aspirin* and *metoclopramide*
Paramax – *paracetamol* and *metoclopramide*
(anti-emetic)

11 ERGOTAMINE
Ergotamine (Dihydergot, Lingraine,
Medihaler-Ergotamine) is a powerful drug
that makes the blood vessels contract. Since
it is expansion of the blood vessels that
causes the pain of migraine (see p128), this
drug can be useful in treating an acute
attack. But if ergotamine is used regularly, the
underlying problem of migraine – failure to
control the expansion and contraction of
blood vessels – could be made worse. Some
patients who have taken ergotamine for many
years find that the drug is actually *causing*
the attacks. *Ergotamine* also has various
side-effects, including nausea, stomach pains
and cramps. Some medicines combine
ergotamine with *caffeine* (Cafergot), or with
caffeine and an anti-emetic, *metoclopramide*
(Migril).
  Because of its many drawbacks,
ergotamine is much less used now. Most
acute attacks of migraine are better treated
with a mixture of pain-killer, anti-emetic and
sedative.

12 DRUGS THAT CAN PREVENT MIGRAINE ATTACKS
There are various drugs that, taken regularly,
can prevent migraine attacks, or at least
reduce their frequency. Beneficial effects may
not be apparent until they have been taken
for several weeks.
  In conventional migraine treatment, these
are not generally prescribed unless migraines
are fairly frequent and severe, and other
measures have been tried without significant
success. Those 'other measures' might
include reducing stress, avoiding situations
that trigger migraines, and avoiding foods
such as chocolate, cheese, red wine and
citrus fruits (see pp126–9). By extension, it
would seem reasonable to investigate food
intolerance, using an elimination diet, before
starting on (or continuing with) these drugs.

12A Serotonin antagonists
Serotonin, or 5HT, is a chemical messenger
produced by the blood platelets that is known
to play a part in migraine (see p128). Drugs
that block the receptors for serotonin seem to
help prevent migraine. Some of these drugs
also act as antihistamines (see Section 2).
The main drug used is *pizotifen* (Sanomigran)
which is generally safe but can cause weight-
gain and drowsiness in some people.
Methysergide (Deseril) is equally effective, but

it can, very rarely, cause serious side-effects
with lasting damage. Anyone taking it should
have close medical supervision. It is advisable
to stop taking the drug for 1–2 months twice
a year, to check that all is well. Sumatripan
(Imigran) is an injection, given under the skin,
for acute migraine.

12B β-blockers
These drugs block β-receptors for adrenaline,
the hormone that produces the 'flight or fight'
reaction (see p151). Their main use is in other
diseases, principally heart disease, and it is
not entirely clear how they help to prevent
migraine.
  Some of these drugs block the effects of
adrenaline generally and they should not be
taken by asthmatics, since they have the
opposite effect to β2 bronchodilators (see
Section 4A). The ones in question are *nadolol*
(Corgard), *propanolol* (Angilol, Apsolol,
Berkolol, Cardinol, Inderal LA, Propanix) and
timolol (Betim, Blocadren). Others are more
selective, only affecting β-receptors in the
heart, and they can be taken by asthmatics,
although good medical supervision is needed.
The principal drug of this type is *metoprolol*
(Betaloc, Lopresor, Mepranix).
  All these drugs have certain side-effects,
including cold hands and feet, disturbed
sleep, stomach upset and wheezing. If dry
eyes or skin rash develop this should be
reported to the doctor immediately, as it can
indicate a severe reaction to the drug. The
drugs should not be stopped abruptly, but
gradually withdrawn.

12C Clonidine
Clonidine is used to lower blood pressure and
when taken at low dosage (Dixarit) it can
prevent migraine in some patients. It is a
relatively safe drug, but some patients may
suffer from drowsiness, dizziness, dry mouth
or insomnia.

CHECKLIST OF DRUGS
The numbers/letters indicate the section of
this appendix where these drugs are
discussed. Generic names and trade names
are listed separately – check both lists. (See
also index.)

Generic names
acrivastine 2A
adrenaline 4D
alclometasone 5A
aloxiprin 7A
aminophylline 4B
antazoline 6
aspirin 7, 7A, 9, 10A
astemizole 2, 2A
atropine 4B
azapropazone 7C

azatadine 2A
azathioprine 8
beclomethasone 5, 5A
benorylate 7A
betamethasone 5A
brompheniramine 2A
buclizine 10, 10A
budesonide 5
bufexamac 6
butethamate 4C
caffeine 9, 11
cetirizine 2A
chlorpheniramine 2A
choline magnesium trisalicylate 7A
choline theophyllinate 4
clemastine 2A
clobetasol 5A
clobetasone 5A
clonidine 12C
codeine 9, 10A
crotamiton 6
cyclizine 10
cyproheptadine 2A
desonide 5A
desoxymethasone 5A
diclofenac 7C
diflucortolone 5A
diflunisal 7A
dimethindene 2A
diphenylpyraline 2A
ephedrine 3, 4D
ergotamine 11
etodolac 7C
felbinac 7B
fenbufen 7B
fenclofenac 7C
fenoprofen 7B
fenoterol 4A
fluclorolone 5A
flunisolide 5
fluocinolone 5A
fluocortolone 5A
flurandrenolone 5A
flurbiprofen 7B
gold salts 8
halcinonide 5A
hydrocortisone 5, 5A
hydroxychloroquine 8
hydroxyzine 2A
ibuprofen 7B, 9
indomethacin 7C
ipratropium 4C
isoetharine 4A
isoprenaline 4A
ketoprofen 7B
ketotifen 2A
loratidine 2A
mebhydrolin 2A
mefenamic acid 7B
mequitazine 2A
methylprednisolone 5A
methysergide 12A
metoclopramide 10, 10A

metoprolol 12B
nadolol 12B
naproxen 7B
nedocromil sodium 1
orciprenaline 4A
oxatomide 2A
oxitropium 4C
oxymetozaline 3
paracetamol 9, 10A
penicillamine 8
phenindamine 2A
pheniramine 2A
phenylephrine 3, 4D
pirbuterol 4A
piroxicam 7C
pizotifen 12A
prednisolone 5
promethazine 2A
propanolol 12B
pseudoephedrine 3
reproterol 4A
rimiterol 4A
salbutamol 4A
salicylates 7, 7A
salmeterol 4A
salsalate 7A
sodium cromoglycate 1
sulindac 7C
sulphasalazine 8
sumatripan 12A
tenoxicam 7C
terbutaline 4A
terfenadine 2, 2A
theophylline 4B
tiaprofenic acid 7B
timolol 12B
tolmetin 7C
triamcinolone 5A
trimeprazine 2A
triprolidine 2A
xylometazoline 3

Trade names
Actidil 2A
Adcortyl 5B, group 7
Adcortyl with Graneodin 5B, group 8
Aerolin Auto 4A
Afrazine 3
Alcoderm 6A
Alpha Keri 6A
Alphaderm 5B, group 6
Alrheumat 7B
Alupent 4A
Anadin 7A
Angilol 12B
Apsifen 7B
Apsolol 12B
Aquadrate 6A
Artracin 7C
Asmaven 4A
Aspro-Clear 7A
Atarax 2A
Atrovent 4C

Aureocort 5B, group 8
Aveeno 6A
Azamune 8
Balmandol 6A
Balneum 6A
Barquinol 5B, group 2
Becloforte 5
Beconase 5
Becodisks 5
Becotide 5
Benoral 7A
Berkaprine 8
Berkolol 12B
Berotec 4A
Betaloc 12B
Betim 12B
Betnesol 5
Betnovate 5B, group 7
Betnovate C 5B, group 8
Betnovate N 5B, group 8
Betnovate RD 5B, group 7
Biophylline 4B
Blocadren 12B
Bricanyl 4A
Bronchilator 4A
Bronchodil 4A
Brovon 4C
Brufen 7B
Cafergot 11
Calmurid 6A
Calmurid HC 5B, group 6
CAM 4C
Caprin 7A
Carbo-Cort 5, 5B group 3
Choledyl 4B
Clarityn 2A
Clinoril 7C
Cobadex 5B, group 1
Corgard 12B
Cream E45 6A
Daktakort 5B, group 2
Daneral 2A
Dermacare 6A
Dermovate 5B, group 10
Dermovate NN 5B, group 11
Deseril 12A
Dexa-Rhinaspray 3
Dihydergot 11
Dimotane 2A
Dioderm 5B, group 1
Diprobase 6A
Diprobath 6A
Diprosalic 5B, group 9
Diprosone 5B, group 7
Disalcid 7A
Disprin 7A
Distamine 8
Dixarit 12C
Dolobid 7A
Duovent 4A
Ebufac 7B
Econacort 5B, group 2
Eczederm 6A

Efcortelan 5B, group 1
Emulsiderm 6A
Epifoam 5B, group 3
Epogam 6A
Eumovate 5B, group 4
Eurax 6, 6A
Eurax-Hydrocortisone 5B, group 3
Exirel 4A
Fabahistin 2A
Feldene 7C
Fenbid Spansule 7B
Fenopron 7B
Fenostil Retard 2A
Fenox 3
Flexin Continus 7C
Franol 4B
Framycort 5B, group 2
Froben 7B
Fucibet 5B, group 8
Fucidin H 5B, group 2
Gentisone HC 5B, group 2
Gregoderm 5B, group 2
Haelan C 5B, group 5
Haelan X 5B, group 4
Haelan 5B, group 4
Halciderm 5B, group 1
Haymine 3
HC 45 5B, group 1
Hismanal 2, 2A
Histryl Spansule 2A
Humiderm 6A
Hydrocal 5B, group 3
Hydrocortistab 5B, group 1
Hydrocortisyl 5B, group 1
Hydroderm 5B, group 2
Hydromol 6A
Ibugel 7B
Ibuleve 7B
Imbrilon 7C
Imigran 12A
Immunoprin 8
Imuran 8
Inderal LA 12B
Indocid 7C
Indolar 7C
Indomod 7C
Intal, Intal Compound 1
Keri 6A
Labophylline 4B
Lacticare 6A
Lanacort 5B
Laraflex 7B
Larapam 7C
Lasma 4B
Ledercort 5B, group 7
Lederfen 7B
Lidifen 7B
Lingraine 11
Lipobase 6A
Locobase 6A
Locoid C 5B, group 8
Locoid 5B, group 7
Locoid Lipocream 5B, group 7

Lodine 7C
Lotriderm 5B, group 8
Maxivent 4A
Medihaler-Duo 4A
Medihaler-Ergotamine 11
Medihaler-Iso 4A
Metosyn 5B, group 7
Midrid 10A
Migraleve 10, 10A
Migravess 10A
Migril 10, 11
Mildison Lipocream 5B, group 1
Miol 6A
Mobiflex 7C
Modrasone 5B, group 1
Monovent 4A
Motrin 7B
Myocrisin 8
Nalcrom 1
Napratec 7B
Naprosyn 7B
Neo-Medrone 5B, group 2
Nerisone 5B, group 7
Nerisone Forte 5B, group 10
Nu-Seals 7A
Nuelin 4B
Nurofen 7B
Nutraplus 6A
Nycopren 7B
Nystadermal 5B, group 8
Nystaform HC 5B, group 2
Oilatum Emollient 6A
Opticrom 1
Optimine 2A
Orudis 7B
Oruvail 7B
Otrivin-Antistin 3
Otrivine 3
Oxivent 4C
Palaprin 7A
Paramax 10A
Parfenac 6
Parfenac 6A
Paxofen 7B
Paynocil 7A
Pecram 4B
Pendramine 8
Periactin 2A
Peveryl TC 5B, group 8
Phenergan 2A
Phyllocontin Continus 4B
Piriton 2A
Plaquenil 8
Ponstan 7B
Preferid 5B group 7
Primalan 2A
Pro-Actidil 2A
Pro-Vent 4B
Proflex 7B
Progesic 7B
Propaderm 5B, group 7
Propaderm A 5B, group 8
Pulmadil 4A

Pulmicort 5
Quinocort 5B, group 2
R.B.C. 6, 6A
Resiston-one 1
Rheumox 7C
Rhinocort 5
Rhumalgan 7C
Ridaura 8
Rimasal 4A
Rynacrom, Rynacrom Compound 1
Sabidal 4B
Salazopyrin 8
Salbulin 4A
Salbuvent 4A
Sanomigran 12A
Semprex 2A
Sential 5B, group 3
Serevent 4A
Siopel 6A
Slo-Phyllin 4B
Solmin 7A
Sprilon 6A
Stiedex LP 5B, group 4
Stiedex 5B, group 7
Stiedex LP N 5B, group 5
Sudafed Plus 3
Sudocrem 6A
Surgam 7B
Synalar 5B, group 7
Synalar 1:4 5B, group 4
Synalar C 5B, group 8
Synalar Cream 1:10 5B, group 1
Synalar Gel 5B, group 7
Synalar N 5B, group 8
Synflex 7B
Syntaris 5
Tarcortin 5B, group 3
Tavegil 2A
Tedral 4B
Terra-Cortril 5B, group 2
Terra-Cortril-Nystatin 5B, group 2
Theo-Dur 4B
Theodrox 4B
Uniphyllin Continus 4B
Thephorin 2A
Thovaline 6A
Tilade 1
Timodine 5B, group 2
Tinset 2A
Tolectin 7C
Topilar 5B, group 7
Traxam Gel 7B
Tri-Adcortyl 5B, group 8
Tri-Cicatrin 5B, group 2
Tridesilon 5B, group 7
Trilisate 7A
Triludan 2, 2A
Trimovate 5B, group 5
Ultrabase 6A
Ultradil 5B, group 4
Ultralanum plain 5B, group 4
Unguentum-Merck 6A
Vallergan 2A

Ventide 4A
Ventodisks 4A
Ventolin 4A
Vibrocil 2, 3
Vioform-hydrocortisone 5B, group 2
Vista-Methasone 5
Volmax 4A
Volmaran 7C
Voltarol 7C
Zaditen 2A
Zirtek 2A

APPENDIX IX
Nutritional supplements

For a general supplement, suitable for adults and the elderly with minor nutritional deficiencies, see p339. A general supplement such as this is not suitable for everyone, and if you have been eating a very inadequate diet, or have serious symptoms that you think might be due to nutritional deficiencies, then you should seek specialist help. For some patients a full nutritional analysis may be needed (see p270) to identify the particular nutrients that are in short supply. Where there are serious deficiencies, treatment should be carried out by a nutritional specialist, because the level of one vitamin or mineral can affect the level or absorption of another. Specialist treatment includes repeated monitoring of nutrient levels to see how they respond to the supplement and making the appropriate adjustments.

Zinc supplements
If you think you may be deficient in zinc (see p272) it is worth trying a zinc supplement to see if this produces an improvement. A dose of 20–40 mg of elemental zinc per day is recommended, and even if you are not deficient this dose is most unlikely to do any harm. Zinc sulphate tablets are widely obtainable from chemists. The amount of elemental zinc per tablet should be given on the label.
   Take the supplement last thing at night, preferably without any late-night snacks or milky drinks, as zinc supplements are not well absorbed if taken with food. You may need to take the supplement for a month or more before any good effects are obvious.

Supplements and the Pill
A special type of supplement is recommended for anyone currently taking the Pill, or stopping the Pill (see p270).
   The supplement given below is designed for those who have *minor* health problems. Some women experience more serious nutritional deficiencies as a result of taking the Pill and they will need specialist help of the kind described above. Women coming off the Pill usually need to take the supplement for two to three months. You should consult your doctor before taking the supplement.
   This supplement is not obtainable in a single combined tablet, but the different vitamins and minerals can all be purchased from specialist suppliers such as Nature's Best (address on p339).

Vitamin B	110–50 mg
Vitamin B2	10–50 mg
Vitamin B3	10–50 mg
Vitamin B5	50–100 mg
Vitamin B6	50–100 mg
Vitamin B12	200–400 mcg (µg)
Folic acid	400mcg–2mg
Inositol	50–75 mg
Vitamin C	250–2000 mg (or more)
Vitamin E	50–200 IUs
Magnesium	100–200 mg (or more)
Zinc	5–15 mg (or more)
Manganese	3–5 mg

The supplement should not contain Vitamin A or copper. Iron should be included only if a blood test indicates anaemia.

(Adapted from *Nutritional Medicine* by Dr Stephen Davies and Dr Alan Stewart, with permission.)

APPENDIX X
Useful Addresses

Inclusion of an organization in this list does not necessarily mean that the authors agree with all the policies or opinions advanced by that organization. In the same way, we give no general endorsement of the commercial companies included – they may sell other items, besides those for which they are listed here, which we believe to be ineffectual or even damaging if used wrongly. Readers are advised to be sceptical about the claims made for some products, such as nutritional supplements and herbal medicines. Buying from a reputable company is advisable.

FOOD

Baby foods

Nutricology
PO Box 191
Corio
Victoria 3214
Australia
Telephone 052 757045
A mail-order service run by a pharmacist with extensive knowledge of intolerance to foods and vitamin preparations. Free catalogue of books, vitamins, etc.

Foods for special diets

Nutricia Dietary Products Ltd.
494-496 Honeypot Lane
Stanmore
Middlesex HA7 1JH
Telephone 081 951 5155
(For the address in Australia, see p337 under *Foods by post*.)
Produce a variety of gluten-free and low-protein products under the Glutafin, Loprofin and Rite Diet brand names. Also provide products which are free of wheat starch, milk, lactose, egg and soya. These products are available from pharmacies and in many health food shops. A mail-order service is also available.

The Cantassium Company
225 Putney Bridge Road
London SW15 2PY
Telephone 081 874 1130
Fax 081 871 0066
Sell a range of gluten-free, lactose-free flours, under the name Trufree. Some of the flours are free of all cereal grains. They also produce a free leaflet showing the ingredients of all flours, and a recipe book, price £4.95. These flours are available on prescription to

those with coeliac disease. They can also be bought without prescription at most chemists, although they will not be on display. They also publish a free booklet 'Getting Safely Started – The Trufree Handbook for Coeliacs and Gluten-free/Wheat-free Dieters', available on request.

General Designs Ltd
PO Box 38E
Worcester Park
Surrey KT4 7LX
Produces gluten-free bread and pastas made with rice flour.

The following companies' products are available in most healthfood stores. However, most shops do not stock the full range of goods produced. It may be worth writing in to discover what is available. Your local shop may be able to order items that you would find useful.

Meridian Foods Ltd.
Corwen
Clwyd LL21 9RT
Telephone 0490 3151
Produce a range of spreads including almond butter, cashew butter, hazel butter, sunflower spread, tahini (sesame seeds) and carob-hazelnut spread (substitute for chocolate spread). Also various oils, including grapeseed oil, safflower oil and walnut oil. Organic sunflower oil and olive oil. Will identify local stockists for anyone who cannot find their products.

Trustin Health
Chase Road
Northern Way
Bury St Edmunds
Suffolk IP32 6NT
Telephone 0284 766265
Food distributor stocking foods produced by a number of British and Continental companies, including Granose and Meridian. Supply a wide range of flours (including gram flour, maize flour, buckwheat flour and soya flour), grains (including millet, buckwheat, wild rice and tapioca), nuts (including pistachios, pine nuts and pecans), seeds (such as pumpkin seeds and sunflower seeds), beans, lentils and chickpeas.

They also stock egg replacer, egg-free salad dressing, powdered goat's milk, concentrated soya milk, coffee substitutes, gluten-free flour and a wide range of herbal teas. Their Swiss vegetable bouillon is a yeast-free substitute for stock cubes.

They supply various organic foods, including: flour, rice 'cakes' (crispbread), wheat 'cakes', biscuits, raisins, apple juice, carrot juice, sauerkraut, vinegar, soya-based

meals, lentil spread, chickpea spread and tofu spread.

This company cannot supply foods by post but can identify local stockists.

Be-well Nutritional Products Ltd
20 King Street Ind. Estate
Langtoft
Nr. Peterborough PE6 9NF
Telephone 0778 560 868
Produce a range of dried 'instant meals' without using preservatives or other additives. Some are free of wheat and soya (*eg* lentil and barley pilaf). Also manufacture an organic cereal beverage – Moccava – which has a coffee-like taste. Obtainable from health-food shops. Send for a full product list and local stockists.

Van den Berghs and Jurgens Ltd.
Sussex House
Burgess Hill
West Sussex RH15 9AW
Telephone 0444 246300
Market milk-free, egg-free and gluten-free products, including milk-free margarine. Produce lists available.

Organic and pesticide-free produce

Thorson's Organic Consumer Guide by Jackie Gear and David Mabey, price £5.75, covers the case for organic farming and food, and lists most organic suppliers and restaurants in the UK. It is available from book shops, or direct from the Henry Doubleday Research Association (address in next section, add 50 pence for postage).

Soil Association
Organic Food and Farming Centre
86 Colston Street
Bristol BS1 5BB
Telephone 0272 290661
Operates an approval scheme for organic growers and meat producers. Their symbol can only be used on food if it has been produced to the association's high standards. They publish regional lists (£2 each) and a national list (£10) of their approved growers. Prices include postage.

The Real Meat Company
Easthill Farm
Heytesbury
Warminster BA12 OHR
Telephone 0985 40436
Markets meat and eggs which have been produced by non-intensive farming methods. The farms supplying them do not spray herbicides on their pastures. Concentrated feeds are used, but these do not contain antibiotics, growth promoters or recycled

animal products. Antibiotics are only used occasionally, for the specific treatment of disease. Also produce pies, burgers and sausages with no preservatives or artificial colouring. The only additive they allow is nitrate (saltpetre) in bacon. Sell through a number of butchers shops. Can also supply meat anywhere in mainland Britain by courier in insulated containers. Write for a list of outlets/mail-order form enclosing an s.a.e. .

Real Foods Trading Ltd.
14 Ashley Place
Edinburgh EH6 5PX
Telephone 031 554 4321
Supply a wide range of organic foods (flour, fruit, nuts, grains, pasta, oils etc.) also wines and beers. Can deliver throughout the UK, or supply by post.

Organic Wine Company
P.O. Box 81
High Wycombe
Buckinghamshire HP13 5QN
Telephone 0494 446557
Sells a wide range of organically produced wines, mostly French and German, by mail-order. Some wines that are completely free of sulphur dioxide are also available, and wines with very low residual sugar, which may be useful to anyone on a low-sugar diet. Also imports organic olive oil and sells organic beers and fruit juices.

Other sources of organic food will be found in the previous section (*Foods for special diets*). Although at present, the range of organic/pesticide-free foods available is fairly limited, the situation is changing all the time as more items become available. New producers of organic food often advertise in the Henry Doubleday Research Association newsletter (address in next section). If you are looking for a particular item without success, and the major stockists (see above) are unable to help, try writing to:

Organic Farmers and Growers Ltd
Abacus House
Station Yard
Needham Market
Ipswich
Suffolk IP6 8AT

Growing your own

Henry Doubleday Research Association
Ryton-on-Dunsmore
Coventry CV8 3LG
Telephone 0203 303517
HDRA produces a huge range of books, booklets and information leaflets on all aspects of organic growing. Carries out research into organic growing and publishes an informative quarterly newsletter for members. Well worth joining if you are interested in growing food organically, even on a small scale. Basic techniques can also be seen at their demonstration garden. Send an s.a.e. for further details.

The Soil Association (address above) carries a comprehensive stock of books on organic growing. Free list available in return for an s.a.e.

Foods by post or delivery

Natural Foods Ltd.
Unit 14
Hainault Industrial Estate
Hainault Road
Leytonstone
London E11
Telephone 081 539 1034
Home delivery service of a huge range of food and beverages, many organic, in London and parts of the Home Counties.

Foodwatch International Ltd.
9 Corporation Street
Taunton
Somerset TA1 4AJ
Telephone 0823 325022
Specialize in supplying foods for those with food sensitivity. Their extensive stock includes most of the standard alternative foods, plus many unusual items not generally available elsewhere.

Gluten-free and grain-free flours, gluten-free pasta, pastry-mix and pancake-mix; wheat-and yeast-free bread mix

Wheat flour (wholemeal or white) with no additives

Buckwheat (whole and flour), millet (whole and flour), sorghum, chestnut flour, banana flour, arrowroot, yam flour, tapioca, amaranth, spelt

Nuts and seeds. Dried fruits with no sulphur dioxide or mineral oil added

Cashew spread, almond spread, sunflower spread

Peas, beans and lentils

Soya milk (including sugar-free brands), goat's cheese, dried goat's milk, skimmed goat's milk

Milk-free margarine, egg-replacer and egg-white replacer

Carob powder, herb teas, coffee substitutes

Sucrose-free jellies and ice-cream mix

Artificial sweetener for use in cooking

Yeast-free vegetable extract for stock

Natural food colourings

Sweets made with natural colours, milk-free chocolate

Some organic foods

Taheebo (pau d'arco) tea

Cookbooks and other books
Water filters, cleaning supplies, toothpaste
Pillow cases, mattress covers, duvet covers,
   paints, timber

Real Foods Trading Ltd. supply organic foods
and drinks by post. See p336.

Country Harvest Products
2A/23 Koornang Road
Carnegie
Victoria 3163, Australia
Telephone 03 563 6538
Manufacture and supply gluten-free foods
('Country Harvest') and other products
suitable for those with food sensitivity; by mail
order and to retailers. Product list available.

National Dietary Supplies
2A/23 Koornang Road
Carnegie
Victoria 3163, Australia
Telephone 03 563 6538
Supply gluten-free foods and other products
suitable for those with food sensitivity.
Product list and mail-order form available.

Allergy Aid Centre
1st Floor
Pran Central
325 Chapel Street
Prahran
Victoria 3181, Australia
Telephone 03 529 7348
Supply some foods suitable for those with
food sensitivity. They also sell bedding, water
filters, face masks, cosmetics, toothpaste,
deodorant, cleaning materials, furniture and
carpets, all designed for allergic individuals.

GUT FLORA TREATMENT

Sugar-free foods

A heat-stable artificial sweetener, suitable for
use in cakes, biscuits and other cooked
foods, is sold by Foodwatch International. In
general, diabetic foods are suitable for a no-
sugar diet, and these are available from good
chemists and healthfood shops. Most
healthfood shops stock peanut butter with no
added sugar, and this is usually suitable for
such a diet, but check the label for other
forms of sugar (see p302). Jams, baked
beans and other products labelled 'no added
sugar' usually contain concentrated apple
juice and are actually very sugary.
   Wines that are virtually sugar-free can be
bought from The Organic Wine Company
(address on p336).

Yoghurt culture

Smallholding Supplies
Pike's Farmhouse

East Pennard
Shepton Mallet
Somerset BA4 6RR
Telephone 074 986 688
Sell yoghurt culture by post, as well as
inexpensive yoghurt-making equipment.

Taheebo or pau d'arco tea (see p194) is sold
by Foodwatch International (address above,
under *Foods by post*).

CLOTHING

Cotton On
29 North Clifton Street
Lytham
Lancs FY8 5HW
Telephone 0253 736611
Supplies attractive pure cotton clothing for
eczema sufferers, with no chemical finishes or
non-cotton trimmings. The dyes used are
non-irritant. Mostly for children, but some
adult clothes as well. Their range includes
mitten-pyjamas, which lessen the damage
done by scratching at night. They sell by mail
order only and their catalogue is free.

BEDDING AND MATTRESSES

These products are available free of VAT for
those who have a proven allergy to house-
dust mite.

Green Farm Catalogue
Burwash Common
East Sussex TN19 7LX
Telephone 0435 882482
Sell lambswool-filled duvets and pillows in
pure cotton cases, suitable for those who are
sensitive to both feathers and synthetic fibres.
Also a duvet filled with 100 per cent silk.

Allergy Relief Products
39 Spring Crescent
Portswood
Southampton SO2 1FZ
Telephone 0703 ~~586709~~ 332 91. 09
Fax 0703 676226
Produces microporous barrier covers against
house-dust mite allergens, for all mattresses
and bedding, at realistic prices.

Allerayde
21 North End
Farndon
Newark
Notts NG24 3SX
Telephone 0636 ~~72636~~ 613444.
Fax 0636 72636
Sell microporous covers to retain dust-mite
allergens, for mattress and all bedding.

Allergy Aid Centre, Australia
(address on p337, under *Foods by post*)
Sell bedding, beds and mattresses. Ask for
their catalogue.

AIRBORNE ALLERGENS AND POLLUTANTS

Air filters

Air filters are not the first measure that should
be taken against any airborne allergen.
Mattress and bedding covers are more
effective against dust-mite, for example, and
other measures (see p69) should also be
tried. With other airborne allergens, removing
the source of the allergen, followed by careful
cleaning, is usually more effective and less
costly than buying an air filter. However, a
filter can be useful against pollen if simply
keeping the windows closed is ineffective (the
windows must remain closed even with the
filter on). If you cannot bear to part with the
family pet, despite allergic reactions, a filter
may be of some help, but cleaning measures
are also essential to reduce the reservoir of
allergens in the carpets and upholstery.
Allerayde (address in previous section) sell a
high-quality filter, the Enviracaire, which has
been tested and shown to help allergy
sufferers in certain circumstances. This filter
represents the best value for money of those
currently available.

Beta Plus Ltd.
177 Haydons Road
Wimbledon
London SW19 8TB
Telephone 081 543 1142
Stock a range of air purifiers. The equipment
can be seen in their showrooms, or can be
supplied by post. Also supply air conditioning.

The Healthy House
Cold Harbour
Ruscombe
Stroud
Glos GL6 4DA
Telephone 0453 752216
Fax 0453 753533
Provide services on all aspects of the home
environment, including organic paint, VDU-
screen covers, linoleum (a 100 per cent
natural product), mite-proof bedding covers,
air and water filters and full-spectrum lights.
Catalogue available.

See also: *Vacuum cleaners*, p338.

WATER FILTERS

See Appendix VII, p317.

CLEANING SUPPLIES

Vacuum cleaners

These products are available free of VAT for
those who have a proven allergy to house-
dust mite.

Medivac
Bollin House
Riverside Works
Manchester Road
Wilmslow
Cheshire SK9 1BE
Telephone 0625 539401
Fax 0625 539507
Produces a high-quality stainless steel
vacuum cleaner designed for those allergic to
house-dust mite or pollen. Normal vacuum
cleaners expel many of the tiny particles they
pick up through the bag, but this machine
does not. Medivac also produce an electronic
dust monitor that can be fitted to the machine
to show when cleaning is complete. Other
products include ionizers and a special
dehumidifier and air filter for those with
allergies to house-dust mite. A range of
hypoallergenic bedding that can be washed
in a domestic washing machine (to kill house-
dust mites) is also available.

Allerayde (address on p337) sell a vacuum
cleaner, the Nilfisk, which retains very small
allergenic particles such as those produced
by house-dust mites. This company also sells
filter pads, called Vacu-Filt, which can be
fitted to an existing vacuum cleaner. They
represent a much cheaper solution, although
they may not be quite as effective. The pads
should be fitted over joints in the machine,
and over the switch unit, as well as covering
the exhaust.

Detergents and other cleaning materials

Faith in Nature,
Unit 5, Kay Street,
Bury
Lancs BL9 6BU
Telephone 061 764 2555
Fax 061 762 9129
Produces a range of 'Clear Spring' cleaning
products, primarily designed to be
biodegradable, but which may prove useful in
other ways. Their washing-up liquid has no
artificial perfumes or foam boosters. They
also sell a liquid substitute for washing
powder which contains no enzymes and
leaves little residue in the clothes, so is less
likely to cause irritation to eczema sufferers.
'Clear Spring' dishwasher liquid and rinse aid
also available, both non-perfumed. All
products available via mail order.

Ecover
Mouse Lane
Steyning
West Sussex BN44 3DG
Telephone 0903 879077
Produces a range of cleaning materials, with
the emphasis on biodegradability. However,
they use no enzymes, synthetic perfumes or
colourings, so they may also be useful to
those with eczema or chemical sensitivity.
Their toilet cleaner and bathroom cleaner
contain no chlorine bleach.

In Australia, the Allergy Aid Centre (address
on p337, under *Foods by post*) supplies the
Herbonics range of soaps, shampoos and
detergents, designed for those with allergies
and chemical sensitivities.

Gloves

Anyone sensitive to rubber gloves should try
PVC gloves instead. The best type are
'Glovlies' which have a cotton lining; they are
available in most chemists. Boots the
Chemists also produce their own brand of
PVC glove with a flock lining.

Treatments for house-dust mite

These products are available free of VAT for
those who have a proven allergy to house-
dust mite.

Crawford Pharmaceuticals
71A High Street
Stony Stratford
Milton Keynes
Bucks MK11 1BA
Telephone 0908 262346
Fax 0908 567730
Produce a spray containing benzyl benzoate
that kills house-dust mites; known as
Acarosan spray. The treatment has to be
repeated twice a year. Thorough vacuum
cleaning should be carried out afterwards,
and the allergy sufferer should be out of the
house throughout. The treatment cost for
two rooms is about £70 per year. Also
produce a test kit for assessing the levels of
dust-mite allergen. Both are available mail-
order.

Actomite spray, a mite-killing spray
containing synthetic pyrethroids, is widely
available in chemists' shops. Treatment has
to be repeated four times a year. Again,
thorough vacuum cleaning is needed
afterwards, and the allergy sufferer must not
be present. The treatment cost for two rooms
is about £80 per year.

Nitroboost
395a Hardgate
Aberdeen AB1 6BW
Telephone 0224 574705
Can carry out liquid nitrogen treatments
anywhere in Britain or Northern Ireland. The
fee includes thorough vacuum-cleaning of
the house afterwards. The liquid nitrogen
does not damage fabrics, and leaves no
harmful residue at all, just nitrogen gas,
which makes up 80 per cent of the air we
breathe normally. The treatment should be
repeated twice a year. Annual costs are £300–
£400.

CENTRAL HEATING

Church Hill Systems Ltd.
Frolesworth
Lutterworth
Leics LE17 5EE
Telephone 0455 202314
Produce a central heating system that does
not use gas, coal or oil, suitable for those
sensitive to fumes from these fuels. The
system utilizes a well-insulated water tank
that is heated by cheap electricity at night
and then supplies the radiators the following
day. Running costs compare favourably with
conventional central heating systems.

COSMETICS

Almay
225 Bath Road
Slough
Bucks SL1 4AU
Telephone 0753 523971
This company specializes in producing
cosmetics for sensitive skins. Almay
Hypoallergenic offers a comprehensive range
of skincare, suncare and cosmetic products.
As well as being unperfumed, they are free of
ingredients that are known to act as irritants,
and only include minimal amounts of
preservative and antioxidants. The company
also produces a lanolin-free range of
products for those allergic to lanolin. The
products are stocked in most large chemists
and department stores, and the company can
identify local stockists for anyone who has
difficulty in finding them. A complete list of
ingredients for all products is available to
dermatologists.

Allergy Aid Centre, Australia
(address on p337, under *Foods by post*)
Supplies several different brands of cosmetics
designed for those with allergies. Also soaps
and a wide range of other goods.

BREAST-FEEDING

All these are voluntary groups, funded by donations. When writing to them, please enclose a large, stamped self-addressed envelope to save them time and money.

Association of Breast-feeding Mothers (ABM)
26 Holmeshaw Close
London SE26 4TH
Telephone 081 778 4769
Can provide telephone numbers of local counsellors who have personal experience of breast-feeding and thorough training. A monthly newsletter, leaflets, library and breast-pump hire scheme are among the other services offered by ABM. They also sell breastfeeding accessories.

National Childbirth Trust
Alexandra House
Oldham Terrace
Acton
London W3 6NH
Telephone 081 992 8637
A national charity which produces leaflets on breast-feeding in various languages, and organizes a network of trained counsellors with personal experience of breast-feeding. They also sell breast-feeding accessories and can help with breast pumps.

Nursing Mothers' Association of Australia
5 Glendale Street
Nunawading
Victoria 3131
Telephone 03 877 5011
The main organization for the promotion of breast-feeding in Australia. Publishes various useful pamphlets and has many local groups all over the country offering counselling, discussion groups and newsletters.

La Leche League New Zealand
PO Box 13383
Wellington 4
New Zealand
Part of the international La Leche League which aims to promote breast-feeding.

Parents' Centres New Zealand Inc.
PO Box 17351
Wellington
New Zealand
Deals with all aspects of pregnancy, childbirth and child-rearing, including breast-feeding. Can put you in touch with your nearest group.

NUTRITIONAL DEFICIENCIES

Nature's Best Health Products
PO Box 1
Tunbridge Wells
Kent TN2 3EQ
Telephone 0892 534143
Produce a vitamin-and-mineral supplement, Health Insurance Plus, formulated by a doctor to be suitable for adults and elderly people with mild deficiencies in a range of nutrients. It is free of yeast, wheat, gluten, milk, corn, soya, artificial colourings and preservatives. They can also supply individual nutrients where required and can give expert advice on nutritional supplements. This company's products are available by mail order only.

Biolab Medical Unit
9 Weymouth Street
London W1N 3FF
Telephone 071 636 5959
Offers comprehensive nutritional testing and treatment for diseases in which nutrition plays a part. Patients must be referred by their GP.

In New Zealand, write to the Allergy Awareness Association for reputable suppliers of nutritional supplements. (Address on p340.)

COUNSELLING AND PSYCHOTHERAPY

When writing to any of these organizations, please enclose a large, stamped self-addressed envelope to save them time and money.

National Council of Psychotherapists and Hypnotherapy Register
46 Oxey Road
Oxey
Watford WD1 4QQ
Telephone 0923 227772
Can supply the names of reputable psychotherapists and hypnotherapists.

British Society of Medical and Dental Hypnosis, Metropolitan Branch
42 Links Road
Ashstead
Surrey KT21 2HJ
Telephone 0372 273522
Can supply the names of medically qualified hypnotherapists.

Westminster Pastoral Foundation
23 Kensington Square
London W8 5HN
Telephone 071 937 6956
Trains counsellors to help with personal problems. Payment is according to means. There are some centres outside London, and counsellors working in their own homes. The London office can put people in touch with their nearest counsellors.

British Association for Counselling
1 Regent Place
Rugby CV21 2PJ

Maintains a directory of counsellors and psychotherapists and can supply a list of those in a given area. Includes details of professional qualifications and general approach to counselling for each individual listed. Those on the list have to comply with a code of ethics.

Co-counselling International
Westerly
Prestwick Lane
Chiddingfold
Surrey GU8 4XW
Can put you in touch with your nearest co-counselling teacher or contact person. See p161 for details of this form of counselling.

SUPPORT AND INFORMATION GROUPS

All these are voluntary groups, funded by donations. When writing to them, please enclose a large, stamped self-addressed envelope to save them time and money.

The National Society for Research into Allergy
PO Box 45
Hinckley
Leics LE10 1JY
Telephone 0455 851546
Members receive a quarterly magazine, and can obtain advice on practical matters, including sources of alternative foods, recipes and air filtration.

Action Against Allergy
24–26 High Street
Hampton Hill
Middlesex TW12 1PD
A registered charity campaigning for greater medical recognition of allergy and food intolerance. Also offers advice. Action Against Allergy stocks a very wide range of books on allergy and intolerance, including many not published in Britain.

ACTA (Australian Chemical Trauma Alliance)
c/o Diana Crumpler
RSD Tennyson
Victoria 3572
Australia
Telephone 05 488 2350
Founded to serve the interests of those whose health has been affected by exposure to chemicals.

Allergy Association Australia
PO Box 298
Ringwood
Victoria 3134
Australia
Telephone 03 888 1382
A self-help group concerned with

environmental illness, including food allergy and intolerance and chemical sensitivity. Services include a journal, telephone contacts, members' handbook, lending library, store discounts and seminars.

Allergy Recognition and Management
PO Box 2
Sandy Bay
Tasmania 7005
Telephone 002 282554
Have just published a new edition of the society's cookbook for the allergy-afflicted, entitled *A Bore? A Chore? Or a Challenge?* Price $10 (Australian dollars), postage and packing.

Allergy Awareness Association
PO Box 120701
Penrose
Auckland 6
New Zealand

SUPPORT GROUPS DEALING WITH SPECIFIC PROBLEMS

All these are voluntary groups, funded by donations. When writing to them, please enclose a large, stamped self-addressed envelope to save them time and money.

National Asthma Campaign
Providence House
Providence Place
London N1 0NT
Telephone 071 226 2260
Also has an asthma helpline on 0345 010203. The line is open 1pm to 9pm Monday to Friday, and is only charged as a local call.

Asthma Society of Ireland
24 Anglesea Street
Dublin 2
Telephone 01 716 551

National Eczema Society
Irish Office
Carmichael House
North Brunswick Street
Dublin 7

National Eczema Society
4 Tavistock Place
London WC1H 9RA
Telephone 071 388 4097

National Association for Colitis and Crohn's Disease
98a London Road
St Albans
Herts AL1 1NX
Telephone 0727 44296

Hyperactive Children's Support Group
71 Whyke Lane
Chichester
West Sussex PO19 2LD
Telephone 0903 725182
(Tue–Fri 10am–1pm)
Can offer very useful support to the parents
of hyperactive children through a network of
local groups. However, they emphasise the
Feingold Diet as the prime method of
treatment, and we would strongly advise
parents to read p213 for a critical assessment
of this approach. We believe that a greater
number of children will benefit by following
the sort of treatment programme outlined in
this book, than by following the Feingold Diet.

Wellington Hyperactivity Association
93 Waipapa Road
Hataitai
Wellington 3
New Zealand
Telephone 04 386 2514

Hyperactivity Association (NSW)
15/29 Bertram Street
Chatswood
New South Wales 2067
Telephone 02 411 2186
Support for people with behaviour problems,
food sensitivites and learning problems.

MEDICAL TREATMENT

The National Society for Research into Allergy
(address in previous section)
A registered charity which can put patients in
touch with reputable doctors offering
treatment privately.

Environmentally controlled units

The Airedale Allergy Centre
Elmsley Street
Steeton
Keighley
West Yorkshire BD20 6SB
Telephone 0535 656013
The only environmentally controlled unit in
Britain at the present time. Treats patients with
chemical sensitivity or food sensitivity. Can
accept patients referred to the Airedale
Hospital Trust under the NHS.

FURTHER READING

If you have difficulty in obtaining any of these
books, write to Action Against Allergy (UK) or
Allergy Aid Centre (Australia) addresses on
pp340 and 337.

Chapter 1
For more on the early development of the
clinical ecology movement in America, see
Allergies: Your Hidden Enemy by Theron G.
Randolph and Ralph W. Moss, published by
Thorsons, £7.95.

Chapters 2–4
For comprehensive information about
hayfever, perennial rhinitis and asthma, and
detailed advice on eliminating or avoiding
airborne allergens, see *The Complete Guide
to Hayfever* by Dr Jonathan Brostoff and
Linda Gamlin, published by Bloomsbury
Publishing, 1993.
For further advice on the management of
asthma, see *The Allergy and Asthma
Reference Book* by Dr H. Morrow Brown,
published by Harper and Row, 1985/Crowood
Press, 1989.

Chapter 6
For those with some medical knowledge, who
are interested in the controversies, *Food
Intolerance*, edited by John Dobbing, makes
fascinating reading. Eleven doctors with a
wide range of views on the subject were
invited to submit a chapter each. After each
one, the comments of the other contributors
are given, followed by the author's reply.
Published by Baillière Tindall, 1987.

Chapter 8
Not All in the Mind by Dr Richard Mackarness
is still available from Pan Books, price £3.50,
and makes interesting reading, although it is
now twelve years since it was first published.
Hypnotherapy by Dr Ruth Lever is a useful
introduction for anyone considering this form
of treatment. Published by Penguin, £3.95.

Chapter 9
Allergies Your Hidden Enemy (see above)
gives an account of Dr Randolph's
pioneering work in the field of chemical
sensitivity.
The Food Magazine, published quarterly by
The London Food Commission (88 Old St,
London EC1V 9AR) covers recent research
and developments in the field of food
additives, pesticide residues, water quality etc.
The same organization has produced
detailed reports on food additives and

pesticides, which anyone with a special interest in this area may find useful. *Additives: a Guide for Everyone* by Dr Erik Millstone and John Abraham is an authoritative guide to the safety of additives. Published by Penguin, 1988.

Chapter 11
An excellent book dealing with food intolerance in babies and children is *Food for Thought* by Maureen Minchin, published in Australia by Unwin Paperbacks, and in the UK by Oxford University Press, second edition 1986, price £4.95. This book is recommended to anyone with a colicky baby, and to those who need advice about breast-feeding.

For the parents of hyperactive children, *Allergies and the Hyperactive Child* by Doris J. Rapp offers a practical, balanced approach to the topic and is very readable. It is published by Simon and Schuster, New York, but can be obtained from Action Against Allergy (address on p340), £8.95. Dr Rapp's latest book on the subject, *Is This Your Child?*, is also recommended.

Chapter 14
For those concerned about possible nutritional deficiencies *Nutritional Medicine* by Dr Stephen Davies and Dr Alan Stewart offers an up-to-date assessment of the available evidence and gives sensible advice. Published by Pan Books, 1987, price £3.95.

Chapter 15
The Foodwatch Alternative Cookbook by Honor Campbell will prove useful if you are trying to cook without wheat or milk, while *The Allergy Cookbook* by Stephanie Lashford gives recipes for egg-free, milk-free and corn-free diets. Both published by Ashgrove Press, £4.95. The former is also available from Foodwatch International, address on p336. Two books written by Dr John Hunter, Dr Virginia Alun Jones and Elizabeth Workman (a dietician) also contain many useful recipes. Some are free from milk, eggs and wheat, others are free from just one or two of these foods. The book also includes useful information on nutrition. The titles are: *The Allergy Diet* and *The Food Intolerance Diet Cookbook*, both published by Macdonald, £3.95.
Food Intolerance by Robert Buist, published by Harper & Row in Australia includes some interesting recipes for cooking without wheat or milk, and advice on using alternative foods.
Food and Nutrition in Australia edited by Wahlquist, published by Cassell, 1983, may also be of interest.

General
Doctors seeking further information on food sensitivity are referred to:
Food Allergy and Intolerance edited by Jonathan Brostoff and Stephen Challacombe, published by Baillière Tindall, 1987, price £75.00.
Clinical Reactions to Food edited by M.H. Lessof, published by Wiley, 1983.
Food Allergy: New Perspectives edited by John W. Gerrard, published by Charles C. Thomas, Illinois, 1980.
Food Allergy edited by R.K. Chandra, published by Nutrition Research Education Foundation, Newfoundland, Canada, 1987.
Food and the Gut edited by J.O. Hunter and V. Alun Jones, published by Baillière Tindall, 1985.
Food Allergy and Food Intolerance – Nutritional Aspects and Development edited by J.C. Somogyi, H.R. Muller and Th. Ockhuiizen, published by Karger, 1991.
Food Allergy – Adverse Reactions to Foods and Food Additives edited by D.D. Metcalfe, H.A. Sampson and R.A. Simon, published by Blackwell Scientific Publications, 1991.

The British Society for Allergy and Environmental Medicine is an organization for doctors interested in food intolerance, chemical sensitivity and related matters. For further information, doctors can contact:

Mrs Ina Mansell (Secretary)
British Society for Allergy and Environmental Medicine
Acorns
Romsey Road
Cadnam
Southampton SO4 2NN
Please note that the society cannot deal with any enquiries from the general public.

Index

Where there are several entries on a subject, the **bold** figure indicates the main entry.
Illustrations are indicated by figures in *italic*.
For drugs, also see the index on pp329–333.
For food relationships, see the index on pp306–7.